Big Data for eHealth Applications

Big Data for eHealth Applications

Editors

Stefano Silvestri
Francesco Gargiulo

MDPI • Basel • Beijing • Wuhan • Barcelona • Belgrade • Manchester • Tokyo • Cluj • Tianjin

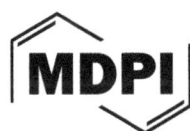

Editors
Stefano Silvestri
Institute for High
Performance Computing and
Networking ICAR
National Research Council of
Italy (CNR)
Rome
Italy

Francesco Gargiulo
Institute for High
Performance Computing and
Networking ICAR
National Research Council of
Italy (CNR)
Rome
Italy

Editorial Office
MDPI
St. Alban-Anlage 66
4052 Basel, Switzerland

This is a reprint of articles from the Special Issue published online in the open access journal *Applied Sciences* (ISSN 2076-3417) (available at: https://www.mdpi.com/journal/applsci/special_issues/Big_Data_eHealth).

For citation purposes, cite each article independently as indicated on the article page online and as indicated below:

LastName, A.A.; LastName, B.B.; LastName, C.C. Article Title. *Journal Name* **Year**, *Volume Number*, Page Range.

ISBN 978-3-0365-5053-4 (Hbk)
ISBN 978-3-0365-5054-1 (PDF)

© 2022 by the authors. Articles in this book are Open Access and distributed under the Creative Commons Attribution (CC BY) license, which allows users to download, copy and build upon published articles, as long as the author and publisher are properly credited, which ensures maximum dissemination and a wider impact of our publications.

The book as a whole is distributed by MDPI under the terms and conditions of the Creative Commons license CC BY-NC-ND.

Contents

About the Editors vii

Preface to "Big Data for eHealth Applications" ix

Stefano Silvestri and Francesco Gargiulo
Special Issue on Big Data for eHealth Applications
Reprinted from: *Appl. Sci.* **2022**, *12*, 7578, doi:10.3390/app12157578 1

Stefano Silvestri, Francesco Gargiulo and Mario Ciampi
Iterative Annotation of Biomedical NER Corpora with Deep Neural Networks and Knowledge Bases
Reprinted from: *Appl. Sci.* **2022**, *12*, 5775, doi:10.3390/app12125775 7

Shareeful Islam, Spyridon Papastergiou, Eleni-Maria Kalogeraki and Kitty Kioskli
Cyberattack Path Generation and Prioritisation for Securing Healthcare Systems
Reprinted from: *Appl. Sci.* **2022**, *12*, 4443, doi:10.3390/app12094443 27

Marek Wyszyński, Michał Grudziński, Krzysztof Pokonieczny and Marek Kaszubowski
The Assessment of COVID-19 Vulnerability Risk for Crisis Management
Reprinted from: *Appl. Sci.* **2022**, *12*, 4090, doi:10.3390/app12084090 49

Mayara Khadhraoui, Hatem Bellaaj, Mehdi Ben Ammar, Habib Hamam and Mohamed Jmaiel
Survey of BERT-Base Models for Scientific Text Classification: COVID-19 Case Study
Reprinted from: *Appl. Sci.* **2022**, *12*, 2891, doi:10.3390/app12062891 77

Flora Amato, Walter Balzano and Giovanni Cozzolino
Design of a Wearable Healthcare Emergency Detection Device for Elder Persons
Reprinted from: *Appl. Sci.* **2022**, *12*, 2345, doi:10.3390/app12052345 97

Maria-Alexandra Pană, Ștefan-Sebastian Busnatu, Liviu-Ionut Serbanoiu, Electra Vasilescu, Nirvana Popescu, Cătălina Andrei and Crina-Julieta Sinescu
Reducing the Heart Failure Burden in Romania by Predicting Congestive Heart Failure Using Artificial Intelligence: Proof of Concept
Reprinted from: *Appl. Sci.* **2021**, *11*, 11728, doi:10.3390/app112411728 109

Radko Mesiar and Ayyub Sheikhi
Nonlinear Random Forest Classification, a Copula-Based Approach
Reprinted from: *Appl. Sci.* **2021**, *11*, 7140, doi:10.3390/app11157140 123

Manuel Casas M., Roberto L. Avitia, Jugal Kalita, Jose Antonio Cardenas-Haro, Marco A. Reyna and Miguel E. Bravo-Zanoguera
A Novel Unsupervised Computational Method for Ventricular andSupraventricular Origin Beats Classification
Reprinted from: *Appl. Sci.* **2021**, *11*, 6711, doi:10.3390/app11156711 135

Min-Wei Huang, Chien-Hung Chiu, Chih-Fong Tsai and Wei-Chao Lin
On Combining Feature Selection and Over-Sampling Techniques for Breast Cancer Prediction
Reprinted from: *Appl. Sci.* **2021**, *11*, 6574, doi:10.3390/app11146574 155

Prayitno, Chi-Ren Shyu, Karisma Trinanda Putra, Hsing-Chung Chen, Yuan-Yu Tsai, K. S. M. Tozammel Hossain, Wei Jiang and Zon-Yin Shae
A Systematic Review of Federated Learning in the Healthcare Area: From the Perspective of Data Properties and Applications
Reprinted from: *Appl. Sci.* **2021**, *11*, 11191, doi:10.3390/app112311191 . . . . **165**

About the Editors

Stefano Silvestri

Stefano Silvestri (PhD) is a researcher at the Institute for High Performance Computing and Networking of the National Research Council of Italy (CNR-ICAR) and is an adjunct professor of computer science at University of Campania "L. Vanvitelli". He received his MSc degree in electronical engineer at University of Naples "Federico II" and his PhD in information and communication technology and engineering at University of Naples "Parthenope". His main research interests are in the areas of artificial intelligence, machine/deep learning, smart health, natural language processing, and big data analytics. He has participated in several national and international research projects, and he has authored and co-authored more than 30 scientific articles in peer-reviewed journals and conference proceedings. Moreover, he was a member of the program committee of several international conferences and workshops and is a guest editor of international journals.

Francesco Gargiulo

Francesco Gargiulo (PhD) received his MSc degree (cum laude) in telecommunication engineering and his PhD degree in information and automatic engineering from the University of Naples Federico II, in 2006 and 2009, respectively. He is currently a technological researcher with the Institute for High Performance Computing and Networking, National Research Council, Italy (ICAR-CNR). He has been involved in different national and European projects. He has authored numerous peer-reviewed articles in international journals and conference proceedings. His current research interests include e-Health, big data analytics, natural language processing, artificial intelligence, and deep learning. he has been on the program committee of international conferences and workshops and, moreover, is currently a member of the editorial board of some international journals.

Preface to "Big Data for eHealth Applications"

In the last few years, the rapid growth of the available digitised medical data has opened new challenges for the scientific research community in the healthcare informatic field. In this scenario, the constantly increasing volume of medical data, as well as the complexity and heterogeneity of this kind of data, requires innovative big data analytics methods for extracting valuable insights from them, and, at the same time, these new approaches must also guarantee the required levels of privacy and security. These solutions must provide effective and efficient tools to support the daily routine of physicians, medical professionals, and policy makers, improving the quality of the healthcare systems. The recent pandemic emergency has made the need for new big data approaches for the processing of such data more urgent.

Stefano Silvestri and Francesco Gargiulo
Editors

Editorial

Special Issue on Big Data for eHealth Applications

Stefano Silvestri * and Francesco Gargiulo *

Institute for High Performance Computing and Networking, National Research Council of Italy, Via Pietro Castellino, 111, 80131 Naples, Italy
* Correspondence: stefano.silvestri@icar.cnr.it (S.S.); francesco.gargiulo@icar.cnr.it (F.G.)

Citation: Silvestri, S.; Gargiulo, F. Special Issue on Big Data for eHealth Applications. *Appl. Sci.* 2022, 12, 7578. https://doi.org/10.3390/app12157578

Received: 22 July 2022
Accepted: 26 July 2022
Published: 28 July 2022

Publisher's Note: MDPI stays neutral with regard to jurisdictional claims in published maps and institutional affiliations.

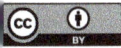

Copyright: © 2022 by the authors. Licensee MDPI, Basel, Switzerland. This article is an open access article distributed under the terms and conditions of the Creative Commons Attribution (CC BY) license (https://creativecommons.org/licenses/by/4.0/).

1. Introduction

In the last few years, the rapid growth in available digitised medical data has opened new challenges for the scientific research community in the healthcare informatics field. In this scenario, the constantly increasing volume of medical data, as well as the complexity and heterogeneity of this kind of data require innovative approaches based on Big Data Analytics (BDA) and Artificial Intelligence (AI) methods for extracting valuable insights [1–5], and at the same time, these new approaches must also guarantee the required levels of privacy and security [6]. These solutions must also provide effective and efficient tools for supporting the daily routine of physicians, medical professionals, and policy makers, improving the quality of healthcare systems. Finally, they should leverage the huge amount of information buried under these Big Data [7], exploiting, in this way, their full potential.

Furthermore, new heterogeneous and extensive COVID-related datasets have been collected during the recent pandemic and have often been made available to the scientific community. In this case, the need for new and specific Big Data approaches for processing such data makes exploiting these data and providing new and innovative approaches for facing the COVID-19 pandemic more urgent [8–10].

In this Special Issue, some innovative applications, tools, and techniques specifically tailored to address issues related to the eHealth domain by leveraging BDA methodologies are presented. Moreover, these techniques are also presented in this Special Issue, given the definition of complex systems and architectures for the eHealth domain fundamentally based on the combination of Internet of Things (IoT) devices and Artificial Intelligence (AI) methods. Finally, the Cyber Security (CS) for eHealth topic is also addressed given the significant increase in cyber threats in the healthcare sector during the last few years.

2. Big Data for eHealth Applications

In light of the above, this Special Issue was introduced to collect the latest research on relevant topics and, more importantly, to address present challenges with using Big Data for eHealth applications. Moreover, it considered AI and/or IoT-based technologies, the combined use of which can lead to the definition and implementation of effective and innovative solutions [11]. Finally, CS techniques for the eHealth domain were also taken into account.

There are 10 contributions selected for this Special Issue, representing innovative applications in the areas mentioned above from original contributions of researchers with broad expertise in various and multidisciplinary fields, considering the medical, informatics, and engineering fields. The Special Issue includes the following papers:

- Iterative Annotation of Biomedical NER Corpora with Deep Neural Networks and Knowledge Bases [12]
- Cyberattack Path Generation and Prioritisation for Securing Healthcare Systems [13]
- The Assessment of COVID-19 Vulnerability Risk for Crisis Management [14]
- Survey of BERT-Base Models for Scientific Text Classification: COVID-19 Case Study [15]
- Design of a Wearable Healthcare Emergency Detection Device for Elder Persons [16]

- Reducing the Heart Failure Burden in Romania by Predicting Congestive Heart Failure Using Artificial Intelligence: Proof of Concept [17]
- Nonlinear Random Forest Classification, a Copula-Based Approach [18]
- A Novel Unsupervised Computational Method for Ventricular and Supraventricular Origin Beats Classification [19]
- A Systematic Review of Federated Learning in the Healthcare Area: From the Perspective of Data Properties and Applications [20]
- On Combining Feature Selection and Over-Sampling Techniques for Breast Cancer Prediction [21]

The aforementioned papers refer to the following main topics within the healthcare scenario: (i) COVID-19 datasets and models [14,15], (ii) large dataset annotation [12], (iii) cyber security [13], (iv) federated learning [20], (v) smart biomedical systems and devices [16], and (vi) artificial intelligence approaches [17–19,21].

More in detail, in [12], a methodology for reducing the manual effort needed to annotate a biomedical-named entity recognition (B-NER) corpus was presented, exploiting both active learning and distant supervision, respectively, based on Deep Learning models (e.g., Bi-LSTM, word2vec FastText, ELMo, and BERT) and biomedical knowledge bases to speed up the annotation task. The proposed approach is also able to limit class imbalance issues. The results showed that this method allows us to annotate an effective and large B-NER corpus with a fraction of the time required by a fully manual annotation, addressing the lack of annotated corpora in the biomedical domain [22]. The authors also analysed the most effective embedding model to represent the input words [23] and the applicability of this approach to other domains.

In [13], a novel methodology for the cyberattack path discovery to ensure security within the healthcare ecosystem is presented. This approach is based on the Common Vulnerability Scoring System (CVSS), so that base metrics and exploitability features can be used to determine and prioritise the possible attack paths based on the threat actor capability, asset dependency, and target user profile and evidence of indicator of compromise. The work includes a real example from the healthcare use case to demonstrate the methodology used for attack path generation. The result from the studied context, which processes Big Data from healthcare applications, shows that the uses of various parameters such as CVSS metrics, threat actor profile, and the indicator of compromise are able to generate realistic attack paths. In this way, healthcare practitioners can be supported in identifying the controls that are required to secure the overall healthcare ecosystem.

The authors of [14] presented a methodology that is used determine COVID-19 vulnerability risk and its change over time in association with the state health care system, turnover, and transport to support the crisis management decision-making process. In detail, this method aims to determine the COVID-19 Vulnerability Index (CVI) based on the selected criteria. The risk assessment was carried out with methodology that includes the application of a multi-criteria analysis and spatio-temporal aspects of available data. Particularly, the Spatial Multicriteria Analysis (SMCA) compliant with the Analytical Hierarchy Process (AHP), which incorporated selected population and environmental criteria were used to analyse the ongoing pandemic. The influence of combining several factors in an analysis of the pandemic was illustrated, and the static and dynamic factors to COVID-19 vulnerability risk were determined to prevent and control the spread of COVID-19 at the early stages of the pandemic. As a result, areas with a certain level of risk in different periods of time were determined. Furthermore, the number of people exposed to a COVID-19 vulnerability risk was presented with time. The results obtained proved that the this approach can support the decision-making process by showing the area where preventive actions should be considered.

In [15], a new pre-trained neural language model based on the BERT model [24] was introduced. This model was named CovBERT, and it was specifically designed to improve the overall review task performances on the COVID-19 literature with respect to the classic BERT model. CovBERT was pretrained on a very large corpus formed by scientific publications in the biomedical domain related to COVID-19. The CovBERT was tested on the classification task of short texts of biomedical articles. The obtained results demonstrated significant improvements. In addition, the authors also made a COVID-19 corpus available, entitled *COV-Dat-20*.

The authors of [16] proposed a wearable system that takes advantage of sensors embedded in a smart device to collect data for movement identification (running, walking, falling, and daily activities) of an older adult user in real-time. To provide high efficiency in fall detection, the sensor readings were analysed using a neural network. If a fall is detected, an alert is sent though a smartphone connected via Bluetooth. The proposed system was tested in both inside and outside environments, and the results of the experiments showed that it is extremely portable and is able to provide high success rates in fall detection in terms of accuracy and loss.

In [17], a noncontact system that can predict heart failure exacerbation through vocal analysis was studied and implemented. The system was designed to evaluate the voice characteristics of every patient, used to identify variations using a Machine Learning-based approach. The authors collected voice data from real hospitalised patients since their admission to a hospital, when their general status was critical, until the day of discharge, when they were clinically stable. Each patient was classified adopting the New York Heart Association Functional Classification (NYHA) classification system for heart failure in order to include them in different stages based on their clinical evolution. Different ML algorithms were tested, namely Artificial Neural Networks (ANN), Support Vector Machine (SVM), and K-Nearest Neighbours (KNN), trained on voice data. The experiments demonstrated that the KNN obtained the best results and was able to correctly classify the NYHA stages of the patients exploiting only their voice recording, with an accuracy of 0.945.

In [18], a study on the copula-based approach to selecting the most important features for a Random Forest classification was used to classify a label-valued outcome. The methodology was simulated on a real dataset of COVID-19 and diabetes. In detail, based on associated copulas between these features, the authors carried out this feature selection and then embedded the selected features into a Random Forest algorithm to classify a label-valued outcome. This algorithm allowed us to select the most relevant features when the features are not necessarily connected by a linear function, and it can stop the classification when the desired level of accuracy is reached. The experimental assessment successfully applied the proposed method on a simulation study as well as a real dataset of COVID-19 and for a diabetes dataset.

The study presented in [19] focused on a new unsupervised algorithm that adapts to every patient using the heart rate and morphological features of the ECG beats to classify beats between supraventricular origin and ventricular origin in order to predict arrhythmia. The results of the experiments performed obtained F-scores equal to 0.88, 0.89, and 0.93 for the ventricular origin beats for three popular ECG databases and around 0.99 for the supraventricular origin for the same databases, comparable with supervised approaches presented in other works, opening a new path to making use of ECG data to classify heartbeats without the assistance of a physician.

The work presented in [20] is a review paper, where a comprehensive and up-to-date review of research employing Federated Learning in healthcare applications was provided. Moreover, the paper highlighted a set of recent challenges from a data-centric perspective in Federated Learning, such as data partitioning characteristics, data distributions, data protection mechanisms, and benchmark datasets, was evaluated. Finally, several potential challenges and future research directions in healthcare applications were pointed out.

In [21], the imbalanced class problem was addressed, in particular for breast cancer prediction datasets. The authors presented a methodology that used a combination of the Information Gain (IG) and Genetic Algorithm (GA) feature selection methods and the Synthetic Minority Over-sampling TEchnique (SMOTE) to overcome this issue. The experimental results based on two breast cancer datasets showed that the combination of feature selection and over-sampling outperformed the single usage of either feature selection and over-sampling for the highly class imbalanced datasets. In particular, performing IG first and SMOTE second is the better choice. For other datasets with a small class imbalance ratio and a smaller number of features, performing SMOTE is enough to construct an effective prediction model.

3. Future in Big Data for eHealth Applications

Although this Special Issue is now closed, more in-depth studies in Big Data Analytics applications developed explicitly for eHealth are expected. The outcomes of the research published in this Special Issue provided some new solutions in this area but also highlighted some of the still open issues that must be addressed to fully exploit Big Data in the healthcare domain in the future.

In detail, the presented papers underlined the need for extensive collections of biomedical annotated data, allowing for the training of high-performance ML and DL models to support physicians in their daily work. ML and AI approaches will support the daily routine of physicians and medical practitioners, but their extensive use will also raise privacy and security issues. It is also clear that the integration among IoT devices and sensors, AI and ML models, and Big Data approaches will be more pervasive for developing eHealth complex systems in the future. Adopting specifically pretrained neural language models will enable the researchers to define more intelligent systems for analysing large natural language clinical documents, fully exploiting their informative content. Finally, the large and heterogeneous data analyses related to COVID-19 can provide innovative pathways, more profound knowledge, and innovative approaches to address the risks of the current pandemic.

Author Contributions: Conceptualization: S.S. and F.G.; writing: S.S. and F.G.; reviewing and editing: S.S. and F.G. All authors have read and agreed to the published version of the manuscript.

Funding: This research received no external funding.

Acknowledgments: This Special Issue would not have been possible without the contributions of the authors, the reviewers, and the dedicated editorial team of *Applied Sciences*. We congratulate all authors on their research. Moreover, we take this opportunity to express our sincere gratefulness to all reviewers. Finally, we express our gratitude to the editorial team of *Applied Sciences* and give a special thanks to Assistant Editor, for her continuous support.

Conflicts of Interest: The authors declare no conflict of interest.

References

1. Lv, Z.; Qiao, L. Analysis of healthcare big data. *Future Gener. Comput. Syst.* **2020**, *109*, 103–110. [CrossRef]
2. Cozzoli, N.; Salvatore, F.P.; Faccilongo, N.; Milone, M. How can big data analytics be used for healthcare organization management? Literary framework and future research from a systematic review. *BMC Health Serv. Res.* **2022**, *22*, 1–14. [CrossRef]
3. Karatas, M.; Eriskin, L.; Deveci, M.; Pamucar, D.; Garg, H. Big Data for Healthcare Industry 4.0: Applications, challenges and future perspectives. *Expert Syst. Appl.* **2022**, *200*, 116912. [CrossRef]
4. Luchini, C.; Pea, A.; Scarpa, A. Artificial intelligence in oncology: Current applications and future perspectives. *Br. J. Cancer* **2022**, *126*, 4–9. [CrossRef] [PubMed]
5. Busnatu, S.; Niculescu, A.G.; Bolocan, A.; Petrescu, G.E.D.; Păduraru, D.N.; Năstasă, I.; Lupușoru, M.; Geantă, M.; Andronic, O.; Grumezescu, A.M.; et al. Clinical Applications of Artificial Intelligence—An Updated Overview. *J. Clin. Med.* **2022**, *11*, 2265. [CrossRef] [PubMed]
6. Ciampi, M.; Sicuranza, M.; Silvestri, S. A Privacy-Preserving and Standard-Based Architecture for Secondary Use of Clinical Data. *Information* **2022**, *13*, 87. [CrossRef]
7. Silvestri, S.; Esposito, A.; Gargiulo, F.; Sicuranza, M.; Ciampi, M.; De Pietro, G. A Big Data Architecture for the Extraction and Analysis of EHR Data. In Proceedings of the 2019 IEEE World Congress on Services (SERVICES), Milan, Italy, 8–13 July 2019; IEEE: Piscataway, NJ, USA, 2019; Volume 2642-939X, pp. 283–288. [CrossRef]
8. Alsunaidi, S.J.; Almuhaideb, A.M.; Ibrahim, N.M.; Shaikh, F.S.; Alqudaihi, K.S.; Alhaidari, F.A.; Khan, I.U.; Aslam, N.; Alshahrani, M.S. Applications of Big Data Analytics to Control COVID-19 Pandemic. *Sensors* **2021**, *21*, 2282. [CrossRef] [PubMed]
9. Lin, L.; Hou, Z. Combat COVID-19 with artificial intelligence and big data. *J. Travel Med.* **2020**, *27*, taaa080. [CrossRef] [PubMed]

10. Catelli, R.; Gargiulo, F.; Casola, V.; De Pietro, G.; Fujita, H.; Esposito, M. Crosslingual named entity recognition for clinical de-identification applied to a COVID-19 Italian data set. *Appl. Soft Comput.* **2020**, *97*, 106779. [CrossRef] [PubMed]
11. Ciampi, M.; Coronato, A.; Naeem, M.; Silvestri, S. An intelligent environment for preventing medication errors in home treatment. *Expert Syst. Appl.* **2022**, *193*, 116434. [CrossRef]
12. Silvestri, S.; Gargiulo, F.; Ciampi, M. Iterative Annotation of Biomedical NER Corpora with Deep Neural Networks and Knowledge Bases. *Appl. Sci.* **2022**, *12*, 5775. [CrossRef]
13. Islam, S.; Papastergiou, S.; Kalogeraki, E.M.; Kioskli, K. Cyberattack Path Generation and Prioritisation for Securing Healthcare Systems. *Appl. Sci.* **2022**, *12*, 4443. [CrossRef]
14. Wyszyński, M.; Grudziński, M.; Pokonieczny, K.; Kaszubowski, M. The Assessment of COVID-19 Vulnerability Risk for Crisis Management. *Appl. Sci.* **2022**, *12*, 4090. [CrossRef]
15. Khadhraoui, M.; Bellaaj, H.; Ammar, M.B.; Hamam, H.; Jmaiel, M. Survey of BERT-Base Models for Scientific Text Classification: COVID-19 Case Study. *Appl. Sci.* **2022**, *12*, 2891. [CrossRef]
16. Amato, F.; Balzano, W.; Cozzolino, G. Design of a Wearable Healthcare Emergency Detection Device for Elder Persons. *Appl. Sci.* **2022**, *12*, 2345. [CrossRef]
17. Pană, M.A.; Busnatu, S.S.; Serbanoiu, L.I.; Vasilescu, E.; Popescu, N.; Andrei, C.; Sinescu, C.J. Reducing the Heart Failure Burden in Romania by Predicting Congestive Heart Failure Using Artificial Intelligence: Proof of Concept. *Appl. Sci.* **2021**, *11*, 11728. [CrossRef]
18. Mesiar, R.; Sheikhi, A. Nonlinear Random Forest Classification, a Copula-Based Approach. *Appl. Sci.* **2021**, *11*, 7140. [CrossRef]
19. Casas, M.M.; Avitia, R.L.; Cardenas-Haro, J.A.; Kalita, J.; Torres-Reyes, F.J.; Reyna, M.A.; Bravo-Zanoguera, M.E. A Novel Unsupervised Computational Method for Ventricular and Supraventricular Origin Beats Classification. *Appl. Sci.* **2021**, *11*, 6711. [CrossRef]
20. Prayitno; Shyu, C.R.; Putra, K.T.; Chen, H.C.; Tsai, Y.Y.; Hossain, K.S.M.T.; Jiang, W.; Shae, Z.Y. A Systematic Review of Federated Learning in the Healthcare Area: From the Perspective of Data Properties and Applications. *Appl. Sci.* **2021**, *11*, 11191. [CrossRef]
21. Huang, M.W.; Chiu, C.H.; Tsai, C.F.; Lin, W.C. On Combining Feature Selection and Over-Sampling Techniques for Breast Cancer Prediction. *Appl. Sci.* **2021**, *11*, 6574. [CrossRef]
22. Silvestri, S.; Gargiulo, F.; Ciampi, M.; De Pietro, G. Exploit Multilingual Language Model at Scale for ICD-10 Clinical Text Classification. In Proceedings of the 2020 IEEE Symposium on Computers and Communications (ISCC), Rennes, France, 7–10 July 2020; IEEE: Piscatway, NJ, USA, 2020; pp. 1–7. [CrossRef]
23. Silvestri, S.; Gargiulo, F.; Ciampi, M. Improving Biomedical Information Extraction with Word Embeddings Trained on Closed-Domain Corpora. In Proceedings of the 2019 IEEE Symposium on Computers and Communications (ISCC), Barcelona, Spain, 29 June–3 July 2019; IEEE: Piscatway, NJ, USA, 2019; pp. 1129–1134. [CrossRef]
24. Devlin, J.; Chang, M.W.; Lee, K.; Toutanova, K. BERT: Pre-training of Deep Bidirectional Transformers for Language Understanding. In Proceedings of the 2019 Conference of the North American Chapter of the Association for Computational Linguistics: Human Language Technologies, Minneapolis, MN, USA, 2–7 June 2019; ACL: Minneapolis, MN, USA, 2019; Volume 1, pp. 4171–4186. [CrossRef]

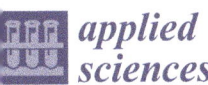

Article

Iterative Annotation of Biomedical NER Corpora with Deep Neural Networks and Knowledge Bases

Stefano Silvestri *,†, Francesco Gargiulo † and Mario Ciampi

Institute for High Performance Computing and Networking of National Research Council, ICAR-CNR, Via Pietro Castellino 111, 80131 Naples, Italy; francesco.gargiulo@icar.cnr.it (F.G.); mario.ciampi@icar.cnr.it (M.C.)
* Correspondence: stefano.silvestri@icar.cnr.it
† These authors contributed equally to this work.

Abstract: The large availability of clinical natural language documents, such as clinical narratives or diagnoses, requires the definition of smart automatic systems for their processing and analysis, but the lack of annotated corpora in the biomedical domain, especially in languages different from English, makes it difficult to exploit the state-of-art machine-learning systems to extract information from such kinds of documents. For these reasons, healthcare professionals lose big opportunities that can arise from the analysis of this data. In this paper, we propose a methodology to reduce the manual efforts needed to annotate a biomedical named entity recognition (B-NER) corpus, exploiting both active learning and distant supervision, respectively based on deep learning models (e.g., Bi-LSTM, word2vec FastText, ELMo and BERT) and biomedical knowledge bases, in order to speed up the annotation task and limit class imbalance issues. We assessed this approach by creating an Italian-language electronic health record corpus annotated with biomedical domain entities in a small fraction of the time required for a fully manual annotation. The obtained corpus was used to train a B-NER deep neural network whose performances are comparable with the state of the art, with an F1-Score equal to 0.9661 and 0.8875 on two test sets.

Keywords: biomedical NER; corpus annotation; distant supervision; active learning; deep learning

1. Introduction

Nowadays, a huge amount of digitised information is produced in clinical and healthcare domains. A large part of this data is formed by or contains natural language (NL) texts, such as electronic health records (EHRs), diagnoses, medical reports, or patient summaries. Extracting and analysing the information in these documents has a great potential for caregivers and policy makers, making possible to support and improve the quality of the healthcare [1,2]. On the other hand, this huge amount of NL text can be processed only through Natural Language Processing (NLP) systems able to automatically extract the required information. An essential NLP task for the Information Extraction (IE) from clinical and biomedical NL documents is the biomedical named entity recognition (B-NER) [3], namely the identification and the classification of words and multi-word expressions belonging to the biomedical domain. The information through NER can be leveraged for many purposes, ranging from primary and secondary use analyses [4] to the support for the standardisation and interoperability of clinical data [5].

Deep learning (DL)-based NER methodologies are actually the best performing approaches in terms of realising NER systems [6–8], but they actually have two main limits: they are strictly language- and domain-dependent and they need a large annotated corpus to train a deep neural network (DNN) with optimal results. The lack of annotated corpora is one of the open issues related to automatic clinical document analysis [9]. An annotated corpus can be obtained only through laborious and costly work performed by domain experts, who must manually analyse and annotate a large number of documents, following precise guidelines in order to produce a high-quality corpus [10,11]. Thus, not many annotated corpora are freely available, especially in the clinical domain and in languages different from English. Some methods have been proposed in the literature trying to overcome the lack of these important resources by using unsupervised machine-learning (ML) [12–14] or rule-based (RB) approaches [15–17], but in both cases the quality of the results is not comparable with that obtained through the manual efforts of domain experts. Other recent works have leveraged cross-language approaches [18,19], but in these cases annotated training and test sets in at least one language are required, in addition to knowledge bases or multi-lingual language models. Methodologies able to ease the work of the experts in the realisation of annotated corpora are required to narrow the gap between automatic and manual annotation, to the end of speeding up the manual annotation process, lowering its cost and reducing the needed efforts [20].

Interesting approaches for the annotation of corpora in an easier and less costly way are based on active learning (AL) and distant supervision (DS). Active learning [21] is an iterative annotation process supported by an ML model. In the first step of this approach, a small dataset extracted from a bigger corpus must be manually annotated. This set is then used to train a machine-learning classifier, to the end of annotating automatically the rest of the corpus. Among these automatic annotations, a human oracle must select the samples with presumably high utility to improve the classifier training, eventually correcting wrong predictions caused by an incomplete or small available dataset. More complex methodologies have been also proposed to improve the selection of the new samples [22]. The selected new samples are then added to the annotated training set and the ML model is retrained, improving the overall classification results in the prediction phase of the unannotated corpus. This process can be iterated until stop criteria or optimal performances are reached. AL methods can generate annotated corpora with less human efforts, but often the data are biased, depending on the method used for the new samples' selection during each iteration and on the content of the original corpus [23].

Distant supervision [24] is a completely automatic approach and exploits the knowledge extracted from knowledge bases (KBs) such as thesauri or a dictionary, assuming that if a string in text is included in a KB, then that string can be automatically annotated as an entity. This approach has no human cost, but the resulting corpus usually suffers from incomplete and noisy annotations. Incomplete annotations are named entities not listed in the KB, which will not be automatically annotated in the training corpus. On the other hand, a noisy annotation is a partial identification of a named entity, due to the presence in the KB of only an entity part (e.g., missing some words of that entity) or due to slight differences between the entity listed in the thesaurus and the one in the corpus (e.g., the use of a synonym of one of the words in multi-word entity, or a plural version of the same word).

In this paper a methodology that leverages both AL and DS for the annotation of B-NER clinical corpora is proposed, addressing some of the issues of both approaches to improve the quality and the speed of the annotation process. Firstly, an AL-based annotation is performed, exploiting a deep-learning NER architecture as an automatic classifier. Then, biomedical KBs are used for DS annotation and dataset expansion through data augmentation, with the purpose of mitigating the class imbalance problems [25] that could affect the annotations obtained through AL. In the experimental assessment the contribution of different pretrained Word Embedding (WE) models trained on a closed biomedical domain corpus as input of the DNN is also analysed, in particular comparing the contribution of word2vec [26], FastText [27] and ELMo [28] with a fine-tuned BERT model [29] pretrained on a general domain corpus. The proposed approach was used to easily and rapidly create an Italian language B-NER annotated corpus with very little effort with respect to a fully manual annotation procedure. The obtained corpus was evaluated on the aforementioned B-NER task, achieving performances comparable with the state of the art, as demonstrated in the experimental assessment.

In summary, the main contributions of this paper are:

- An automatic annotation methodology for B-NER corpora based on AL and DS techniques;
- An analysis of the contribution of different clinical closed-domain WE models (including word2vec, FastText and ELMo models), compared to a fine-tuned BERT model trained on a general-domain document collection;
- The annotation of an Italian clinical B-NER corpus.

The paper is organised as follows: in the next Section 2, an overview of the recent related works is presented, mainly focusing on methods for the annotation of texts from clinical and biomedical domains. Then, the details of the proposed approach are described in Section 3. In Section 4, the experimental assessment and the obtained results are shown and discussed and, finally, in Section 5 the final considerations, conclusions and future works are highlighted.

2. Related Works

Many methodologies devoted to the support of the annotation of an NER corpus have been proposed in recent years. Some studies are related to the guidelines for manual annotation of large corpora [10,11], which are very important for ensuring that the domain experts will follow the same approach during the annotation process. Besides them, many automatic and semi-automatic methods based on active learning and distant supervision have been presented. In [30], several AL algorithms were implemented to produce and assess corpora for a clinical text classification task in detail to determine the assertion status of clinical concepts. The results demonstrated that AL strategies are able to generate better classification models than the passive learning method such as random sampling. In [20,22], different sample selections for AL methods devoted to the clinical concept extraction task were proposed and evaluated, demonstrating their effectiveness in terms of building effective and robust ML models, reducing the time and the efforts involved in manual annotation. The authors of [31] described an AL method for the annotation of a corpus formed by MEDLINE abstracts annotated with pathological named entities. They proposed two different annotations, namely a short annotation that maps well defined diseases, and a long annotation that describes longer statements related to pathological phenomena and observations. Then, they defined an AL approach, which introduces a sampling bias by focusing on the most uncertain annotation samples, generating the annotated corpus. A clustering-based AL approach for B-NER is described in [32]. A document vector representation is obtained through TF-IDF; shared nearest neighbour (SNN) clustering is used to select documents with higher informative content during the iterations of AL, following the assumption that documents sharing similar named entities provide less information to the ML classifier. This AL method achieved a sensible improvement compared with random selection.

The authors of [33] presented a method to support the annotation of proteins, leveraging and ensemble learning together with WE, recurrent convolutional neural network, logistic regression and support vector machine models to effectively classify whether the title of a journal publication provides the information needed to show that experimental evidence of protein function for a given protein annotation is presented in the publication, reducing the manual effort only to a simple final confirmation. Their approach proved to outperform the transformer-based BioBERT model [34] fine-tuned on the same data.

The work described in [35] investigates whether conditional random fields (CRF) can be efficiently trained for NER in German texts, by means of an iterative procedure combining self-learning with a manual annotation—active learning—component, which leverages a CRF-based annotation and a manual correction to iteratively increase and improve the available dataset. Their results showed that their approach enabled the training of more accurate models with the annotation of fewer, more relevant data points, which are most helpful for modelling training.

In [36], the authors described an approach to deploy an annotated corpus for NER with minimal data and a light effort from experts combining both statistical and rule-based approaches. The authors of [24] proposed a novel approach to mitigate the incomplete and noisy annotations obtained from automatic annotation through DS. This approach is based on an instance selector, exploiting reinforcement learning. The selector chooses sentences from a candidate dataset to expand training data, improving the performances of a DL NER architecture. The instance selector is trained on a reward provided by the NER tagger. The authors of [37] provided a tool which is able to leverage and integrate the information from many available biomedical knowledge bases with the purpose, among the other things, of creating and annotating new corpora. In [38], the authors presented a method to reduce human efforts for the annotation of a clinical text classification corpus, exploiting weak supervision and deep representation. In detail, they annotated training data using KBs and a rule-based approach, and then they used WEs as deep representation features as input to different ML models. They proved that this approach is very effective when used to train a convolutional neural network, but needs many training samples and suffers when applied in multi-class problems. Other methods to annotate a corpus through DS using domain KBs and rule-based approaches are discussed in [15,16]. In these latter cases, the results are strongly dependent on the predefined rule set and the considered KBs.

In [39], a semi-supervised self-learning technique is presented to extend an Arabic sentiment annotated corpus with unlabeled data. In detail, a long short term memory (LSTM) neural network is used to train a set of models on a manually labeled dataset. These models were then used to extend the original corpus, ensuring an improvement in the Arabic sentiment classification task. In [40], an approach to automatically annotate EHRs is described. First, a DS based on KBs is used to create an annotated training set. Then, a weighted function of WEs was used to create a sentence-level vector representation of relevant expressions, which are used to train an ML classifier, with the purpose of assessing the presence, absence, or risk of urinary incontinence and bowel dysfunction. The resulting model outperformed a other rule-based models for annotation with a significant margin. In [41], the authors described an approach for the annotation of a B-NER corpus, exploiting an automatic translator and knowledge bases, such as UMLS or ICD9, which contain lists of medical domain terms. They first used automatic translators to convert the English language annotated corpus into Italian. Then KBs were used to address the limits of the machine translations when applied to the specific lexicon from the biomedical domain, improving in this way the quality of the obtained corpus. In [42], the authors proposed a method to enhance the performance of a DL biGRU-CRF model devoted to clinical named-entity recognition in the French language, exploiting medical terminologies. Regardless, we also compared the results of the proposed approach with a fine-tuned BERT model pretrained on a generic domain Italian corpus, leveraging it for both the AL phase, as well as for the analysis of the performances of the annotated biomedical NER corpus.

3. Methodology

The proposed annotation methodology can be split into two main phases: an iterative active learning phase, followed by a distant supervision phase.

3.1. Active Learning

In the preliminary step of the methodology, human experts have manually annotated a small number of documents extracted from an unannotated corpus. A small part of these annotated documents is used as a training set of a DL model, whereas the remaining annotated samples are used as a test set during all iterations of the AL phase, with the purpose of assessing the improvement obtained in each step and providing a stop criterion when no more performance increment is observed. The few samples of the training set can lead to poor performances in the DL model; on the other hand, the reduced time and efforts for the annotation of a small fraction of the whole corpus make this process affordable. At this point, experts will not annotate more documents, but they must simply review a subset of new documents from the whole dataset automatically annotated through DL, eventually correcting the wrong or missing predictions. These new annotated samples are then added to the training set, in order to retrain the ML model with higher precision thanks to a larger training set. The same procedure, namely the selection and review/correction of new AL-annotated samples and the retraining of the DL model, must be iterated until no further improvements of the ML results are observed. Figure 1 illustrates a schematic representation of the proposed AL-based annotation procedure.

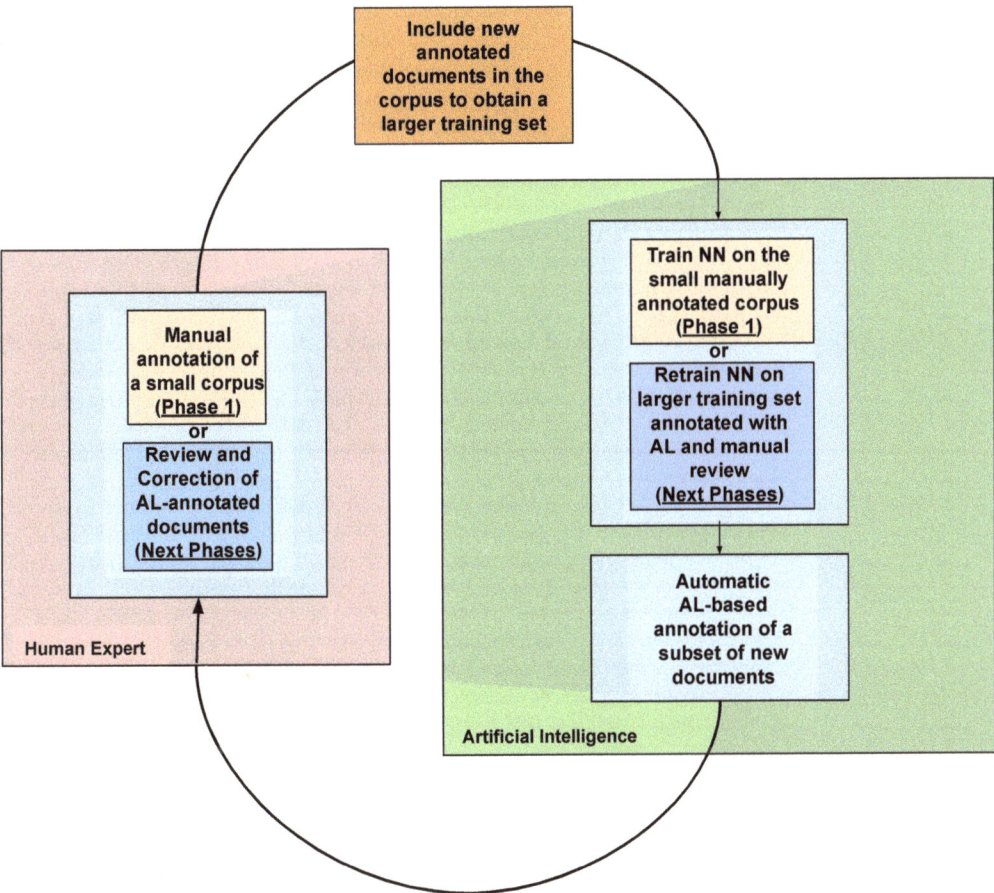

Figure 1. Schematic representation of the active learning annotation procedure.

The iterative AL annotation, followed by a manual review of the data, improves the quality of the obtained results with respect to a single-step AL annotation, because the effort of the human experts allows to correct any missing or wrong annotation obtained after each AL phase.

The selection of new samples from the dataset that will be annotated by the ML system is demanded of the domain experts without further support of automatic algorithms, such as those done in more complex AL approaches [22]. An improvement of the performance of the automatic annotation system is obtained using WE models trained on a biomedical closed domain corpus, as explained in Section 3.1.1. Deep neural network architectures are actually the state-of-the-art approaches for the B-NER task [3]. Thus, a DNN architecture for NER is used as an automatic ML classifier in the AL procedure. We adopted the classic DNN model presented in [43], known as Bi-LSTM CRF. This architecture is formed by the following layers: a bidirectional long short term memory (Bi-LSTM) character embedding layer, concatenated with a pretrained WE layer, a Bi-LSTM layer for words and a conditional random field (CRF) layer, counting in total 166,082,553 parameters. The Bi-LSTM CRF model offers both good performance and reasonable training times. Moreover, the BERT model [29,34] pretrained on a general domain was also considered, in comparison with the Bi-LSTM CRF architecture.

3.1.1. Closed Domain Embedding Models

As mentioned above, the proposed methodology requires the preliminary training of an ML model in order to start the iterative AL process. In this first step, a manually annotated training set that counts few examples is used. While it does not require a long time to be manually annotated, its limited number of samples limits the performances of the ML system trained on it. In order to mitigate this issue, we represented the input text using WE models pretrained on biomedical-domain document collections [44], improving in this way the performance of the NER DNN. A higher precision of the results during the AL phase can provide a substantial help to the experts, further reducing the efforts required for the selection and correction of new samples. In particular, following the results described in [44–46], we conducted experiments with several WE models specifically trained on a biomedical closed-domain corpus. For this purpose, a further collection of documents related to the biomedical domain were collected in order to train the embedding models (see Section 4.3 for further details on this corpus). Five different WE models are tested: two word2vec (W2V) models [26], two fastText (FT) models [27], considering in both cases skip-gram and cbow algorithms, and ELMo [28], a contextual embedding model, pretrained on the Italian language biomedical domain, following the same approach presented for the BioELMo model in English [47].

We analysed the performance of these embedding models when used to represent the text in the first layer of the adopted DNN architecture, during the training of the AL model in the preliminary step of the proposed method, when only a small manually annotated training set is available. All embedding models during the subsequent steps of the proposed methodology are also tested to better underline their contribution when a larger training set is available. Finally, the results are compared with models trained on a very large Italian language general domain corpora: a word2vec model [48], provided by ISTI-CNR (the model is publicity available at https://github.com/MartinoMensio/it_vectors_wiki_spacy, accessed on 6 June 2022), and a BERT model [29], fine tuned on the B-NER task, as better explained in Section 3.1.2.

3.1.2. Fine-Tuned BERT Model

As explained above, we also adopted in our experimental assessment a BERT model [29], with the main purpose of comparing the performance of the Bi-LSTM CRF model with WEs trained on a biomedical closed-domain corpus, with a fine-tuned BERT model pretrained on a general domain corpus. In particular, we adopted the *bert-base-italian-xxl-uncased* model from the MDZ Digital Library team (dbmdz) BERT Italian model (https://huggingface.co/dbmdz/bert-base-italian-cased, accessed on 6 June 2022). This model is based on the *BERT-base* architecture, which is formed by a stack of 12 layers of decoder-only transformers [49], 768 hidden dimensional states and 12 attention heads. This model was pretrained on a very large general domain Italian corpus, whose size is 81 GB and counts 13,138,379,147 tokens, exploiting the masked language modelling approach, which consists in randomly applying a mask on a fraction of the words in the training corpus, encoding in this way information of the sentences from both directions and training at the same time the model to predict the masked words.

The transformer-based language models, such as BERT, allow for the transfer learning of the knowledge acquired through the pretraining on large corpora, as well as for the fine-tuning of the model on other tasks. Several pretrained BERT models are available in the literature due to the long time and computational resources required for the pretraining phase, as well as due to the need for collecting sufficiently large document collections. For these reasons, we were not able to pretrain the BERT model on a biomedical closed-domain document corpus, neither a biomedical domain Italian language pretrained BERT model is available.

3.2. Distant Supervision Dataset Augmentation

Corpora annotated using ML-based methods are often affected by the problem of skewed class distribution [23]. An imbalanced class in the training set could limit the performance of a DNN trained with such corpora [50]. Undersampling or oversampling can help to mitigate the class imbalance problem [51], but undersampling can also lower the overall performances, deleting samples of all classes. With the purpose of improving the quality of the annotated corpus and resolving some of the problems related to class imbalance, a distant supervised annotation and augmentation after the AL phase is proposed. In detail, the annotated corpus is augmented with new samples belonging to the imbalanced classes, obtained through DS-exploiting domain KBs. The KB must contain a list of entities of the same class that must be augmented.

The dataset augmentation after the AL annotation is performed as follows. The sentences containing at least one entity belonging to the imbalanced classes are extracted from the corpus. Then, new sentences are obtained by substituting the named entities in these sentences with new entities of the same class randomly extracted from the respective KB. The process is iterated until a sufficient number of new sentences is obtained; that is, the respective class is less imbalanced, and, at the same time, all the entities from the KBs have been considered. In this way, we also include new entities in the dataset, in addition to reducing the class imbalance. Moreover, the augmentation process also oversamples the entities belonging to not imbalanced classes, providing in general more samples for all classes. As demonstrated by the results described in Section 4, this improves the overall performance, not only in the cases of imbalanced classes. Finally, the obtained new sentences are randomly reinserted in the corpus.

The whole proposed annotation methodology, including both iterative AL and DS phases, is represented in the block diagram depicted in Figure 2.

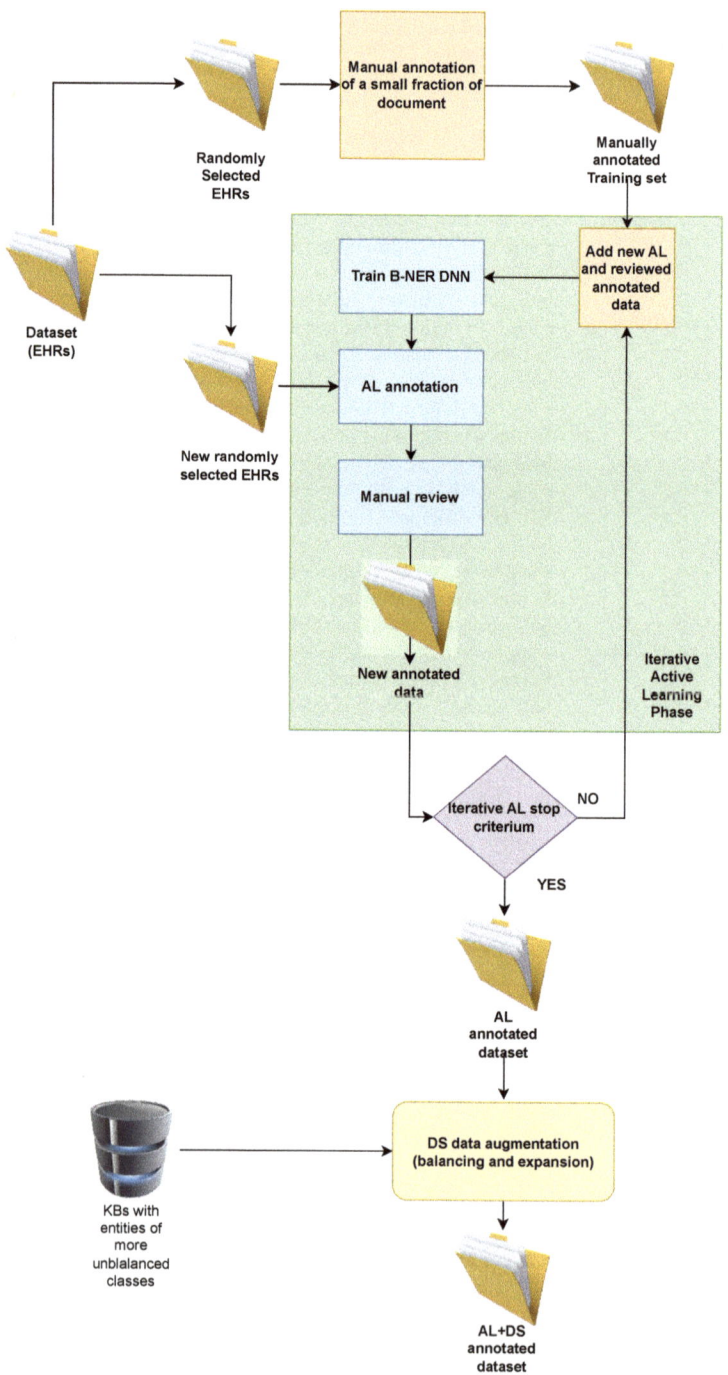

Figure 2. Schematic representation of the active learning annotation procedure.

4. Experimental Assessment and Discussion

In this section, in the following, after a description of the features of the original dataset and the details of the obtained annotated corpus, the performances of the DNN trained using the self-made corpus will be discussed, measured in terms of precision, recall and F1-score and considering also the contribution of the closed-domain WE models.

4.1. B-NER Annotated Corpora

The original unannotated dataset is formed by the narrative parts of NL text extracted from a set of 1011 anonymized EHRs in the Italian language, which has a total word count of 1,657,970. In detail, the dataset contains EHRs acquired from the eHealth systems of some different hospitals in Italy. As mentioned above, the EHRs had been previously anonymized and they are related to patients admitted to different departments of the hospitals. The content of these documents is relatively homogeneous, containing the clinical diary of the patients, where the causes of the admission to the hospitals, the diseases, the prognosis, the follow-ups, the exams, the procedures and the prescriptions are described. Some sample sentences extracted from two different EHRs (translated into English) are reported below.

- *Found sub-capital fracture and dislocation of left shoulder and contusion of right hip caused by accidental fall at home.*
- *Tomorrow follow-up exams.*
- *Patient admitted to cardiology from 9 February to 19 February due to episodes of arrhythmia, likely secondary to chronic renal failure.*

Eight different named-entity classes are identified, as shown in Table 1, following UMLS semantic types [52] and considering at the same time possible real-world applications of the trained ML models [2].

Table 1. Entity classes with corresponding acronyms and examples. The English translation of the examples is in italics between parentheses.

Class Type	Acronym	Examples
Diseases and Symptoms	DIS	Febbre (*Fever*), pressione alta (*High blood pressure*), cirrosi epatica (*liver cirrhosis*)
Drug names	DRU	Paracetamolo (*Paracetamol*), antibiotico (*antibiotic*)
Departments	DEP	Ortopedia (*Orthopedics*), pronto soccorso (*emergency room*)
Therapeutic procedures and Medical Instruments	THE	Ecografo (*ultrasound scanner*, profilassi antitrombotica (*thrombosis prophilaxis*), stent (*stent*)
Body Parts	BOD	Piede destro (*right foot*), testa dell'omero (*humeral head*), fegato (*liver*)
Measures	MEA	30 cc, 12 mm, 120 bpm
Dates	DAT	23 giugno 2012 (*23 June 2012*), oggi (*today*), ore 12:30 (*12:30*)
Diagnostic procedures or lab tests	ANA	Radiografia (*radiography*), valutazione cardiologica (*cardiac assessment*), glicemia (*glycaemia*), coronarografia (*angiography*)

As explained in Section 3.1, in the preliminary step of the annotation process a small set of documents formed by the text extracted from 25 randomly selected EHRs was manually annotated by two domain experts. The annotation procedure was conducted according to predefined guidelines, which describe general and specific annotation rules. The labelling process followed the *IOB* notation [53], i.e., each token belonging to an entity is labelled with the corresponding class adding the prefix *B* (Begin) if it is the first token of the entity, the prefix *I* for all subsequent tokens of the same multi-word entity and the tag *O* (Outside) if the token does not belong to an entity. The result of the manual annotation is a small dataset, which counts 7421 tokens and 1963 named entities, as shown in the first row of Table 2. The experts worked for approximately eight hours to produce this dataset, including the discussion about conflicts and disambiguation of the conflicting annotations. To the end of providing a stop criterion for the iterative AL phase (see Section 3.1), a further test set, which counts 21,133 tokens, was also manually annotated.

Table 2. Number of words and annotated entities in each step of the iterative AL annotation procedure.

Step	Word Number	Entity Number
1	7421	1963
2	20,083	5621
3	32,856	9285
4	78,449	21,914
5	133,200	37,029
6	201,956	55,601
7	304,797	60,669

This small dataset is used to train the DNN Bi-LSTM-CRF [43] architecture. This DL model has been used to automatically annotate new documents randomly extracted from the whole dataset, starting the iterative AL phase. In each iteration, the human experts had to review the correctness of the annotations produced by the DL model, eventually correcting the wrong or the missing ones. They worked each step for approximately eight hours, but, in this case, they were able to annotate wider datasets, thanks to the reduced effort provided by the partial annotation of the data, as shown in Table 2. The new data obtained in each iteration were added to the training set, producing a larger dataset, which was used to retrain the DL model. The same process was iterated and at each step the experts were able to speed up the annotation process, producing at the same time an increasing number of annotations thanks to the higher precision of the DL model trained on a larger and more complete dataset (see Table 2 for the details). The iterative AL process was stopped after seven iterations (see Section 4.3) when no more notable performance improvements of the ML model were observed. At the end of the AL phase, a corpus counting 304,798 words and 60,669 entities was annotated.

The results shown in Table 2 demonstrate that the proposed approach allows one to obtain a sensitive improvement of the time required for the annotation, with respect to a fully manual process. In the first preliminary step, a human expert was able to annotate a document collection formed by almost 8000 words in about 8 h, with a rate of 1000 words per hour. The dataset obtained through the AL phase counts 304,797 words: considering the same annotation rate of the preliminary step, the fully manual annotation of this dataset would have required about 300 h. The proposed AL process required seven steps where the experts reviewed and corrected the annotations of the new data obtained from the DNN for about 8 h for each step, with a total manual effort of 56 h. Moreover, the process required an average training time of the DNN equal to 1.5 h for each iteration (the training time increases with larger training sets) on the hardware used for the experimental assessment (see Section 4.2). In summary, the proposed iterative AL phase required in total about 66 h, allowing one to obtain an annotated dataset in almost 1/5 of the time required by a fully manual annotation.

Table 3 shows the distribution of the classes in the dataset obtained at the end of the AL phase. We note that there are very few examples of DEP (Departments) and DRU (Drugs) classes. This skewed class distribution can limit the performances of the ML systems, in particular for these two specific classes (see next Table 7). Then, in order to mitigate the skewed class distribution, the annotated corpus was automatically augmented using DS with our proposed approach, exploiting knowledge sources related to the more imbalanced classes, such as a complete list of drugs and pharmaceutical substances extracted from the Pharmaceutical Reference Book officially maintained by the Agenzia Italiana del Farmaco (https://farmaci.agenziafarmaco.gov.it/bancadatifarmaci/cerca-farmaco, accessed on 6 June 2022), the Italian government agency in charge for drug administration, and a list of medical departments was obtained from the main Italian medical centre (hospitals, clinical facilities, etc.) websites. These two KBs were used to expand the corpus, applying the data augmentation/oversampling, as described in Section 3.2. The final resulting annotated corpus has a total word count equal to 1,699,028 and a total entity count equal to 424,776. In Table 3, it is shown that the distribution of the samples after the DS augmentation clearly reduces the original skewness.

Table 3. Number of entities in the annotated corpus before and after the application of DS entity expansion.

Class Type	Entity Number	
	No Expansion	Expansion
MEA	12,168	65,668
DRU	2046	45,336
DEP	1099	25,469
THE	8170	46,900
BOD	11,423	33,203
DIS	31,179	125,059
DAT	4933	34,263
ANA	12,258	48,878
Total	60,669	424,776

The final corpus was split into a training set and a test set, randomly selecting about 15% of the data for the test and the remaining data for the training. In this way, the entity classes, respectively, in the training set and the test set are distributed as shown in Table 4. The test set was used to assess the performance of the DNN with the annotated corpus.

Table 4. Number of entities in the final annotated corpus, split into test set and training set.

Class Type	Entity Number	
	Test Set	Training Set
MEA	9458	56,210
DRU	6624	38,712
DEP	3860	21,609
THE	6859	40,041
BOD	4539	28,664
DIS	17,354	107,705
DAT	4920	29,343
ANA	7055	41,823
Total	60,669	364,107

Finally, a further test set was also manually annotated by the domain experts, extracting documents from a different medical domain document collection, with the purpose of assessing the quality of the corpus obtained with the proposed methodology. The aforementioned document collection, named hereinafter *out-of-corpus*, is formed by short medical notes and diagnoses from various medical departments and counts 15,728 words and 3816 entities. A common problem of the Bi-LSTM CRF B-NER architecture is that it often fails to generalise to out of vocabulary words, namely words that do not appear in the training set [54]. Thus, we tested the DL model also on the out-of-corpus test set, which contains many named entities not present in the original dataset.

4.2. Hardware

The AL phase requires the availability of hardware equipped with GPUs capable of training the DNN in a reasonable time. The hardware used in our experiments was a dual CPU Intel Xeon E5-2630, clocked at 2.2 GHz, with 256 GB of RAM and 1TB SDD, equipped with four Nvidia Titan X 1080 GPU with 11 GB of VRAM. With this system, the average time required to train the DNN during each iteration of the AL phase was about 1.5 h, considering that the training time increases with the size of the dataset.

4.3. Performances

To verify the effectiveness of the annotated corpus, we evaluated the performance of the same DNN used in the AL phase, trained on the obtained corpus. As explained above, we also tested different WE models to represent the input of the DNN, whose details are reported below.

Firstly, we considered a word2vec model [26] trained on a general domain Italian language corpus, hereinafter called *W2V ISTI*, formed by a Wikipedia dump and a collection of 31,432 novels [48]. This document collection is very large (242,261,172 sentences and 2,534,600,769 words), and its content is related to many knowledge fields. The training parameters used for this model are: skip-gram algorithm, vector size 300, window size 10 and negative samples 10.

Then, a more specific biomedical closed domain text corpus, hereinafter *BIO-Corpus*, was used to train the embedding models. This corpus was created considering different biomedical sources, in detail: (i) a dump of a selection of Italian Wikipedia pages related to medicine, biology, healthcare and other similar domains, following the procedure and the tools described in [45]; (ii) the text extracted from the package leaflets of all drugs available in Italy, downloading all pdf files from Agenzia Italiana del Farmaco (AIFA) and extracting the corresponding text exploiting Apache Tika (https://tika.apache.org/, accessed on 6 June 2022) and some specific Python scripts; (iii) the text extracted from the Italian Medical Dictionary of the *Corriere della Sera* (https://www.corriere.it/salute/dizionario/, accessed on 6 June 2022) through a set of custom web scraping Python scripts; and (iv) the text extracted from other Italian biomedical documents freely available online, such as scientific papers, presentations, technical reports and other things, exploiting also in this case Tika pipelines and Python scripts. The BIO-corpus is made up of 2,160,704 sentences and 511,649,310 words and it was used as a training set for five different WE models: two word2vec (W2V) [26] models and two FastText (FT) models [27], considering in both cases skip-gram and cbow algorithms and setting the vector size equal to 300, the window size equals to 10, the negative samples equals to 10 and, in the case of FastText embeddings, the char n-gram size varying from 3 to 6, as well as one contextual embedding model based on ELMo [28]. These latter models trained on the BIO-Corpus were called, respectively, *W2V cbow, W2V skip, FT cbow, FT skip* and *ELMo*.

Finally, we also tested the obtained annotated corpus by fine-tuning the BERT model pretrained on a very large general domain corpus, previously described in Section 3.1.2.

Table 5 shows the results obtained on the manually annotated test set (see Section 3.1) in the preliminary step of the AL phase when the DNN has been trained with few manually annotated data. The results are in terms of F1-Score, precision and recall averaged over all classes. It is possible to observe that *ELMo* embeddings trained on the BIO-Corpus and used to represent the input to the DNN obtain performances sensibly higher than the other cases, despite a training set with few samples. This can provide substantial help to the experts during the next steps of the AL phase, further reducing the effort in the correction of wrong predictions.

Thus, this model was selected for further steps of the AL phase for the annotation of the B-NER corpus, as well as the input layer of the DNN used to test the effectiveness of the annotated corpus. Moreover, the experiments also considered the fine tuning of the BERT model pretrained on a general domain document collection, that being the current reference model for NER tasks in the literature and because it obtained performances comparable to the ELMo case in the preliminary step of the proposed approach.

Table 5. Results in terms of F1-Score, precision and recall averaged on all classes obtained during the first training of the DNN of the AL phase, using different pretrained embedding models.

WE Model	F1-Score	Precision	Recall
W2V ISTI	0.4520	0.5274	0.4624
W2V cbow	0.3905	0.4764	0.3738
W2V skip	0.4734	0.6062	0.4131
FT cbow	0.3758	0.3976	0.4478
FT skip	0.4611	0.4438	0.4913
ELMo	0.6900	0.6758	0.7078
BERT	0.6787	0.6557	0.7034

The AL-based iterative annotation stopped when no further improvements to the results were obtained. Seven iterations are considered empirically sufficient to produce in the AL phase an annotated corpus with 304,977 words and 60,669 entities. Table 6 shows the performance improvements obtained in the test set at each step of the iterative AL procedure, using the ELMo model with BiLSTM CRF and the BERT model. As shown in Table 6, increasing the size of the annotated corpus during the steps of the iterative AL phase improved the performances of both the ELMo and the BERT experiments. We also note that the ELMo model pretrained on the biomedical domain corpus performs slightly better when fewer data in the training set are available during the first iterations of the procedure, while, when larger training sets are obtained during the AL phases, the BERT model pretrained on a general domain corpus obtains slightly better results. In any case, both models obtain comparable performances, demonstrating that a simpler neural language model, such as ELMo, pretrained on the biomedical domain corpus obtains performances comparable with the ones produced by a more complex DNN, such as BERT, pretrained on a general domain corpus. Then, we focused the next phase of the experimental assessment only on the ELMo model, investigating the contribution of the DS data augmentation phase.

Table 6. Performance of the best performing DNNs (ELMo Bi-LSTM CRF and BERT fine tuned) at each step of the AL phase of the annotation procedure, in terms of precision, recall and F1-Score averaged over all classes.

Iteration Step	ELMo BiLSTM-CRF			BERT Fine Tuned		
	Precision	Recall	F1-Score	Precision	Recall	F1-Score
1	0.6758	0.7078	0.6900	0.6557	0.7034	0.6787
2	0.7195	0.7504	0.7346	0.7187	0.7517	0.7349
3	0.7269	0.7567	0.7406	0.7252	0.7638	0.7440
4	0.7364	0.7697	0.7522	0.7449	0.7738	0.7590
5	0.7552	0.7743	0.7646	0.7581	0.7849	0.7712
6	0.7629	0.7767	0.7695	0.7639	0.7915	0.7775
7	0.7635	0.7889	0.7760	0.7790	0.8001	0.7893

In Table 7, the results of the ELMo experiment obtained in the last step of the AL phase are highlighted, showing the precision, recall and F1-Score obtained for each class of the dataset. Observing at the same time the left column of Table 3, where the number of entities of each class are shown, and Table 7, with the results obtained by the DNNs trained on the corpus obtained at the end of the AL phase, it is possible to note that the worst performances were obtained in the cases of the entities belonging to the more imbalanced classes, namely DRU (Drugs) and DEP (Departments), also limiting the average results.

Table 7. Performance of the ELMo Bi-LSTM CRF at the last step of the AL phase of the annotation procedure, in terms of precision, recall and F1-Score for each class.

Entity Type	Precision	Recall	F1-Score
MEA	0.8436	0.8599	0.8517
DRU	0.8085	0.3576	0.4959
DEP	0.1845	0.1404	0.1595
THE	0.5668	0.8459	0.6788
BOD	0.8283	0.8949	0.8603
DIS	0.8316	0.9125	0.8702
DAT	0.8905	0.9492	0.9189
ANA	0.8145	0.9137	0.8612
Average	0.7635	0.7889	0.7760

We introduced the DS data augmentation phase in order to limit this issue. After the expansion and the balancing of the training set using the second part of the proposed approach, where new sentences are obtained leveraging DS with domain KBs containing lists of entities of two more imbalanced classes, the performance of the ELMo DNN trained on the training set obtained with both the AL and DS phases are sensibly improved, as shown in Table 8. In this case, we reported only the results obtained by the best performing model, which was the Bi-LSTM CRF architecture with the ELMo embeddings. This behaviour is expected, due to overfitting issues of the BERT model trained on very large datasets [55].

In particular, comparing the obtained results for DRU and DEP classes in Table 8, where the DS augmentation for balancing and expansion were applied for the annotation of the training set after the AL, with the results achieved in the same class types shown in Table 7, where only the AL is performed, it is possible to observe that the DS augmentation applied to the most unbalanced classes DEP and DRU provided a sensible performance boost. Moreover, we can also note an improvement in all the other classes thanks to the oversampling performed during the DS data augmentation.

Table 8. Results obtained by the ELMo Bi-LSTM CRF trained with the final annotated corpus (AL and DS augmentation) in terms of precision, recall and F1-Score for each class.

Entity Type	Precision	Recall	F1-Score
MEA	0.9636	0.9675	0.9655
DRU	0.9863	0.9893	0.9878
DEP	0.9878	0.9860	0.9869
THE	0.9609	0.9636	0.9622
BOD	0.9203	0.9262	0.9232
DIS	0.9595	0.9634	0.9615
DAT	0.9783	0.9809	0.9796
ANA	0.9647	0.9718	0.9682
Average	0.9642	0.9679	0.9661

To the end of further verifying the effectiveness of the final obtained annotated corpus, we also tested the DNN models on the out-of-corpus test set, previously described in Section 4.1. This additional manually annotated test set was extracted from a different document collection, which contains many entities not present in the dataset used to build and annotate the training set. Table 9 shows the results obtained by the ELMo BiLSTM CRF architecture trained on the final annotated corpus and tested on the out-of-corpus test set. It is worth noting that, despite a slight performance drop, the DNN model still performs at a good level, assessing the effectiveness of the obtained annotated training corpus.

Table 9. Results in terms of precision, recall and F1-Score averaged on all classes obtained with the DNN with ELMo embeddings trained on the final annotated corpus and tested on the out-of-corpus test set.

Entity Type	Precision	Recall	F1-Score
MEA	0.9374	0.9051	0.9210
DRU	0.6429	0.8824	0.7438
DEP	0.9000	1.000	0.9474
THE	0.7983	0.8559	0.8261
BOD	0.9112	0.8701	0.8902
DIS	0.8475	0.9278	0.8858
DAT	0.5608	0.9222	0.6975
ANA	0.9364	0.8805	0.9076
Average	0.8809	0.8986	0.8875

In summary, these results demonstrate that the DS data augmentation phase is capable of further improving the quality of the dataset obtained from the previous iterative AL phase, mitigating the issues of the AL related to unbalanced classes and out-of-corpus named entities.

Finally, the next Table 10 reports the metrics averaged on all classes obtained by each considered DNN model, namely the Bi-LSTM CRF with the various considered WE models as input layer and the fine-tuned BERT model, trained on the final annotated dataset (AL and DS) and tested on the out-of-corpus test set. The purpose of this last experiment is to evaluate the contribution of different neural language models on a corpus containing many named entities not present in the training set. The results in Table 10 show that the WE model trained on a biomedical closed-domain document collection (W2V cbow, W2V skip, FT cbow and FT skip) provides sensible improvements with respect to the W2V ISTI model, trained on a general domain corpus. We also note that the WEs trained using the skipgram algorithm provide improved performance with respect to the cbow algorithm. The ELMo model produces the best performance, but the simpler W2V skip model also obtains good results, although it does not reach the performance obtained by more complex ELMo and BERT architectures. As in the previous case, the performances of the BERT model are limited by the overfitting issues, although we adopted a drop-out rate equal to 0.7 to limit them, following the literature [55].

Table 10. Results in terms of F1-Score, precision and recall obtained by the DNN on the out-of-corpus test set, using different pretrained WE models.

WE Model	Precision	Recall	F1-Score
W2V ISTI	0.7794	0.7714	0.7714
W2V cbow	0.8047	0.8000	0.8010
W2V skip	0.8676	0.8464	0.8545
FT cbow	0.8164	0.8143	0.8125
FT skip	0.8367	0.8107	0.8213
ELMo	0.8809	0.8986	0.8875
BERT	0.7356	0.7246	0.7301

5. Conclusions

This paper presented an approach based on both active learning and distant supervision, which makes the manual annotation of a corpus for biomedical named entity recognition (B-NER) a less costly process, reducing the efforts needed by human experts. In detail, the method is based on a first AL phase, where a DNN architecture for NER composed of a BiLSTM-CRF is used to support the manual annotation. When no further improvements are achieved by the AL-based process, the corpus is augmented using DS, exploiting domain KBs, in order to mitigate the class imbalance. Finally, an assessment of the utility of using a WE model trained on a closed domain document collection as input for the DNN was carried out, considering word2vec, FastText and ELMo embeddings, and also comparing the obtained results with the fine tuned BERT model pretrained on a very large general domain document collection.

The approach was tested by creating an Italian language B-NER corpus used to train different B-NER DNNs. The experiments demonstrated that the obtained corpus is capable of training a B-NER DNN with very good performance, allowing one to annotate an NER corpus in a fraction of the time required for a fully manual annotation. Moreover, they showed that the pretraining of the ELMo contextual embedding model on a biomedical closed domain corpus allows one to obtain results comparable with the more complex BERT architecture pretrained on a very large general domain document collection, which demands more computational resources.

The proposed annotation methodology can facilitate the development and the implementation of AI-powered information extraction and indexing systems, improving the management of large natural language document collections, as well as supporting the analysis and the extraction of knowledge from such documents. On the other hand, a limit of the proposed approach is that KBs in the domain and the language of the annotations must be available to apply the DS phase. Moreover, the method is not fully automatic, requiring in any case human supervision, as well as a fully manual annotation in the preliminary phase. It also requires the availability of DL-dedicated hardware to carry out the AL phase in a reasonable time. Finally, the training of the NLM (in particular, the BERT-based models) requires the collection of a very large closed-domain unannotated document corpus, which in some cases may not be easy to obtain.

In future work, the B-NER DL model trained on the obtained annotated corpus on more out-of-corpus documents, such as medical tweets or scientific papers, assessing the effectiveness of the proposed annotation methodology will be evaluated. Moreover, we want to collect a very large biomedical closed domain corpus in order to pretrain a domain-specific Italian biomedical BERT model, following the BioBERT [34] approach, in order to further test the proposed annotation approach.

Finally, the presented annotation methodology could be applied to other languages and domains in order to demonstrate its general validity. In particular, the same approach was also developed, tailored and tested for the annotation of a cyber security (CS) English NER corpus, exploited for an innovative ML-based threat assessment methodology [56] proposed in the EC-funded AI4HEALTHSEC project (https://www.ai4healthsec.eu, accessed on 6 June 2022). In this case, a large document collection was previously extracted from a CS news website, allowing for the creation of an unannotated training set for the neural language models, while CAPEC (https://capec.mitre.org, accessed on 6 June 2022) and CPE (https://nvd.nist.gov/products/cpe, accessed on 6 June 2022) KBs were used in the DS phase for the annotation of CS threats and the corresponding assets. Moreover, a CS closed-domain BERT model was also exploited, confirming the effectiveness of the use of a closed-domain transformer-based NLM.

Author Contributions: Conceptualization, S.S. and F.G.; methodology, S.S. and F.G.; software, S.S. and F.G.; validation, S.S., F.G. and M.C.; formal analysis, S.S. and F.G.; investigation, S.S. and F.G.; resources, S.S., F.G. and M.C. ; data curation, S.S. and F.G.; writing—original draft preparation, S.S. and F.G.; writing—review and editing, S.S., F.G. and M.C.; visualization, S.S. and F.G.; supervision, M.C.; project administration, M.C.; funding acquisition, M.C. All authors have read and agreed to the published version of the manuscript.

Funding: This research was partially funded by the European Commission, grant number 883273, AI4HEALTHSEC—A Dynamic and Self-Organized Artificial Swarm Intelligence Solution for Security and Privacy Threats in Healthcare ICT Infrastructures.

Institutional Review Board Statement: Not applicable.

Informed Consent Statement: Not applicable.

Data Availability Statement: Not applicable.

Acknowledgments: The authors would like to thank Simona Sada and Giuseppe Trerotola for the technical and administrative support.

Conflicts of Interest: The authors declare no conflict of interest. The funders had no role in the design of the study; in the collection, analyses, or interpretation of data; in the writing of the manuscript, or in the decision to publish the results.

References

1. Yadav, P.; Steinbach, M.; Kumar, V.; Simon, G.J. Mining Electronic Health Records (EHRs): A Survey. *ACM Comput. Surv.* **2018**, *50*, 1–40. [CrossRef]
2. Silvestri, S.; Esposito, A.; Gargiulo, F.; Sicuranza, M.; Ciampi, M.; De Pietro, G. A Big Data Architecture for the Extraction and Analysis of EHR Data. In Proceedings of the 2019 IEEE World Congress on Services (SERVICES), Milan, Italy, 8–13 July 2019; Volume 2642-939X; pp. 283–288. [CrossRef]
3. Shickel, B.; Tighe, P.; Bihorac, A.; Rashidi, P. Deep EHR: A Survey of Recent Advances in Deep Learning Techniques for Electronic Health Record (EHR) Analysis. *IEEE J. Biomed. Health Inform.* **2018**, *22*, 1589–1604. [CrossRef] [PubMed]
4. Abadeer, M. Assessment of DistilBERT performance on Named Entity Recognition task for the detection of Protected Health Information and medical concepts. In Proceedings of the 3rd Clinical Natural Language Processing Workshop, Online, 16–20 November 2020; pp. 158–167. [CrossRef]
5. Oemig, F.; Blobel, B. Natural Language Processing Supporting Interoperability in Healthcare. In *Text Mining: From Ontology Learning to Automated Text Processing Applications*; Biemann, C., Mehler, A., Eds.; Springer International Publishing: Cham, Switzerland, 2014; pp. 137–156. [CrossRef]
6. Yadav, V.; Bethard, S. A Survey on Recent Advances in Named Entity Recognition from Deep Learning models. In Proceedings of the 27th International Conference on Computational Linguistics, Melbourne, Australia, 15–20 July 2018; pp. 2145–2158.
7. Lewis, P.; Ott, M.; Du, J.; Stoyanov, V. Pretrained Language Models for Biomedical and Clinical Tasks: Understanding and Extending the State-of-the-Art. In Proceedings of the 3rd Clinical Natural Language Processing Workshop, Online, 16–20 November 2020; pp. 146–157. [CrossRef]
8. Weber, L.; Sänger, M.; Münchmeyer, J.; Habibi, M.; Leser, U.; Akbik, A. HunFlair: An easy-to-use tool for state-of-the-art biomedical named entity recognition. *Bioinformatics* **2021**, *37*, 2792–2794. [CrossRef]
9. Xiao, C.; Choi, E.; Sun, J. Opportunities and challenges in developing deep learning models using electronic health records data: A systematic review. *JAMIA* **2018**, *25*, 1419–1428. [CrossRef] [PubMed]
10. Patel, P.; Davey, D.; Panchal, V.; Pathak, P. Annotation of a Large Clinical Entity Corpus. In Proceedings of the 2018 Conference on Empirical Methods in Natural Language Processing, Brussels, Belgium, 31 October–4 November 2018; pp. 2033–2042.
11. Xia, F.; Yetisgen-Yildiz, M. Clinical corpus annotation: Challenges and strategies. In Proceedings of the Third Workshop on Building and Evaluating Resources for Biomedical Text Mining (BioTxtM'2012) in conjunction with the International Conference on Language Resources and Evaluation (LREC), Istanbul, Turkey, 21–27 May 2012.
12. Alicante, A.; Corazza, A.; Isgrò, F.; Silvestri, S. Unsupervised entity and relation extraction from clinical records in Italian. *Comput. Biol. Med.* **2016**, *72*, 263–275. [CrossRef] [PubMed]
13. Wangpoonsarp, A.; Shimura, K.; Fukumoto, F. Unsupervised Predominant Sense Detection and Its Application to Text Classification. *Appl. Sci.* **2020**, *10*, 6052. [CrossRef]
14. Nadif, M.; Role, F. Unsupervised and self-supervised deep learning approaches for biomedical text mining. *Briefings Bioinform.* **2021**, *22*, 1592–1603. [CrossRef]
15. Ghiasvand, O.; Kate, R.J. Learning for clinical named entity recognition without manual annotations. *Inform. Med. Unlocked* **2018**, *13*, 122–127. [CrossRef]
16. Diomaiuta, C.; Mercorella, M.; Ciampi, M.; Pietro, G.D. A novel system for the automatic extraction of a patient problem summary. In Proceedings of the 2017 IEEE Symposium on Computers and Communications (ISCC), Heraklion, Greece, 3–6 July 2017; pp. 182–186. [CrossRef]
17. Hammami, L.; Paglialonga, A.; Pruneri, G.; Torresani, M.; Sant, M.; Bono, C.; Caiani, E.G.; Baili, P. Automated classification of cancer morphology from Italian pathology reports using Natural Language Processing techniques: A rule-based approach. *J. Biomed. Inform.* **2021**, *116*, 103712. [CrossRef]
18. Silvestri, S.; Gargiulo, F.; Ciampi, M.; De Pietro, G. Exploit Multilingual Language Model at Scale for ICD-10 Clinical Text Classification. In Proceedings of the 2020 IEEE Symposium on Computers and Communications (ISCC), Rennes, France, 7–10 July 2020; pp. 1–7. [CrossRef]
19. Suárez-Paniagua, V.; Dong, H.; Casey, A. A multi-BERT hybrid system for Named Entity Recognition in Spanish radiology reports. In Proceedings of the Working Notes of CLEF 2021—Conference and Labs of the Evaluation Forum, Bucharest, Romania, 21–24 September 2021; Faggioli, G., Ferro, N., Joly, A., Maistro, M., Piroi, F., Eds.; CEUR-WS.org: Bucharest, Romania, 2021; Volume 2936, *CEUR Workshop Proceedings*; pp. 846–856.
20. Kholghi, M.; Sitbon, L.; Zuccon, G.; Nguyen, A. Active learning reduces annotation time for clinical concept extraction. *Int. J. Med. Inform.* **2017**, *106*, 25–31. [CrossRef]
21. Cohn, D.A.; Ghahramani, Z.; Jordan, M.I. Active Learning with Statistical Models. *J. Artif. Intell. Res.* **1996**, *4*, 129–145. [CrossRef]

22. Kholghi, M.; Sitbon, L.; Zuccon, G.; Nguyen, A.N. Active learning: A step towards automating medical concept extraction. *JAMIA* **2016**, *23*, 289–296. [CrossRef]
23. Tomanek, K.; Hahn, U. Reducing class imbalance during active learning for named entity annotation. In Proceedings of the 5th International Conference on Knowledge Capture (K-CAP 2009), Redondo Beach, CA, USA, 1–4 September 2009; pp. 105–112. [CrossRef]
24. Yang, Y.; Chen, W.; Li, Z.; He, Z.; Zhang, M. Distantly Supervised NER with Partial Annotation Learning and Reinforcement Learning. In Proceedings of the 27th International Conference on Computational Linguistics, Santa Fe, NM, USA, 20–26 August 2018; pp. 2159–2169.
25. Li, Q.; Mao, Y. A review of boosting methods for imbalanced data classification. *Pattern Anal. Appl.* **2014**, *17*, 679–693. [CrossRef]
26. Mikolov, T.; Chen, K.; Corrado, G.; Dean, J. Efficient Estimation of Word Representations in Vector Space. In Proceedings of the International Conference on Learning Representations ICLR 2013, Scottsdale, AZ, USA, 2–4 May 2013.
27. Bojanowski, P.; Grave, E.; Joulin, A.; Mikolov, T. Enriching Word Vectors with Subword Information. *Trans. Assoc. Comput. Linguist.* **2017**, *5*, 135–146. [CrossRef]
28. Peters, M.; Neumann, M.; Iyyer, M.; Gardner, M.; Clark, C.; Lee, K.; Zettlemoyer, L. Deep Contextualized Word Representations. In Proceedings of the 2018 Conference of the North American Chapter of the Association for Computational Linguistics: Human Language Technologies, Volume 1 (Long Papers), Melbourne, Australia, 15–20 July 2018; pp. 2227–2237. [CrossRef]
29. Devlin, J.; Chang, M.W.; Lee, K.; Toutanova, K. BERT: Pre-training of Deep Bidirectional Transformers for Language Understanding. In Proceedings of the 2019 Conference of the North American Chapter of the Association for Computational Linguistics: Human Language Technologies, Volume 1 (Long and Short Papers), Minneapolis, MI, USA, 2–7 June 2019; pp. 4171–4186. [CrossRef]
30. Chen, Y.; Mani, S.; Xu, H. Applying active learning to assertion classification of concepts in clinical text. *J. Biomed. Inform.* **2012**, *45*, 265–272. [CrossRef]
31. Hahn, U.; Beisswanger, E.; Buyko, E.; Faessler, E. Active Learning-Based Corpus Annotation—The PathoJen Experience. In Proceedings of the AMIA 2012, American Medical Informatics Association Annual Symposium, Chicago, IL, USA, 3–7 November 2012.
32. Han, X.; Kwoh, C.K.; Kim, J. Clustering based active learning for biomedical Named Entity Recognition. In Proceedings of the 2016 International Joint Conference on Neural Networks (IJCNN), Vancouver, BC, Canada, 24–29 July 2016; pp. 1253–1260. [CrossRef]
33. Tao, J.; Brayton, K.A.; Broschat, S.L. Automated Confirmation of Protein Annotation Using NLP and the UniProtKB Database. *Appl. Sci.* **2021**, *11*, 24. [CrossRef]
34. Lee, J.; Yoon, W.; Kim, S.; Kim, D.; Kim, S.; So, C.H.; Kang, J. BioBERT: A pre-trained biomedical language representation model for biomedical text mining. *Bioinformatics* **2019**. btz682, [CrossRef] [PubMed]
35. Alves-Pinto, A.; Demus, C.; Spranger, M.; Labudde, D.; Hobley, E. Iterative Named Entity Recognition with Conditional Random Fields. *Appl. Sci.* **2022**, *12*, 330. [CrossRef]
36. Gabbard, R.; DeYoung, J.; Lignos, C.; Freedman, M.; Weischedel, R. Combining rule-based and statistical mechanisms for low-resource named entity recognition. *Mach. Transl.* **2018**, *32*, 31–43. [CrossRef]
37. Kanterakis, A.; Kanakaris, N.; Koutoulakis, M.; Pitianou, K.; Karacapilidis, N.; Koumakis, L.; Potamias, G. Converting Biomedical Text Annotated Resources into FAIR Research Objects with an Open Science Platform. *Appl. Sci.* **2021**, *11*, 9648. [CrossRef]
38. Wang, Y.; Sohn, S.; Liu, S.; Shen, F.; Wang, L.; Atkinson, E.J.; Amin, S.; Liu, H. A clinical text classification paradigm using weak supervision and deep representation. *BMC Med. Inform. Decis. Mak.* **2019**, *19*, 1. [CrossRef] [PubMed]
39. Al-Laith, A.; Shahbaz, M.; Alaskar, H.F.; Rehmat, A. AraSenCorpus: A Semi-Supervised Approach for Sentiment Annotation of a Large Arabic Text Corpus. *Appl. Sci.* **2021**, *11*, 2434. [CrossRef]
40. Banerjee, I.; Li, K.; Seneviratne, M.; Ferrari, M.; Seto, T.; Brooks, J.D.; Rubin, D.L.; Hernandez-Boussard, T. Weakly supervised natural language processing for assessing patient-centered outcome following prostate cancer treatment. *JAMIA Open* **2019**. [CrossRef] [PubMed]
41. Attardi, G.; Cozza, V.; Sartiano, D. Annotation and Extraction of Relations from Italian Medical Records. In Proceedings of the 6th Italian Information Retrieval Workshop, Cagliari, Italy, 25–26 May 2015.
42. Lerner, I.; Paris, N.; Tannier, X. Terminologies augmented recurrent neural network model for clinical named entity recognition. *J. Biomed. Inform.* **2020**, *102*, 103356. [CrossRef]
43. Lample, G.; Ballesteros, M.; Subramanian, S.; Kawakami, K.; Dyer, C. Neural Architectures for Named Entity Recognition. In Proceedings of the 2016 Conference of the North American Chapter of the Association for Computational Linguistics: Human Language Technologies, San Diego, CA, USA, 12–17 June 2016; pp. 260–270. [CrossRef]
44. Silvestri, S.; Gargiulo, F.; Ciampi, M. Improving Biomedical Information Extraction with Word Embeddings Trained on Closed-Domain Corpora. In Proceedings of the 2019 IEEE Symposium on Computers and Communications (ISCC), Barcelona, Spain, 29 June–3 July 2019; pp. 1129–1134. [CrossRef]
45. Alicante, A.; Corazza, A.; Isgrò, F.; Silvestri, S. Semantic Cluster Labeling for Medical Relations. In Proceedings of the third International Conference Innovation in Medicine and Healthcare 2016, Puerto de la Cruz, Spain, 15–17 June 2016; pp. 183–193. doi: [CrossRef]

46. Kameswara Sarma, P.; Liang, Y.; Sethares, B. Domain Adapted Word Embeddings for Improved Sentiment Classification. In Proceedings of the Workshop on Deep Learning Approaches for Low-Resource NLP, Melbourne, Australia, 15–20 July 2018; pp. 51–59.
47. Jin, Q.; Dhingra, B.; Cohen, W.; Lu, X. Probing Biomedical Embeddings from Language Models. In Proceedings of the 3rd Workshop on Evaluating Vector Space Representations for NLP, Minneapolis, MN, USA, 2–7 June 2019; pp. 82–89. [CrossRef]
48. Berardi, G.; Esuli, A.; Marcheggiani, D. Word Embeddings Go to Italy: A Comparison of Models and Training Datasets. In Proceedings of the 6th Italian Information Retrieval Workshop, Cagliari, Italy, 25–26 May 2015.
49. Vaswani, A.; Shazeer, N.; Parmar, N.; Uszkoreit, J.; Jones, L.; Gomez, A.N.; Kaiser, L.; Polosukhin, I. Attention is All you Need. In Proceedings of the Annual 31st Conference on Neural Information Processing Systems, Long Beach, CA, USA, 4–9 December 2017; pp. 5998–6008.
50. Buda, M.; Maki, A.; Mazurowski, M.A. A systematic study of the class imbalance problem in convolutional neural networks. *Neural Netw.* **2018**, *106*, 249–259. [CrossRef]
51. Han, W.; Huang, Z.; Li, S.; Jia, Y. Distribution-Sensitive Unbalanced Data Oversampling Method for Medical Diagnosis. *J. Med. Syst.* **2019**, *43*, 39:1–39:10. [CrossRef]
52. Bodenreider, O. The unified medical language system (UMLS): Integrating biomedical terminology. *Nucleic Acids Res.* **2004**, *32*, D267–D270. [CrossRef]
53. Tjong, E.F.; Sang, K.; Veenstra, J. Representing Text Chunks. In Proceedings of the Ninth Conference of the European Chapter of the Association for Computational Linguistics, Bergen, Norway, 8–12 June 1999.
54. Wang, X.; Zhang, Y.; Ren, X.; Zhang, Y.; Zitnik, M.; Shang, J.; Langlotz, C.; Han, J. Cross-type biomedical named entity recognition with deep multi-task learning. *Bioinformatics* **2019**, *35*, 1745–1752. [CrossRef]
55. Wang, Y.; Liu, F.; Verspoor, K.; Baldwin, T. Evaluating the Utility of Model Configurations and Data Augmentation on Clinical Semantic Textual Similarity. In Proceedings of the 19th SIGBioMed Workshop on Biomedical Language Processing, Online, 9 July 2020; pp. 105–111. [CrossRef]
56. Islam, S.; Papastergiou, S.; Silvestri, S. Cyber Threat Analysis Using Natural Language Processing for a Secure Healthcare System. In Proceedings of the 27th IEEE Symposium on Computers and Communications (ISCC 2022), Rhodes Island, Greece, 29 June–3 July 2022, to be published.

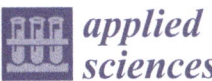

Article

Cyberattack Path Generation and Prioritisation for Securing Healthcare Systems

Shareeful Islam [1,*,†], Spyridon Papastergiou [2,†], Eleni-Maria Kalogeraki [2,†] and Kitty Kioskli [3,4]

1 School of Computing and Information Science, Anglia Ruskin University, Cambridge CB1 1PT, UK
2 Department of Informatics, University of Piraeus, 185 34 Piraeus, Greece; paps@unipi.gr (S.P.); elmaklg@unipi.gr (E.-M.K.)
3 Institute of Analytics and Data Science (IADS), School of Computer Science and Electronic Engineering, University of Essex, Essex CO4 3SQ, UK; kitty.kioskli@essex.ac.uk
4 Trustilio B.V., 1017 HL Amsterdam, The Netherlands
* Correspondence: shareeful.islam@aru.ac.uk
† Focal point, Belgium.

Abstract: Cyberattacks in the healthcare sector are constantly increasing due to the increased usage of information technology in modern healthcare and the benefits of acquiring a patient healthcare record. Attack path discovery provides useful information to identify the possible paths that potential attackers might follow for a successful attack. By identifying the necessary paths, the mitigation of potential attacks becomes more effective in a proactive manner. Recently, there have been several works that focus on cyberattack path discovery in various sectors, mainly on critical infrastructure. However, there is a lack of focus on the vulnerability, exploitability and target user profile for the attack path generation. This is important for healthcare systems where users commonly have a lack of awareness and knowledge about the overall IT infrastructure. This paper presents a novel methodology for the cyberattack path discovery that is used to identify and analyse the possible attack paths and prioritise the ones that require immediate attention to ensure security within the healthcare ecosystem. The proposed methodology follows the existing published vulnerabilities from common vulnerabilities and exposures. It adopts the common vulnerability scoring system so that base metrics and exploitability features can be used to determine and prioritise the possible attack paths based on the threat actor capability, asset dependency and target user profile and evidence of indicator of compromise. The work includes a real example from the healthcare use case to demonstrate the methodology used for the attack path generation. The result from the studied context, which processes big data from healthcare applications, shows that the uses of various parameters such as CVSS metrics, threat actor profile, and Indicator of Compromise allow us to generate realistic attack paths. This certainly supports the healthcare practitioners in identifying the controls that are required to secure the overall healthcare ecosystem.

Keywords: healthcare ecosystem; medical devices; cyberattack path; vulnerability; exploitability

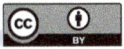

1. Introduction

The healthcare sector is becoming more digitally connected due to the advancement of technology, and so the potential risk of a cyber incident will increase. The connectivity of medical devices with other software and information communication technology (ICT) infrastructures poses potential risks. There is increasing concern that the connectivity of these medical devices will directly affect healthcare service delivery and patient safety, which is unique compared to traditional computing systems [1]. Research studies have shown that the number of hacking incidents reported in healthcare was 42% more in 2020 [2]. The healthcare information infrastructure is equipped with medical devices that require both physical and cyber interaction, which can create new attacker capabilities [3]. It is necessary to identify the possible attacks and related paths that can pose potential risks within the healthcare context. To our knowledge, this is the first study that focuses on the vulnerabilities related to healthcare devices and their dependencies on other information technology (IT) infrastructures to propagate an attack.

The present paper illustrates an evidence-based attack path discovery method, considering the unique characteristics of the healthcare information infrastructure, such as assets, and its cyber and physical dependencies, vulnerabilities, threat actor and user profile, and indicator of compromise (IoC). There are three main contributions of this work. Firstly, the proposed approach includes a systematic process for attack path identification based on the assets, dependencies, and vulnerabilities. It adopts the existing standards, such as common vulnerabilities and exposures (CVE) and the common vulnerability scoring system (CVSS), to identify and analyse the vulnerabilities relating to the attack paths. These repositories contain huge amounts of data about the vulnerabilities. The identified attack paths are prioritised based on the IoC, which shows the evidence of any attack. Secondly, a knowledge base is developed that consists of rule-based reasoning to identify the possible attack paths. The rules are based on certain conditions that are necessary for a successful attack campaign. This allows us to determine possible attack paths so that appropriate control actions can be taken for securing the system. Finally, a real healthcare use case scenario that processes big data of healthcare applications is considered to validate the applicability of the proposed method. The results show that it is a practical approach for the attack path generation and determine the necessary areas that need adequate protection for the overall cyber security improvement.

2. Related Work

There are a number of studies that focus on attack path discovery. Existing research treats attack path discovery as an important stage focused on identifying and understanding the routes in a network that potential attackers might follow to gain unauthorized access to a system. This section provides an overview of the existing related work.

The attackers first infiltrate vulnerable hosts to access the system and use the previous attack result as a precondition and repeat this process until they achieve the level of control desired. Previous studies [4,5] aimed to evaluate all possible attack paths in a network and to predict future attacks by combining components from a collaborative filtering recommender systems and attack path discovery approaches using Naïve Bayes and random forest. This method searches for all non-circular attack paths that exist between assets that belong to the network and induces a model where an attacker can gain access to information system sources following a directed path. The security weaknesses of an asset follow the vulnerability assessment, conducting a thorough analysis of the existing and potential threat landscape within a network that can be valued. A stochastic analysis is considered for the evaluation of cyberattack paths through sophisticated methods to measure the probability and acceptability of faults [6]. The development of threat scenarios can delineate the underlined threat landscape and thus facilitate the threat knowledge and improve the visualization [7]. Other groups consider Attack Trees or Attack Graphs, which are widely used approaches for considering threat analysis during the risk assessment process. The attack graph network measurement can be classified into structure and probability-based metrices to quantify network security [8] to illustrate the network's agility in taking preemptive measures to respond to attacks and stochastic-based metrices to estimate large nodes of networks. Another work focuses on attack modelling as a useful tool in risk assessment for cyber physical systems based on the attack vector within the technical and operational environment [9]. Attack graphs are considered a series of exploitation of atomic attacks, which can drive the process to an undesirable state and are used for various applications including threat detection and forensic analysis [10].

More recently, research has appeared that focuses on discovering and analysing attack paths using threat intelligence and vulnerability exploitation. The exploration of attacks based on threat intelligence data is collected using cloud-based web service in [11]. The attack surface classification methodology of mobile malware with known threat actors through automated tactics, techniques and procedures (TTP) and IoC analysis is described in [12]. Hence, IoC is considered as a key parameter to analyse the attack surface and attackers' motivations. A further study [13] focuses on just certain parts of the network to identify and generate attack graphs. For instance, in this strategy, they assume that there is a privilege over an asset across the network. If it is accurate, that means that the user gained access to the asset. An attack path discovery in the dynamic supply chain is proposed using the MITIGATE method in [14]. The approach considers a dynamic risk management system to detect the vulnerabilities that can deliver attack paths based on certain criteria. It considers attacker capability, attack path and its length, and knowledge base for analysing the attack paths. Another work proposes a recommended system that focuses on possible methods that can be used to classify future cyberattacks in terms of risk management [15]. This approach considers the exploitability features for attack path generation and uses a multi-level collaborative filtering method to predict the future attacks. Another indicative example for supply chain context is presented by [16], where cyber threat intelligence is integrated into the cyber supply chain for analysing the threats and determining suitable control strategies. An integrated cyber security risk management integrates vulnerability and threat profile for risk management and predication [17]. In particular, various threat actor parameters such as skill, motivation, location and resources are considered important for determining the likelihood of the risks related to a specific threat. A distributed approach for attack path generation based on a multi-agent system is considered by [18]. It follows an in-depth search, where the performance is improved with the use of agents after a specific graph size.

The contributions presented above have greatly contributed to the identification and analysis of attack paths. Several observations have been made based on the existing literature. Firstly, there is a lack of focus on specific vulnerabilities and their exploitability that contribute to the attack path discovery, particularly in the healthcare sector. Additionally, there is also a need to understand the threat actors' profiles in terms of attacker capability and motivation, as well as target user profiles for a successful attack campaign. Healthcare systems consist of interconnected cyber systems and infrastructures at the physical and cyber levels for critical healthcare service delivery [16]. There is a pressing need to understand the possible attack paths and prioritise the paths so that possible control actions can be identified to ensure the security and resilience of healthcare service delivery. The proposed work contributes towards this direction and adopts the widely used CVE vulnerability database and CVSS scoring system to examine the vulnerabilities that exist within the healthcare system.

3. The Proposed Attack Path Discovery

A cyberattack path determines the possible routes that an attacker can propagate to execute an attack. In general, all high-impact cyberattacks have several phases where an attacker conducts lateral movement from the initial point to the target landing point. A healthcare ecosystem by its inherent nature is complex and interconnects with a number of medical and IT assets for service delivery. The attack within the ecosystem can propagate from any initial point to the final target asset depending on the attacker profile and motivation. It is necessary to understand the vulnerabilities within the attack surface to adopt suitable control measures. The proposed method follows the existing attack path discovery methods such as MITIGATE [17], cyber-physical attack paths against critical systems [18], and attack path discovery in a dynamic supply chain context [19] and extends with new parameters and rule sets to formulate the attack paths. Additionally, the proposed method adopts the widely used CVE vulnerability database and CVSS scoring system to examine the vulnerabilities that exist within the healthcare system [20–22]. There is also a need to understand the threat actor profile in terms of attacker capability and motivation for a successful attack campaign. The proposed methodology also adopts the NIST's SP800-30 guideline [23] for profiling the attacker. This section presents an overview of the proposed methodology in terms of the general assumptions and process.

3.1. Assumptions

The proposed attack path discovery method considers the following assumptions:
- The assets within the healthcare ecosystem are dependent upon each other for the healthcare service delivery;
- Each asset may link with single or multiple confirmed vulnerabilities published by the National Vulnerability Database (NVD) or CVE, which are required to be considered for the attack path generation. CVE contains a huge list of published vulnerabilities that assist in determining vulnerabilities related to specific healthcare assets;
- The threat actor needs a certain profile in terms of attacker capability (knowledge and skill) and access vector (local, adjacent, network, and physical) to exploit a vulnerability and discover an attack path;
- Each user within the healthcare system performs certain functionalities based on the roles and responsibilities. Threat actors could take advantage of target user profiles to execute an attack;
- Each attack path includes several variables, such as entry point asset, intermediate point (if any), target point asset, dependencies among the assets, and underlying characteristics of the vulnerability within the assets;
- The methodology follows the CVSS for attack path generation and vulnerability estimation. It mainly considers the base score metric values for generating the attack path.

3.2. Cyberattack Path Generation and Analysis Process

This section presents the attack path generation and analysis process, which consists of seven distinct steps. Each step performs specific functionalities and contributes towards the attack path discovery. It initiates source and target asset identification, followed by the vulnerability chain for a successful attack campaign. An overview of the steps is given below.

Step 1—Identify possible entry points: This initial step identifies the healthcare ecosystem's potential assets that the attacker may consider as an entry point to execute an attack. This can be a medical device and software that runs the device, hardware, or other assets within an ICT infrastructure. A medical device defined by the FDA as software, electronic and electrical hardware, including wireless, is a critical asset for healthcare systems. The entry point is a point of failure where the attack exploits the vulnerability to propagate the target point. Generally, the attacker spends a lot of time trying to understand the existing system, and specifically, the healthcare system consists of several interconnected healthcare and IT devices. Vulnerabilities within these assets can be exploited by an attacker to achieve their intention. Almost every aspect of the network and application has a potential entry point, and securing the weakest link principle should be followed by the healthcare entity in order to make it difficult for an attacker to identify the entry point.

Step 2—Determine asset dependencies: Once the entry point is identified, it is necessary to determine the dependencies of these assets within the healthcare ecosystem. The goal is to focus on the potential cyber interaction of the entry point asset. A cyber dependency of assets is assumed to be a cyber-asset pair (node) interrelation and/or interconnection (edge) aiming to fulfil a healthcare service delivery or specific operation over communication networks. For instance, it is necessary to exchange patient treatment data from various sources for clinical decision making. Such dependency is critical for an attacker to propagate an attack from the entry point to the target point.

Step 3—Identify possible target points: This step aims to identify the possible target points that an attacker strives to reach by following the entry point asset and associated dependencies. An attacker needs to exploit single or multiple vulnerabilities to reach target points to achieve its objective. This includes assets that are compromised at interim stages of an attack campaign. Therefore, the accessibility of a target point depends on the entry point asset, cyber dependencies, and capability of the actor for possible exploitation. This step develops assets' dependency graph that shows assets and their dependencies.

Step 4—Determine entry and target point vulnerabilities: Once the entry and target points are identified, it is necessary to determine the vulnerabilities related to the assets. These vulnerabilities are preconditions based on the attacker's profile for a successful attack path campaign. The goal of this step is to accurately reflect the exploitability level of the identified vulnerabilities and link the vulnerabilities to formulate the vulnerability chain. These vulnerabilities are identified by following the CVE and NVD published vulnerabilities entries. The proposed method follows a rule-based reasoning approach (filters) to produce the chain of sequential vulnerabilities on different assets that arise from consequential multi-step attacks, initiated from the entry points in order to exploit the vulnerabilities. Individual vulnerability is measured by following the CVSS base metrics and possible further exploitation for the vulnerability chain. CVSS allows us to determine the criteria relating to discoverability, exploitability, and reproducibility to materialize a threat relating to the vulnerability. Therefore, the vulnerability chain demonstrates and escalates the attack vector from local to network access or vice versa.

Step 5—Define the threat actor and user profile: A threat actor needs a certain profile to exploit a vulnerability for a successful attack. Depending on the asset dependencies and nature of the vulnerability, the profile may vary. The threat actor profile includes sub-attributes relating to attacker capability (very low, low, moderate, high, and very high) and location (local, adjacent, network, and physical) for an attack campaign by following the NIST SP800-30 guidelines. Additionally, it is also necessary to consider existing users of the healthcare ecosystem and their profiling, which may assist the threat actor to exploit the vulnerability. Depending on the user role and access rights to various systems and other assets, the user profiling can be categorized into three scales of high, medium, and low.

Step 6—Generate attack paths: This step of the described methodology aims to generate the possible attack paths against target point assets. The individual and chain vulnerabilities are examined using a number of parameters, including assets, vulnerabilities, threat actor profiles, and exploitability level, for this purpose. The vulnerability chain demonstrates a series of exploitation of vulnerabilities using appropriate access vectors and escalation of the privilege. We follow the individual and propagated vulnerability level to determine the attack path. This step is iterative to generate the possible attack paths for the chosen healthcare context and the impact of the vulnerability are considered for selecting the appropriate ones.

Step 7—Generate and prioritise an evidence-based vulnerability chain: Once the attack paths are identified, it is necessary to generate the vulnerability chains whose exploitation can lead to possible attack paths on given cyber-dependent assets. It is also necessary to collect the evidence relating to the attack path so that we can prioritise which paths need to be taken into consideration for suitable control measures. This step consists of a number of sub-steps (7.1–7.4):

Step 7.1—Identify the vulnerability chain: The attack path discovery relies on unique characteristics, i.e., entry and target point assets and related vulnerabilities, the threat actor's capability, and asset interdependencies to identify all possible paths that can be exploited to gain access by generating vulnerability chains. At this stage, only the vulnerability chains that are under the attack capability for the exploitation are considered.

Step 7.2—Assess the vulnerability chain: Once all vulnerability chains are identified, it is necessary to assess the vulnerabilities for a given chain. The step considers individual, cumulative and propagation vulnerability values:

The individual vulnerability assessment (IVL): This measures the probability that a threat actor can successfully reach and exploit a specific confirmed vulnerability in a given asset. We follow the Exploit Prediction Scoring System (EPSS) of individual vulnerability and CVSS 3.1 score metrics (if EPSS is not available) to estimate the vulnerability level. Hence, several external sources such CVSS, EPSS, exploit-db are considered for IVL. Table 1 shows the individual vulnerability assessment scales. A list of generic assumptions for calculating the probability is made.

Assumption 1. *If exploitability features (proof-of-concept exploit code or weaponized exploits or arbitrary code execution) are available, then the probability of exploitation for a specific vulnerability is higher than without exploitable features.*

Assumption 2. *If a security control is not defined or there is a lack of evidence about the existing control for a specific vulnerability, then the Attack Complexity (AC) can be low and increase the probability of exploitation. Otherwise, AC should be considered based on the CVSS base metrics.*

Assumption 3. *If the Access Vector (AV) is a physical or adjacent network and the threat actor has a root or user-level access, then the probability of exploitation can be very high or high.*

Table 1. Individual vulnerability assessment.

Vulnerability Scale		Description of Vulnerability Level
Vulnerability Occurrence	Value Range (%)	Description of Successful Exploitation of the Vulnerability
Very High (5)	80–100	>80%
High (4)	60–80	60–80%
Medium (3)	40–60	40–60%
Low (2)	20–40	20–40%
Very low (1)	1–20	<20%

The cumulative chain vulnerability level assessment: This includes the threat actor's exploitation capability to assess a specific vulnerability chain and determines the probability of exploitation for an individual chain. The reason for considering the threat actor's exploitation capability is that the exploitability level of an individual vulnerability may be high, but the threat actor may not have the right capability to exploit the vulnerability due to lack of access vector or attack complexity. Additionally, it is necessary to have knowledge about the specific medical device to exploit a vulnerability related to the medical device. This sub-step measures if a threat actor can successfully reach and exploit each of the vulnerabilities identified in a given vulnerability chain. Figure 1 shows how the threat actor capability is linked to the CVSS metrics and the vulnerability chain. To accomplish this, the calculated individual vulnerability levels and the asset cyber-dependencies produced in the first step and the threat actor profile are considered. Figure 1 also shows that the threat actor capability is linked to the vulnerability chain.

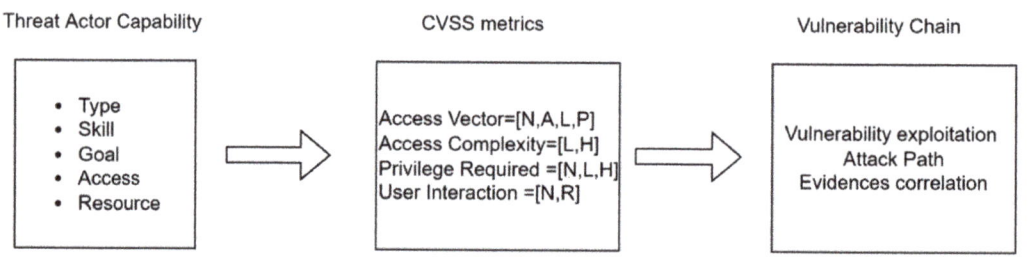

Figure 1. Threat actor capability linking with vulnerability chain.

Table 2 shows the threat actor's exploitation capability, which includes the availability of exploitation features and the required access vector for successful exploitation.

Table 2. Threat actor exploitation capability.

Threat Actor Capability Scale		Description of Scale		
Qualitative Values	Semi-Quantitative Values	Description	Exploitability Features	Metrics
Very High	80–100	TA has a very sophisticated level of expertise and is well-resourced for the required access vector and attack complexity. TA can generate opportunities to support multiple successful, continuous, and coordinated attacks.	Availability of all features = PoC and Weaponized Exploit, arbitrary code execution	PR = required level Entry point asset AV = required level
High	60–80	TA has a sophisticated level of expertise, with significant resources for the required access vector and attack complexity. TA has opportunities to support multiple successful coordinated attacks.	Availability of all features = PoC and Weaponized Exploit, arbitrary code execution	PR = required level Entry point asset AV = required level
Medium	40–60	TA has moderate resources, expertise, and opportunities for the required access vector and attack complexity to support multiple successful attacks.	Availability of some features = PoC and Weaponized Exploit, arbitrary code execution	PR = required level Entry point asset AV = required level
Low	20–40	TA has limited resources, expertise, and opportunities for the required access vector and attack complexity to support a successful attack.	Availability of some features = PoC and Weaponized Exploit, arbitrary code execution	PR = not required level Entry point asset AV = not required level
Very Low	0–20	TA has very limited resources, expertise, and opportunities for the required access vector and attack complexity to support a successful attack.	No Availability = PoC and Weaponized Exploit, arbitrary code execution	PR = not required level Entry point asset AV = not required level

Table 3 presents the cumulative vulnerability level by combining individual vulnerability level and threat actor exploitation capability. The propagated vulnerability assessment estimates how deep into the network an attacker can penetrate if a vulnerability is exploited.

Table 3. Cumulative exploitability vulnerability level.

IVL \ Threat Actor's Exploitation Capability	Very Low	Low	Medium	High	Very High
Very Low	VL	VL	L	L	M
Low	VL	L	L	M	H
Medium	L	L	M	H	H
High	L	M	H	H	VH
Very High	M	H	H	VH	VH

Step 7.3—Gather and correlate evidence: This sub-step aims to collect relevant evidence that is necessary to consider for the attack path. The approach advocates considering the IoC and related point of compromise (PoC) for the gathering and correlating of the evidence. IoC is a commonly used term for cyber threat intelligence, which broadly indicates unusual behaviour in a system and network. IoCs are the artefacts left due to malicious activity, whereas vulnerabilities are possible weaknesses presented within a system that can be exploited by a threat actor. Evidence of IoC specifies that the vulnerability is already exploited, and the system is compromised. Therefore, the early detection of IoC could delimit the damage of any attack. The possible IoC includes hash code, IP addresses, domains, network traffic, unauthorised setting change, log, suspicious activities on accounts. Additionally, healthcare devices can have other indicators, including configuration changes, disconnection of patient monitors, disruption of healthcare services, or amendment of drug level. Figure 2 shows the possible indicator types for the evidence chain generation.

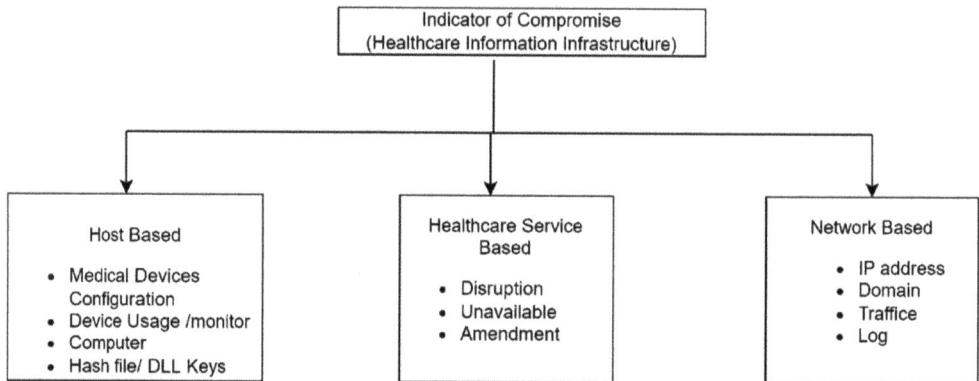

Figure 2. Possible IoCs for healthcare information infrastructure.

Once IoC is gathered, then it is necessary to correlate the evidence using the PoC. A PoC is a specific location such as an asset that is compromised by a threat actor. At this stage, it is necessary to determine the common PoC based on the vulnerability and its exploitability within the overall healthcare information infrastructure. The PoC allows us to correlate the IoC to formulate the evidence-based vulnerability chain and reproduce the attack path. The reproducibility also depends on the threat actor's capability to exploit the related vulnerabilities for a successful attack campaign. It is also necessary to determine the level of exploitability for a specific attack path based on the IoC and threat actor's exploitation capability.

Step 7.4—Prioritise Attack Path: This is the final sub-step of the proposed method that aims to prioritise the attack paths. The reason for prioritising the attack path is that attack path generation may identify a high number of paths, but some of the paths may not be materialized due to various factors such as lack of exploitability feature, threat actor capability, or a number of security measures in place. Therefore, it is necessary to prioritise the attack paths that are relevant to a specific healthcare context based on the evidence and attacker exploitation capability for the attack path reproduction. The proposed approach exploits the chain level for a confirmed event for this purpose. The prioritisation focuses on the evidence chains which have more chances to the confirmed incident and exhibits potential risks.

Figure 3 shows the attack path generation and analysis process by including the seven defined steps. It considers the overall healthcare ecosystem, which consists of healthcare entities, such as hospitals and clinics, medical and IT devices and healthcare processes and services. This allows attackers to identify the possible entry point and target points for any attack.

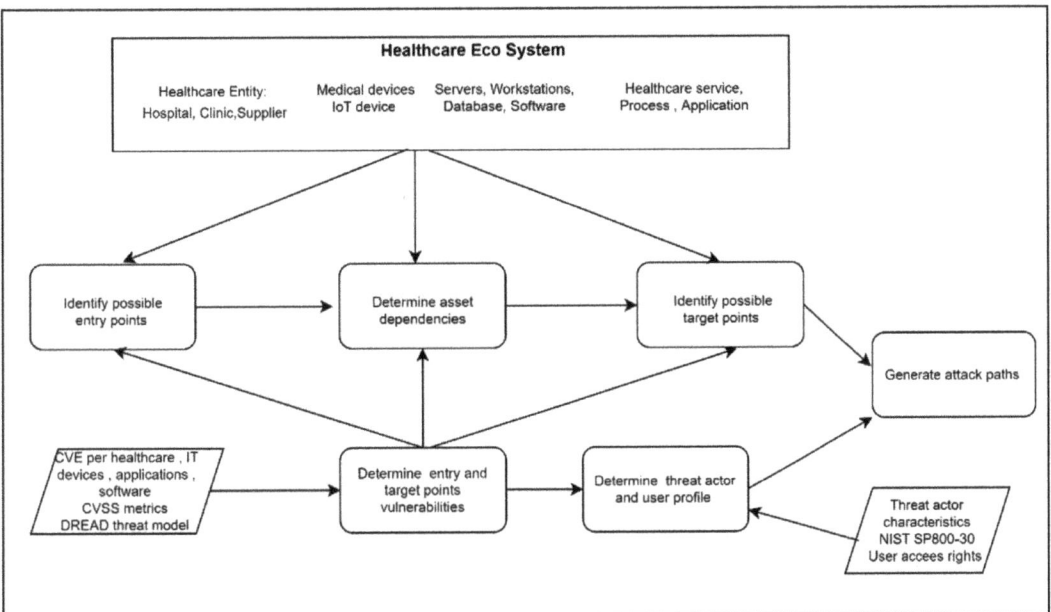

Figure 3. Attack path generation and analysis process.

4. Attack Path Generation Rules

Rule sets are essential for a successful attack campaign. In particular, the propagation rules are the certain conditions that need to be fulfilled to propagate an attack in different phases. The rules provide certain conditions that are necessary to satisfy and exploit a vulnerability based on the attack profile and asset interdependencies. The rules are created based on different parameters such as attack profile, asset dependency, and vulnerability metrics. The rules are independent of the device specification or the IT infrastructure, so there is no need to amend the rule sets due to the evolution of infrastructure or due to new vulnerabilities. To generate these rules, several variables and the knowledge base (KB) are necessary to be defined and understood.

4.1. Variables

The propagation rules determine the possible vulnerabilities that an attacker can exploit for the implementation of a successful attack campaign. Asset dependency, vulnerability exploitability, threat actor profiles and target user profiles are key parameters for propagation rules. A European funded project, named 'A Dynamic and Self-Organized Artificial Swarm Intelligence Solution for Security and Privacy Threats in Healthcare ICT Infrastructures' (AI4HEALTHSEC) [24] works towards developing a solution to enhance the identification and analysis of threats and cyberattacks on healthcare information infrastructures (HCII). The project AI4HEALTHSEC considers a number of attributes for the attack propagation rule set, which are presented below.

Asset dependency: An asset within a healthcare ecosystem may have a number of dependencies in order for the related healthcare service to be delivered within the HCII. For instance, an insulin pump needs to inject insulin into the patient's body. The cyber-asset pair enfolds a source cyber-asset and a destination cyber-asset. There are two infrastructures necessary for the transfer and processing of cyber resources, i.e., communications (transmission of big data and information) and IT (use and processing of big data). The dependency type is capable of defining in which manner a cyber-asset pair is interdependent within the healthcare service. To fulfil this, the following cyber dependency types are considered:

exchanging, storing, controlling, processing, accessing, and installing. Additionally, there are also physical dependencies among the assets when one asset is physically connected with another asset.

Vulnerability exploitability: Each asset includes a single or multiple vulnerabilities that could be exploited for a given attack path to materialize. Additionally, there are dependencies among the assets that allow us to exploit the vulnerabilities from an entry point asset to a target asset. The attacker needs to identify the entry point asset vulnerabilities that could be discovered and exploited to initiate the attack and then use the target point asset vulnerability to complete the attack path. Therefore, there is a dependency among the assets for the attack path generation.

Threat actor profile: The threat actor profile indicates the capability, skills, and motives of an attacker for an attack campaign. Depending on the skill and sophistication, there are variations in the threat actor profile. It is necessary to identify the threat actor profile for the attack path generation. The threat actor profile considers two variables:

- Threat actor capability: Defines the attackers' necessary skill, goals supplication, resources required to execute an attack. It includes five given scales (very low, low, moderate, high, and very high);
- Attack access vector: Define the necessary access path for an attack campaign. There are four different access vectors for executing an attack: **Local**—A vulnerability is exploitable with only local access; **Adjacent**—A vulnerability is exploitable with adjacent network access; **Network**—A vulnerability is exploitable with network access; **Physical**—A vulnerability is exploitable with physical access.

Target user profile: Threat actors are targeting various users for an attack campaign. The AI4HEALTHSEC cyberattack path discovery method considers the target user profile that assists the threat actor to execute the attack. The actors involved in the overall healthcare ecosystem, such as healthcare practitioners, nurses, admin workers and IT service workers, could be targeted by a threat actor. The target user profile considers user context such as knowledge and skill (high, medium, and low) for running various healthcare services, applications, and maintenance operations. Users have different execution rights within the system, e.g., an IT admin has the right to install and update applications and a doctor uses different healthcare applications and devices for the healthcare service delivery.

4.2. Knowledge Base

As stated before, the attack path identification follows certain rules. However, to generate the rules, it is necessary to define the KB as a foundation for the rule set generation. The KB includes a set of predicate symbols to describe a predicate within the rule set. These will mainly constitute domain elements attributes (e.g., the attributes of assets), along with predicates used in the reasoning process. The list is not exhaustive, and the KB and quantifiers can be extended to capture a more complete or different view of the domain.

Symbols: The following symbols are used for the KB rule set generation:

- Vul denotes Vulnerability which links with an asset;
- Asset denotes specific assets of the overall healthcare ecosystem and possible cyber dependencies with other assets including Hosting, ExchangingData, Storing, Controlling, Processing, Accessing, Installing, Trusted, Inclusion, Interaction, and Connected;
- TA and TAP denotes Threat Actor and Threat Actor Profile, respectively with capability VeryHigh, High, Moderate, Low, and VeryLow, threat require for an attack;
- AV denotes Access Vector with Local Network, Adjacent Network, Local and Physical;
- Vuln_PR denotes Privileged Required as a level of privileges, i.e., None, Low, and High, before successfully exploiting a vulnerability by a Threat Actor;
- Vuln_AC denotes Attack complexity in terms of certain conditions, i.e., Low and High, beyond the attacker's control that must exist in order to exploit the attack;
- Vuln_UI denotes the user interaction, i.e., None and Required, excluding the threat actors for an attack;

- TUP denotes the Target User Profile, i.e., High, Medium, and Low, that assists an attacker to execute an attack;
- Vuln_Exp denotes vulnerability exploitability level, i.e., High, Medium, and Low, based on the exploitability properties;
- Vul_Exp_Fea denotes specific exploitability features of the vulnerability.

The following relationship symbols are used for the KB rule set generation:

Connected relation defines the connectivity between two assets due to the dependency or through the related vulnerabilities. Asset dependencies and inherent vulnerabilities within the asset are considered for the connected relation. Additionally, connectivity can be also achieved if the assets are in the same network. The KB for the connected relation is given below.

Connected using assets dependency.

- $\forall asset1, asset2$ ExchangingData(asset1,asset2) $\lor$ Storing(asset1,asset2) $\lor$ Configuring(asset1,asset2) $\lor$ Updating(asset1,asset2) $\lor$ Accessing(asset1,asset2) $\lor$ Installing(asset1,asset2) $\Rightarrow$ Connected (asset1,asset2) $\land$ Connected(asset2,asset1)

Connected using vulnerability.

- $\forall vuln1, vuln2, asset1, asset2$ Connected(vuln1,asset1, vuln2,asset2) $\Rightarrow$ Connected (vuln2,asset2, vuln1,asset1)

Accessible relation denotes threat actors with specific profiles that can access the asset using a specific access vector required for a confirmed vulnerability.

- $\forall vuln, asset, TA$ vuln_AV() $\land$ TAP() $\Rightarrow$ Accessible(vuln,asset,TA)

Exploitable relation denotes threat actors that exploit a specific vulnerability on an asset. The threat actor needs to access the asset for exploitation using the appropriate profile that links with the required base metric values.

- $\forall vuln, asset, TA$ Accessible(vuln,asset,TA) $\land$ (vul_UI() $\lor$ vul_PR() $\lor$ vul_AC()) $\land$ TAP() $\Rightarrow$ Exploitable(vuln,asset,TA)

Attacked relation denotes when a threat actor successfully attacks an asset based on a specific vulnerability exploitation and certain profile. Therefore, threat actor accessibility and vulnerability exploitability are required for an attack.

- $\forall vuln, asset, TA$ Accessible(vuln,asset,TA) $\land$ Exploitable(vuln,asset,TA) $\Rightarrow$ Attacked (vuln,asset,TA)

4.3. Attack Path Generation

4.3.1. Rules Using Access Vector

An existing vulnerability on an asset is accessible by a threat actor based on the possible access vectors such as Network, Adjacent Network, Local, Physical (AV: N/A/L/P).

- If AV is 'Network' (i.e., remotely exploitable), this means both asset and TA are connected to the same network (Internet).
- $\forall vuln, asset, TA,$ locNetwork(TA,loc) $\land$ ConnectsTo(asset,loc) $\land$ Vulnerability(vuln,asset) $\land$ Network(vuln) $\Rightarrow$ Accessible(vuln,asset,TA).

Otherwise, if AV is 'Adjacent Network' (i.e., exploitable over local network) and both asset and TA are connected to the same local network.

- $\forall vuln, asset, TA, loc$ AdjacentNetwork(TA,loc) $\land$ ConnectsTo(asset,loc).
- $\land$ Vulnerability(vuln,asset) $\land$ (AdjacentNetwork(vuln) $\lor$ Network(vuln)) $\Rightarrow$ Accessible(vuln,asset,TA).

4.3.2. Rules Using Base Metrics

The reason for considering vulnerability exploitability is that there are too many confirmed vulnerabilities published each month and it is challenging for healthcare entities to fix all these vulnerabilities. It is necessary to consider the base metrics such as attack vector, attack complexity, privileges required and user interaction for attack path generation. It is worth mentioning that not all vulnerabilities can be easily exploited due to the nature of the specific product, overall system context and threat actor profile. Additionally, vulnerabilities do not always exploit in isolation, and there is a link between the vulnerabilities and healthcare assets for an attack campaign.

4.3.3. Access Vector and Privileges Required

If two vulnerabilities are linked into two different dependent assets, and entry point assets' vulnerability requires AV = N and PR = L and target point assets' vulnerability requires AV = L and PR = N, then TA with AV = N can easily act as a local user to exploit the vulnerability for the target asset. Hence, TA can reach the target asset using the vulnerability of the entry point asset.

Note that if a threat actor obtains (PR = H) for a specific vulnerability on an asset, then TA can exploit the other vulnerabilities on the same asset with lower PR. It implies PR:H $\geq$ PR:L $\geq$ PR:N.

- $\forall$vuln1,asset1,vuln2,asset2, TA(vuln1_AV(N) $\wedge$ vuln1_PR(L)) $\wedge$ (vuln2_AV(N) vuln2_PR(L)) $\Rightarrow$ Accessible(vuln2,asset2,TA).

4.3.4. Target User Profile and User Interaction

Vulnerabilities often require a certain level of user interaction for successful exploitation. AI4HEALTHSEC correlates the target user profile with the user interaction for this purpose. Generally, three types of user profiles (high, medium, and low) exist depending on knowledge, skill, and experience. If a vulnerability needs user interaction and the target user profile is low for that interaction, this indicates that the user has a lack of knowledge about the context. It is assumed that in such a scenario, the threat actor with a very high and high profile (AC = VH/H) can exploit the vulnerability with the required access vector.

- $\forall$vuln,asset,TA Vuln_UI(R) $\wedge$ Vuln_TUP(L) $\wedge$ TA AC(VH or H) $\Rightarrow$ Exploitable (vuln,asset,TA).

4.3.5. Threat Actor Profile and Attack Complexity

If the attack complexity (AC = H) is high, then the threat actor requires a very high or high profile to exploit the vulnerability. For such cases, there are specific conditions beyond threat actor control that are required to be completed before exploitation. A threat actor with very high and high profile is more likely to successfully exploit the vulnerability.

If the threat actor is capable of high AC to trigger an attack on an asset, then it is more likely that the threat actor can exploit also the other low AC on vulnerabilities on the same asset. It implies AC:H $\geq$ AC:L.

- $\forall$vuln,asset, TA Vuln_AC(H) $\wedge$ Vuln_TAP(VH $\vee$ H) $\Rightarrow$ Exploitable(vuln,asset,TA).

4.3.6. Rules Using Vulnerability Exploitability

There are a number of key exploit features, such as proof-of-concept, weaponized, and arbitrary code execution. The exploitability provides the threat actor to reproduce the attack.

4.3.7. Exploitability Level and Threat Actor Profile

If the exploitable level for a vulnerability is high, then a threat actor with any profile can attack the specific asset. Additionally, if a low-profile threat actor can successfully attack an asset, then it is more obvious that a threat actor with any other profile level can also attack the asset.

- $\forall$vuln,asset,TA Accessible(vuln,asset,TA) $\wedge$ Vuln_Exp(H) $\wedge$ Vuln_TAP(VH $\vee$ H VM $\vee$ L $\vee$ VL) $\Rightarrow$ Attacked(vuln,asset,TA).

4.3.8. Proof of Concept Exploit, Weaponized Exploit, Arbitrary Code Execution

There is a strong correlation between the availability of proof of concept and weaponized exploitation for a successful exploitation. Weaponized exploits indicate that the exploit works for every potential threat actor. Additionally, arbitrary code execution also provides more exploitability possibilities.

- $\forall \text{vuln,asset, TA Vuln\_Exp\_Fea(PoC ExploitCode)} \land \text{Vuln\_Exp\_Fea(weaponized exploits)} \lor \text{Vuln\_Exp\_Fea(arbitrary code execution)} \Rightarrow \text{Exploitable(vuln,asset,TA)}$.

5. Evaluation: A Healthcare Scenario

The proposed attack path approach is evaluated using a real healthcare case study scenario. This section presents an overview of the scenario, incorporating the implementation of the attack path process. The studied context may identify the potential attacks and take necessary measures to tackle the attacks and related vulnerabilities. The aims of this evaluation are to: demonstrate the applicability of the proposed attack path generation method into a real healthcare scenario; highlight the usefulness of CVSS metrics and exploitability for attack path generation; and display the benefits of the KB rules and IoC for analysing the attack path.

5.1. Healthcare Use Case Scenario

The chosen scenario is based on a user-centred Digital Health Living lab, which provides a systematic user co-creation and co-production approach while integrating research and innovation processes in a real-life setting [25]. The residents, council, service providers, academic institutions, and technology companies are the key stakeholders within this living lab and are involved in every step of the way, from the creation of a product or service to commercialization. In particular, the related stakeholders contribute to health innovation in a new way, receive the opportunity to help individuals and society and can be key partners in inspiring health innovation based on their needs, perceptions, and user experience. It is an open innovation ecosystem where the living lab acts as a unique test bed for developing and testing prototypes or more mature digital healthcare solutions. The scenario is mainly based on Tier 3 test and trial category according to the UK National Institute for Health and Care Excellence (NICE) for Digital Health Technologies (DHTs). In particular, Tier 3 aims to help people with a diagnosed condition and provides treatment and health management. It includes tools used for treatment and diagnosis, as well as those influencing clinical management through active monitoring or calculation. This may include a symptom tracking function which records patient information and transmits this to the healthcare team for the derivation and the support of the clinical decision.

Every involved stakeholder, such as patients, healthcare practitioners, residents, and service providers, will engage with the living lab within their own infrastructures and network connections. As such, they connect to the internet through their own Wi-Fi (routers) and communicate through emails (PCs) or their mobile devices (mobile phones, tablets, laptops). There is much critical big data involved in the scenario including patient healthcare information, personal information, device usage and connectivity with other devices. Additionally, the living lab includes various patient healthcare devices such as insulin pump, infusion pump and Internet of Things (IoT) devices for healthcare treatment. The scenario presented above is used to demonstrate the proposed methodology. The next section provides a detailed description of the implementation.

5.2. Implementation of the Attack Path Generation

We follow the living lab healthcare scenario to implement the attack path generation (see Figure 4). This section presents the implementation of the attack path generation. Vulnerabilities of healthcare services and systems are the main components for the path generation. In particular, the vulnerabilities in the healthcare sector are unique compared to the other sectors. This is due to the connectivity of different medical devices with the other parts of the network, and these medical devices, in general, have a lack of security measures. Healthcare information infrastructure contains a large number of legacy systems that are hard to replace and threat actors are always looking into this system for potential exploitation. Healthcare practitioners need to collect sensitive patient data, such as personal and financial information, and therefore potential breaches of this data could provide additional benefits to the criminals or inside attackers.

We made several assumptions for the purpose of implementation. In particular, the home patients use an infusion pump and insulin pump for their treatment and the pump is managed and configured by the healthcare practitioner. Additionally, there are IT devices, such as computers, routers, servers and applications software and operating systems, that are required for the overall system infrastructure. Finally, the low cost of IoT devices, such as smart lamps and IP surveillance cameras, in both home and service provider environments are considered. The security of medical devices is critical to protect patient information and to ensure healthcare service delivery since the devices are connected to the internet. These devices are dependent on the other IT devices and network infrastructure to exchange and collate data from various sources for making clinical decisions. There are vulnerabilities due to the interdependencies among the assets from the hardware, software, human, and overall healthcare system context. Compromised healthcare devices can be used to propagate the attack path on the other part of the healthcare information infrastructure. Software is embedded in the devices to assist their functions and operation of the medical devices. Therefore, an attack path can also be initiated and propagated from this embedded software. Additionally, web services are commonly used for interfacing the connected medical devices with the other parts of the system.

A list of assets is identified based on the scenario which consists of medical devices, IT devices, IT infrastructure and applications. These assets are critical for the overall healthcare service delivery and research activities for the living lab. The potential threat actors and user profiles are also considered to demonstrate the attack path. We have extracted a number of vulnerabilities from the CVE database and categorised them based on the assets of the studied scenario. Additionally, CVSS is also considered for the base metrics properties which are necessary for the ruleset. The identified vulnerabilities and base metrics are used to generate the attack paths. The process allows the generation of a possible attack path and the CVSS metrics impact value is considered to select the appropriate ones. The attack path generation is iterative to generate the possible attack paths.

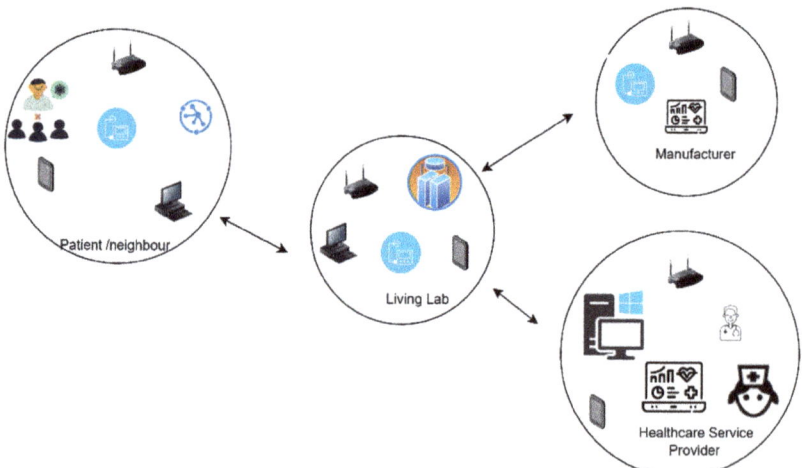

Figure 4. Living lab healthcare scenario.

5.2.1. Identify Entry, Target Point Assets, and Possible Dependencies

This section combines the first three steps of the attack paths, providing a list of assets identified based on the healthcare use case scenario, specifically, the healthcare service delivery and related healthcare information infrastructure. Each device needs an interface such as a wireless or network interface to connect with the other devices. For instance, an insulin pump management system that is physically located at home has one wireless interface to interact with another device interface. Note that we have only considered the devices for the demonstration of the attack path. Entry and Target Point Assets: Medical and IT device:

- **Infusion Pump (A1):** Braun's Infusion System 871305U aims to deliver fluid such as nutrients and medications into the patient's body. Trained healthcare practitioners should program the rate and duration for the medication. The pump stores patient drug information;
- **Insulin pump (A2):** Medtronic MiniMed 508 is one of the most widely used pumps for delivering a specific amount of insulin to the diabetic patient's body. The device is programmed to inject a specific amount of insulin set by the doctor into the patient body. The pump stores patient sensitive insulin information;
- **Insulin management system (A3):** Omnipod DASH Insulin Management System 19191 is a tubeless and wireless system that allows continuous insulin delivery for 3 days. It consists of a pod that is worn directly on the patient's body and a personal diabetic manager which programs and controls the delivery;
- **IoT devices (A4):** There are several IoT devices that are relevant to the scenario. A heartrate monitor (Maxim's 700-MAXREFDES117) can be used to monitor the heart rate (wearable device). Additionally, a smart light system (Philips) is also considered for the healthcare service delivery;
- **Information and communication network (A5):** This includes multiple devices, such as routers, WiFi, switches, wireless interface cards, and others that are responsible for the connection from the device to the network;
- **Computer system (A6):** Windows-based workstation and servers connected to the medical devices, patient interfaces and servers;
- **Rugged tablets (A7):** These tablets are commonly used for patient care applications such as medication alerts and tracking, Electronic Health Records (EHR) support, blood pressure monitoring, and connecting to barcode readers and can directly interface to the other medical equipment. Healthcare practitioners can directly use these tablets for patient treatment.

5.2.2. Information and Software

- **Hospital information management system (A8):** Care 2X software is a patient medical record and staff management system. It supports web-based platforms and a simple user interface. The patient medical record includes patients' identifiable and treatment information;
- **SpaceCom and SpaceStation (A9):** This is the software that operates the infusion pump and resides either on the pump or the space station. Generally, the pump is attached to the space station. We have considered Braun's Infusion System 871305U, which is linked with the SpaceCom 012U000050. SpaceCom is responsible to update two critical functions, i.e., drug library and pump configuration. Drug libraries can prevent incorrect dosing of drugs;
- **Device usage information:** This includes the amount of time used by the patient from the device and the relevant programme data.

5.2.3. Possible Asset Dependencies

The identified assets rarely perform any operation alone. Assets within the healthcare system are connected for a specific service delivery. For instance, the data from the home infusion pump are transferred to the pump server. The server correlates the data for making clinical decisions. The home care service software needs to update the medical device installed into the home healthcare system. The insulin pump needs to inject insulin into the patient's body and is controlled by the software through wireless communication. Therefore, there are different types of dependencies among the assets, which are shown in Table 4.

Table 4. Asset dependency.

Entry Point Asset and Type	Target Point Asset and Type	Dependency Type
A9 (SpaceCom Software)	A1 (Infusion Pump)	Configured_to, Updated_to
A3 (Insulin Management System)	A2 (Insulin Pump)	Configured_to, Updated_to
A8 (Care2X-Hospital Management System)	A6 (Windows System)	Installed_on, Updated_by
A5 (Router)	A6 (Windows System)	Connected_to, Exchange_data
A4 (IoT Device)	A5 (Router)	Connected_to, Exchange_data
A7 (Tablet)	A8 (Care2X-Hospital Management System)	Exchange_data
A9 (SpaceCom Software)	A1 (Infusion Pump)	Configured_to, Updated_to

The asset dependency graph is also presented in Figure 5.

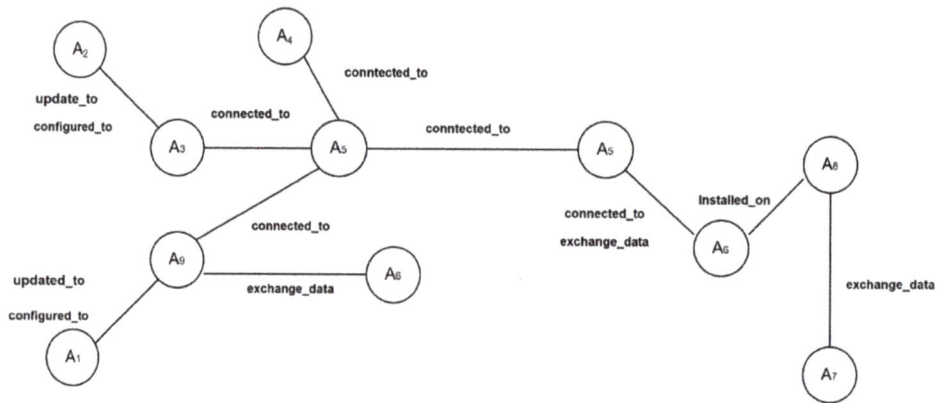

Figure 5. Asset-dependency graph.

5.2.4. Entry and Target Point Vulnerabilities

Once the assets and their dependencies are identified, the next step is to identify the vulnerabilities that can be exploited in order to compromise the assets. As mentioned before, the CVE list is used for vulnerability identification. There are fifteen confirmed recent vulnerabilities considered among those assets which go as follows:

- two vulnerabilities are identified on asset A1;
- one vulnerability is identified on asset A2;
- one vulnerability is identified on asset A3;
- one vulnerability is identified on asset A4;
- three vulnerabilities are identified on asset A5;
- three vulnerabilities are identified on asset A6;
- one vulnerability is identified on asset A7;
- one vulnerability is identified on asset A8;
- two vulnerabilities are identified on asset A9.

Once the vulnerabilities are identified, it is necessary to understand the base nature of exploitability and the base metric for each specific vulnerability. This allows for the analysis regarding how the asset of this scenario can be exploited considering the threat actor profile. Table 5 presents details regarding the identified vulnerabilities.

Table 5. Vulnerabilities and CVSS metrics for each asset.

Asset	Vulnerabilities & Exploitability
A1 = Braun's Infusion Pump	A1,V1 = Lack of input validation provides command line access and privilege escalation. TA requires in the same network as device CVE-2021-33886, A1.V3 = VH(8.8) AV:A/AC:L/PR:N/UI:N/S:U/C:H/I:H/A:H
	A1,V2 = Unrestricted file upload that can overwritten critical files due to privilege escalation CVE-2021-33884, A1.V4 = VH(9.1) CVSS:3.1/AV:N/AC:L/PR:N/UI:N/S:U/C:N/I:H/A:H
A2 = Medtronic MiniMed 508 insulin pump	A2,V1 = lack of security (authentication and authorization) in RF communication protocol with other devices such as blood glucose meter and glucose sensor transmitters. TA requires in the same network as device can inject or intercept data and change pump settings CVE-2019-10964, A2.V1 = VH(8.8) CVSS:3.0/AV:A/AC:L/PR:N/UI:N/S:U/C:H/I:H/A:H
A3 = Insulin Management System	A3,V1 = improper access control in the wireless RF communication protocol allows local TA to intercept or modify insulin data and change pump settings. CVE-2020-10627 A3.V1 = VH(8.1) CVSS:3.1/AV:A/AC:L/PR:N/UI:N/S:U/C:H/I:H/A:N
A4 = IoT device Philips Hue light bulb	A4,V1 = communication protocol can be abused to remotely installed malicious firmware in the light bulb as remote code execution through buffer overflow and spread to other IoT devices that use Zigbee communication protocol. CVE-2020-6007 A4.V1 = H(7.8) CVSS:3.1/AV:A/AC:H/PR:N/UI:R/S:C/C:H/I:H/A:H
A5 = Router (Buffalo, Cisco RV Series—Netgear)	A5,V1 (Buffalo routers) = Bypass authentication procedures on the affected routers though files which do not need authentication and gain root level access. It enables telnet service to connect other devices' control such as IoT Devices. CVE-2021-20090 A5.V1 = VH(9.8) CVSS:3.1/AV:N/AC:L/PR:N/UI:N/S:U/C:H/I:H/A:H
	A5,V2 (Cisco RV series) = Remote TA with administrative privileges inject arbitrary commands into operating system due to lack of input level validation through web-based interface. CVE-2021-4012 A5.V2 = H(7.2) CVSS:3.1/AV:N/AC:L/PR:N/UI:N/S:U/C:H/I:H/A:H
	A5,V3 (Netgear router) = unauthenticated TA can affect the device through buffer overflow attack. CVE-2018-21224 A5.V3 = VH(8.8) CVSS:3.1/AV:A/AC:L/PR:N/UI:N/S:U/C:H/I:H/A:H
A6 = System (Windows Compatible)	A6,V1 = A remote code execution vulnerability allows TA to execute arbitrary code and gain same right as current user. This allows to install program modify files based on the existing user rights. CVE-2019-1236 A6.V1 = H(7.5) CVSS:3.1/AV:N/AC:H/PR:N/UI:R/S:U/C:H/I:H/A:H
	A6,V2 = A remote code execution vulnerability allows TA to execute arbitrary code and gain same right as current user. TA needs control of a server to execute this vulnerability and tricks the user for the to connect the server. CVE-2019-1333 A6.V2 = H(7.5) CVSS:3.1/AV:N/AC:L/PR:N/UI:R/S:U/C:H/I:H/A:H
	A6,V3 = A remote code execution vulnerability allows TA to run arbitrary code with system privilege. TA could install program, amend files, and create new users with full rights. CVE-2021-36958 A6.V3 = H(7.8) CVSS:3.1/AV:L/AC:L/PR:N/UI:R/S:U/C:H/I:H/A:H
A7 = Rugged Tablet (Dell)	A7,V1 = A local TA without the necessity of authentication can exploit this vulnerability and execute arbitrary code in system management mode. CVE-2020-5348 A8.V1 = H(7.8) CVSS:3.1/AV:L/AC:L/PR:L/UI:N/S:U/C:H/I:H/A:H
A8 = web-based hospital management system (Care2X)	A8,V1 = A cross site scripting vulnerability exploited during patient registration. TA can send the XSS payload to this vulnerable parameter and take control of another register user. TA needs victim user interaction Exploitability features = PoC and Weaponized Exploit, CVE-2021-36352 A9.V1 = M(5.4) CVSS:3.1/AV:N/AC:L/PR:L/UI:R/S:C/C:L/I:L/A:N
A9 = SpaceCom	A9,V1 = Lack of authentication for critical space com function allows connection to the pump Exploitability features = PoC and Weaponized Exploit, arbitrary code execution CVE-2021-33882, A1.V1 = VH(8.6) AV:N/AC:L/PR:N/UI:N/S:C/C:N/I:H/A:N
	A9,V2 = Clear text transmission allows TA to snoop network traffic. Exploitability features = PoC and Weaponized Exploit, arbitrary code execution CVE-2021-33883, A1.V2 = H(7.5) AV:N/AC:L/PR:N/UI:N/S:U/C:H/I:N/A:N

5.2.5. Threat Actor and User Profile

The threat actor profile considers capability and attack vectors for exploiting a vulnerability. The threat actors can be external or internal with different motivations such as financial gain, harm to the patient, and/or competitors. In general, a threat actor needs to understand the device-specific verification information, and specifically for the medical devices, it is necessary to understand spectrum, transmission radio frequency, and data structure.

- **Infusion Pump:** TA should have knowledge regarding the access to the local network, CAN bus data structure, escalation of privilege from user access to admin access and the pump configuration;
- **Medtronic Insulin Pumps:** Knowledge regarding how to access the network and intercept radio frequency and the pump configuration;
- **Smart bulb:** Knowledge of smart bulb operation and access point to overtake the bulb control.

Finally, healthcare practitioners and other users need to perform various activities based on the roles for the healthcare service delivery. For instance, a practitioner needs to update the patient's medical records, set insulin levels, and monitor infusion pump activities for the service delivery. Therefore, the practitioner needs to have basic knowledge about how to operate the devices and their security. IT users need to update and manage all devices, including medical and IT, within the network.

5.3. Results: Attack Path Generation

Once the asset dependencies and vulnerabilities are identified, this final step aims to generate the attack path. There are a number of attack paths generated from the source asset to the target asset through the combination of vulnerabilities and dependencies. Note that there can be additional attack paths generated from the scenario, but this section presents only the relevant ones. Additionally, we only considered the three critical target point assets, i.e., infusion pump, insulin pump, and healthcare system, for the attack path generation.

Attack Path—Target Point Infusion Pump: It is assumed that the threat actor (TA) is acting as an outsider without any prerequisite credential (PR:N) and user interaction (UI:N) can gain user level access to the SpaceCom system (A9,V1) through the network (AV:N) and escalate the privileges to gain root access. This allows the TA to communicate with the pump (A1,V1) with no privilege (AV:A) and user interaction (UI:N). The TA can finally manipulate the drug library or pump configuration. The TA can also execute malicious code in the pump's RTOS by accessing the SpaceCom (A9,V2) and executing the code and overwrite the pump (A1,V2) RTOS. Additionally, a TA who is able to access the hospital management system can obtain the patient drug information and further exploit the infusion pump. The TA can also exploit the hue light bulb (A4,V1) to access the home network and then further propagate into the infusion pump. This can happen mainly when the pump is idle or in standby mode. There are four potential attack paths through which the target point infusion pump can be exploited:

A5,V1 → A9,V1 → A1,V1
A9,V2 → A1,V2
A8,V1 → A9,V1 → A1,V2
A4,V1 → A9,V1 → A1,V1

Attack Path—Target Point Insulin Pump: It is assumed that an internal threat actor (i.e., may be an employee) who has access to the insulin management system (A3,V1) using (AV:A/L), unrestricted (user) access (PR:N), basic computer skills (AC:L) and without user interaction (UI:N) exploits the insulin pump (A2,V1). The TA can also exploit the router (A5,V3) through an adjacent network and access the insulin management system (A3,V1) to access the pump (A2,V1). A TA from an adjacent network can take control of the hue lightbulb (A4,V1), become unreachable to the user and send malicious code to other devices and networks. It is assumed that a patient as the user may have a lack of knowledge about the smart bulb operation, which can be exploited by the TA. When the user interacts with the bulb, the TA can take over the control and propagate to the other part of the network. There are three potential attack paths which can exploit the target point insulin pump.

A5,V3 → A3,V1 → A2,V1
A3,V1 → A2,V1
A4,V1 → A3,V1 → A2,V1

Attack Path—Target Point Hospital Management System: It is assumed that a TA with network access through the router (A5,V2) can exploit the healthcare system (A8,V1) that is installed on a Windows-based system (A6,V1). User interaction is necessary to exploit this attack path; therefore, a healthcare practitioner needs to interact with the system for the exploitation. Additionally, such an attack path needs a TA with high skills who needs root level privilege to exploit the router and amend the user rights within the windows system. It allows them to access the hospital management system and add new users and gather sensitive data from the system. Another possibility could be that an internal TA with local access from tablet (A7,V1) may also attempt to exploit the (A9,V1) through the windows system (A6,V3). This path needs a local access vector and user interaction. There are three potential attacks through which the target point infusion pump can be exploited.

A5,V3 → A6,V1 → A8,V1
A5,V3 → A6,V2 → A8,V1
A7,V1 → A6,V3 → A8,V1

5.4. Generate and Prioritise Evidence-Based Vulnerability Chain

We assume that there are two confirmed events that occurred in the studied living lab scenario. The first event occurred in the patient homecare unit, where cyber threats are detected on the home care and the IoCs are analysed. In the current scenario, unauthorized access to the SpaceCom software (PoC = A9) allows the threat actor to access the infusion pump (PoC = A1). The IoCs in this case are the log (IoC1), amendment of drug library (IoC2), pump configuration (IoC3), and obtained pump data (IoC4). This case enfolds a confirmed event of a cyberattack. To discover and produce the potential cyberattack paths for the compromised asset A1, cyber dependency with the infusion pump (A1) is considered, and possible attack paths for A1 are listed. The second event is data leak, where high-profile TAs access the hospital management system (PoC = A8) and collect the data (IoC6) through Windows system (PoC = A6) using IoC5 and IoC7 (user right and install program). Cyber threats are detected in the healthcare service provider infrastructure. Table 6 shows the evidence chain for the identified security incidents.

Table 6. Attack path based on confirmed security events and potential evidence chains.

Security Incident	Attack Path	Evidence Chain
Amendment of drug level and pump configuration	A5,V1 → A9,V1 → A1,V1 A9,V2 → A1,V2 A8,V1 → A9,V1 → A1,V2 A4,V1 → A9,V1 → A1,V1	A5,V1 → A9, IoC1 → A1, IoC2 A9, IoC4 → A1, IoC3 A8,V1 → A9, IoC1 → A1, IoC2 A4,V1 → A9, IoC1 → A1, IoC2
Patient data leak	A5,V3 → A6,V1 → A8,V1 A5,V3 → A6,V2 → A8,V1 A7,V1 → A6,V3 → A8,V1	A5,V3 → A6, IoC5 → A8, IoC6 A5,V3 → A6, IoC7 → A8, IoC6 A7,V1 → A6,V3 → A8, IoC6

To estimate the exploitability for each reconstructed attack path, different attackers' profiles are considered and displayed in Table 7. To estimate the EL per vulnerability, with respect to the analysed IoC, only vulnerabilities of the assets interconnected with the IoCs are considered.

Once the individual vulnerability and TA exploitability level are identified, then it is necessary to determine the probability of an attack path exploitation level. This needs to consider IoCs related to the attack path. Note that the probability of exploitation for a disclosed IoC is the maximum value; therefore, exploitation level for the attack path depends on the vulnerabilities that are not exploited. These values are converted to qualitative values to estimate the attack path exploitability level (APEL) defined in the previous section. This is depicted in Table 8 for APEL. We made a number of assumptions for a given vulnerability based on the CVSS metrics. For instance, attack path 1 in the initial node, A5,V1, and threat actor capability is considered as a medium to exploit the vulnerability. Therefore, the exploitation level for the A5,V1 is H by following Table 8 and APEL for the overall attack path is H. Another example could be attack path 2, where both nodes are exploited; therefore, the APEL should be the maximum value. The TA capability for the A4,V1 is low, A5,V3 is medium A7,V1 is high, and A6,V3 is medium.

Table 7. Individual vulnerability exploitation.

Vulnerability	Asset	Individual Vulnerability Level (IVL)	Threat Actor's Exploitability Level				
			Capability = Very Low (VL)	Capability = Low (L)	Capability = Moderate (M)	Capability = High (H)	Capability = Very High (VH)
V1	A1	IVL(A1,V1) = VH	M	H	H	VH	VH
V2	A1	IVL(A1,V2) = VH	M	H	H	VH	VH
V1	A9	IVL(A9,V1) = VH	M	H	H	VH	VH
V2	A2	IVL(A9,A2) = H	L	M	H	H	VH
V1	A6	IVL(A6,V1) = H	L	L	H	H	VH
V2	A6	IVL(A6,V2) = H	L	L	H	H	VH
V1	A8	IVL(A8,V1) = VH	M	H	H	VH	VH

Table 8. Prioritised attack path.

AP No.	Attack Paths	Evidence Chains	Exploitation Level Chain (ELC)	Exploitation Probability	APEL
1	A5,V1 → A9,V1 → A1,V1	V1 → IoC1 → IoC2	H → IoC1 → IoC2	0.75 × 1 × 1 = 0.75	H
2	A9,V2 → A1,V2	IoC4 → IoC3	IoC4 → IoC3	1 × 1 = 1	VH
3	A8,V1 → A9,V1 → A1,V2	V1 → IoC1 → IoC2	M → IoC1 → IoC2	0.5 × 1 × 1 = 0.5	M
4	A4,V1 → A9,V1 → A1,V1	A4,V1 → A9, IoC1 → A1, IoC2	M → IoC1 → IoC2	0.5 × 1 × 1 = 0.5	M
5	A5,V3 → A6,V1 → A8,V1	A5,V3 → IoC5 → IoC6	H → IoC5 → IoC6	0.75 × 1 × 1 = 0.75	H
6	A5,V3 → A6,V2 → A8,V1	A5,V3 → A6, IoC7 → A8, IoC6	H → IoC7 → IoC6	0.75 × 1 × 1 = 0.75	H
7	A7,V1 → A6,V3 → A8,V1	A7,V1 → A6,V3 → A8, IoC6	H → H → IoC6	0.75 × 0.75 × 1 = 0.56	M

6. Discussion

The purpose of this research was to present the attack path discovery method considering the unique characteristics of the healthcare information infrastructure, such as assets and their cyber and physical dependencies, vulnerabilities, threat actor and user profile, and IoC. A scenario in a real-life healthcare setting has also been used to prove the implementation of the attack path discovery method. The cyber threat landscape is constantly evolving, and threat actors are highly skilled in conducting sophisticated and multiple attacks on a number of infrastructures. They target the initial access point assets and exploit possible vulnerabilities to reach the target point through several intermediate nodes.

Research shows that most studies on cybersecurity in the healthcare field focus on technical aspects [26]. Following this focus on technology, other significant components, such as threat actors' profiles and related psychosocial and behavioural characteristics remain understudied in the field [20]. This comes as a surprise when taking into consideration that most cyberattacks are caused by individuals and the adopted risk mitigation by technological solutions is successful to a limited extent. The core of a sturdy strategy for cyberattacks needs to be human-centric and consider attackers' profiles for ultimate benefit. It is worth noting that attack potentials are positively connected to attackers' profiles, while studying this further would shed light on the early detection, prevention, and protection of cybersecurity incidents within healthcare organizations. Examining involved human aspects is also of paramount importance to further investigate how healthcare professionals understand data privacy and security and its significance. This significance lies on the attitudes towards cyber threats, operations, and related controls.

The proposed methodology provides an understanding of possible entry point assets for the studied context and possible paths to reach the target point asset. It adopts the CVSS metrics and its exploitability feature for a common understanding of how the threat actor can exploit particular attack paths. Additionally, threat actor individual and exploitability capability are also taken into consideration for attack path generation and prioritisation.

Hence, the combination of threat actor capability, i.e., skill, motivation, and location, with the availability of exploitability features justifies the prioritised attack paths. Healthcare information infrastructure is an attractive target for the threat actor due to the potential benefits of obtaining sensitive patient data. In recent years, the value of personal medical data has increased on the black market. Credit card information sells for USD 1–2 on the black market, but personal health information (PHI) can sell for as much as USD 363. Therefore, the proposed attack path discovery and prioritisation provides an effective way to identify the potential attacks and undertake suitable control to tackle the attacks.

Cybersecurity issues should be considered from the design stage of the medical devices, otherwise risks will continue to grow. Medical devices are no longer a standalone component, but they are rather connected with other devices for overall healthcare service delivery. Vulnerabilities in connected devices used in hospital networks would allow attackers to disrupt healthcare service delivery and medical equipment. There is a need for sound and proven cybersecurity approaches for ensuring overall security. Threat actors tend to exploit vulnerabilities within a network and form attack paths from one asset to another until they have reached the asset they wish to harm. The proposed approach assists in identifying the common vulnerabilities that can be exploited within the healthcare context so that the necessary course of action can be taken into consideration.

7. Conclusions

Enhancing the security and resilience of healthcare service delivery is of paramount importance for securing the overall healthcare ecosystem. It is always necessary to ensure the safety of patients' data and secure healthcare service delivery. The proposed approach provides an understanding of the areas that have potential for cyberattacks. This is conducted by looking for existing vulnerabilities and their possible exploitations based on the assets and their dependencies for possible attack path generation. This work contributes to the identification of the vulnerabilities from both healthcare and IT devices and demonstrates how the attack paths can be propagated from a connected medical device to other parts of the system. This can also be possibly achieved in other infrastructures and scenarios, identifying the relevant attack areas and deploying appropriate measures. The novelty of the proposed approach is to analyse the threat actor profile to generate attack paths and use evidence-based vulnerability chain to prioritise the attack path. This allows us to determine the suitable control to tackle the attacks. Finally, the approach is applied to the living lab healthcare scenario, and the results from the studied context identify the possible attack paths based on the asset and related vulnerabilities. These paths are prioritised so that suitable controls can be identified to tackle the attack for secure healthcare service delivery. As part of our future research, we would like to deploy the proposed methodology in different healthcare context and other supply chain system. Additionally, it is necessary to develop a checklist of controls that would link with the attack paths for the overall cyber security improvement.

Author Contributions: Conceptualization, S.I., S.P., E.-M.K. and K.K.; methodology, S.I. and S.P.; validation, S.I. and K.K.; formal analysis, S.I., S.P. and E.-M.K.; investigation, S.I., S.P., E.-M.K. and K.K.; resources, S.I., S.P., E.-M.K. and K.K.; writing—original draft preparation, S.I.; writing—review and editing, S.I. and K.K.; visualization, S.I., S.P., E.-M.K. and K.K.; supervision, S.I.; project administration, K.K.; funding acquisition, S.P. All authors have read and agreed to the published version of the manuscript.

Funding: The research conducted in this paper was triggered by the authors' involvement in the project 'A Dynamic and Self-Organized Artificial Swarm Intelligence Solution for Security and Privacy Threats in Healthcare ICT Infrastructures' (AI4HEALTHSEC) under grant agreement No 883273. The authors are grateful for the financial support of this project that has received funding from the European Union's Horizon 2020 research and innovation programme. The views expressed in this paper represent only the views of the authors and not of the European Commission or the partners in the above-mentioned project.

Conflicts of Interest: The authors declare no conflict of interest. The funders had no role in the design of the study; in the collection, analyses, or interpretation of data; in the writing of the manuscript, or in the decision to publish the results.

References

1. Williams, A.H.P.; Woodward, J.A. Cybersecurity vulnerabilities in medical devices: A complex environment and multifaceted problem. *Med. Devices Evid. Res.* **2015**, *12*, 305–316. [CrossRef] [PubMed]
2. Forbes. Available online: https://www.forbes.com/sites/forbestechcouncil/2021/06/07/increased-cyberattacks-on-healthcare-institutions-shows-the-need-for-greater-cybersecurity/?sh=7b228d895650 (accessed on 5 January 2022).
3. McKee, D.; Laulheret, P. McAfee Enterprise ATR Uncovers Vulnerabilities in Globally Used B. Braun Infusion Pump. Available online: https://www.mcafee.com/blogs/enterprise/mcafee-enterprise-atr/mcafee-enterprise-atr-uncovers-vulnerabilities-in-globally-used-b-braun-infusion-pump/#_Toc76469513 (accessed on 5 January 2022).
4. Hanemann, A.; Patricia, M. Algorithm design and application of service-oriented event correlation. In Proceedings of the 3rd IEEE/IFIP International Workshop on Business-Driven IT Management, Salvador, Brazil, 7 April 2008.
5. Kathleen, J.A.; DuBois, D.A.; Stallings, C.A. *An Expert System Application for Network Intrusion Detection*; No. LA-UR-91-558; CONF-911059-1; Los Alamos National Lab.: Santa Fe, NM, USA, 1991.
6. Chochliouros, I.; Spiliopoulou, A.; Chochliouros, S. Methods for Dependability and Security Analysis of Large Networks. In *Encyclopedia of Multimedia Technology and Networking*; Pagani, M., Ed.; IGI Global: Milan, Italy, 2009; pp. 921–929.
7. Bodeau, D.J.; McCollum, C.D.; Fox, D.B. Cyber Threat Modeling: Survey, Assessment, and Representative Framework. The Homeland Security Systems Engineering and Development Institute (HSSEDI) & MITRE Cooperation. 2018. Available online: https://www.mitre.org/sites/default/files/publications/pr_18-1174-ngci-cyber-threat-modeling.pdf (accessed on 25 January 2022).
8. Frigault, M.; Wang, L. Measuring Network Security Using Bayesian Network-Based Attack Graphs. In Proceedings of the 3rd IEEE International Workshop on Security, Trist and Privacy for Software Applications, Turku, Finland, 28 July–1 August 2008.
9. Kriaa, S.; Bouissou, M.; Piètre-Cambacédès, L. Modeling the Stuxnet attack with BDMP: Towards more formal risk assessments. In Proceedings of the 2012 7th International Conference on Risks and Security of Internet and Systems (CRiSIS), Cork, Ireland, 10–12 October 2012.
10. Jha, S.; Sheyner, O.; Wing, J. Two formal analyses of attack graphs. In Proceedings of the 15th IEEE Computer Security Foundations Workshop. CSFW-15, Cape Breton, NS, Canada, 24–26 June 2002.
11. Al-Mohannadi, H.; Awan, I.; Al Hamar, J. Analysis of adversary activities using cloud-based web services to enhance cyber threat intelligence. *Serv. Oriented Comput. Appl.* **2020**, *14*, 175–187. [CrossRef]
12. Kim, K.; Shin, Y.; Lee, J.; Lee, K. Automatically Attributing Mobile Threat Actors by Vectorized ATT&CK Matrix and Paired Indicator. *Sensors* **2021**, *21*, 6522. [CrossRef] [PubMed]
13. Somak, B.; Ghosh, S.K. An attack graph-based risk management approach of an enterprise. *J. Inf. Assur. Secur.* **2008**, *2*, 119–127.
14. Polatidis, N.; Pavlidis, M.; Mouratidis, H. Cyber-attack path discovery in a dynamic supply chain maritime risk management system. *Comput. Stand. Interfaces* **2017**, *56*, 74–82. [CrossRef]
15. Polatidis, N.; Pimenidis, E.; Pavlidis, M.; Papastergiou, S.; Mouratidis, H. From product recommendation to cyber-attack prediction: Generating attack graphs and predicting future attacks. *Evol. Syst.* **2020**, *11*, 479–490. [CrossRef]
16. Yeboah-Ofori, A.; Islam, S. Cyber security threat modeling for supply chain organizational environments. *Future Internet* **2019**, *11*, 63. [CrossRef]
17. Kure, H.I.; Islam, S.; Mouratidis, H. An integrated cyber security risk management framework and risk predication for the critical infrastructure protection. *Neural Comput. Appl.* **2022**, *1*, 1–31. [CrossRef]
18. Stellios, I.; Kotzanikolaou, P.; Grigoriadis, C. Assessing IoT enabled cyber-physical attack paths against critical systems. *Comput. Secur.* **2021**, *107*, 102316. [CrossRef]
19. Cheung, K.; Bell, M.; Bhattacharjya, J. Cybersecurity in logistics and supply chain management: An overview and future research directions. *Transp. Res.* **2021**, *146*, 102217. [CrossRef]
20. Kioskli, K.; Polemi, N. Psychosocial approach to cyber threat intelligence. *Int. J. Chaotic Comput.* **2020**, *7*, 159–165. [CrossRef]
21. Common Vulnerabilities and Exposures (MITRE). Available online: https://cve.mitre.org/ (accessed on 10 February 2022).
22. CVSS v.2 (FIRST). 2007. Available online: https://www.first.org/cvss/v2/guide (accessed on 15 February 2022).
23. NIST SP 800-30. 2020. Available online: https://www.nist.gov/privacy-framework/nist-sp-800-30 (accessed on 5 February 2022).
24. A Dynamic and Self-Organized Artificial Swarm Intelligence Solution for Security and Privacy Threats in Healthcare ICT Infrastructures. Available online: https://cordis.europa.eu/project/id/883273 (accessed on 5 February 2022).
25. Digital Health Living Lab. Available online: https://www.brighton.ac.uk/research/enterprise/enterprise-projects/brighton-and-hove-digital-health-living-lab.aspx (accessed on 15 February 2022).
26. Kioskli, K.; Fotis, T.; Mouratidis, H. The landscape of cybersecurity vulnerabilities and challenges in healthcare: Security standards and paradigm shift recommendations. In Proceedings of the 16th International Conference on Availability, Reliability and Security, the 1st SecHealth Workshop, Vienna, Austria, 17–20 August 2021; Digital Conference. ACM ICPS: New York, NY, USA, 2021; Volume 136, pp. 1–9.

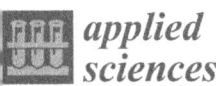

Article

The Assessment of COVID-19 Vulnerability Risk for Crisis Management

Marek Wyszyński *, Michał Grudziński, Krzysztof Pokonieczny and Marek Kaszubowski

Institute of Geospatial Engineering and Geodesy, Faculty of Civil Engineering and Geodesy, Military University of Technology (WAT), 00-908 Warsaw, Poland; michal.grudzinski@student.wat.edu.pl (M.G.); krzysztof.pokonieczny@wat.edu.pl (K.P.); marek.kaszubowski@student.wat.edu.pl (M.K.)
* Correspondence: marek.wyszynski@wat.edu.pl

Abstract: The subject of this article is to determine COVID-19 vulnerability risk and its change over time in association with the state health care system, turnover, and transport to support the crisis management decision-making process. The aim was to determine the COVID-19 Vulnerability Index (CVI) based on the selected criteria. The risk assessment was carried out with methodology that includes the application of multicriteria analysis and spatiotemporal aspect of available data. Particularly the Spatial Multicriteria Analysis (SMCA) compliant with the Analytical Hierarchy Process (AHP), which incorporated selected population and environmental criteria were used to analyse the ongoing pandemic situation. The influence of combining several factors in the pandemic situation analysis was illustrated. Furthermore, the static and dynamic factors to COVID-19 vulnerability risk were determined to prevent and control the spread of COVID-19 at the early stage of the pandemic situation. As a result, areas with a certain level of risk in different periods of time were determined. Furthermore, the number of people exposed to COVID-19 vulnerability risk in time was presented. These results can support the decision-making process by showing the area where preventive actions should be considered.

Keywords: risk management; decision-making; Spatial Multicriteria Analysis; temporal analysis; vulnerability risk; COVID-19

1. Introduction

The end of 2019 brought the outbreak of SARS-CoV-2 followed by introducing a global state of emergency that affected the lives of people around the world [1,2]. For this reason, it became a popular subject of research for scientists from various disciplines. The spatial nature of the pandemic determines the increasing number of articles with the use of spatial data. Among them, the discussion on new challenges in operational crisis management and the role of spatial information and spatial technologies is visible [3].

The search performed on the "crisis management" phrase only in the Web of Science database (WoS) resulted in 59,138 research items (as of 20 October 2021), 5620 of them have been published in 2021, and 4424 were related to the pandemic of COVID-19. This leads to the conclusion that the problem of crisis management is a hot topic of science. In order to identify the ongoing trends in literature, "crisis management spatial analysis" research was performed and the obtained results were presented with the use of Weighted Network Visualization (WNV) shown in Figure 1.

The WNV was prepared with the use of the fractionalization method for normalizing the strength of the links between items [4]. The bigger the label, the higher the weight of certain terms. The colours are determined by the cluster to which the term belongs, while lines represent links: the closer two terms appear, the stronger the correlation between them. For example, Geographic Information System (GIS) is strongly related to "vulnerability", "model", "framework" etc. The homonyms joining were not performed.

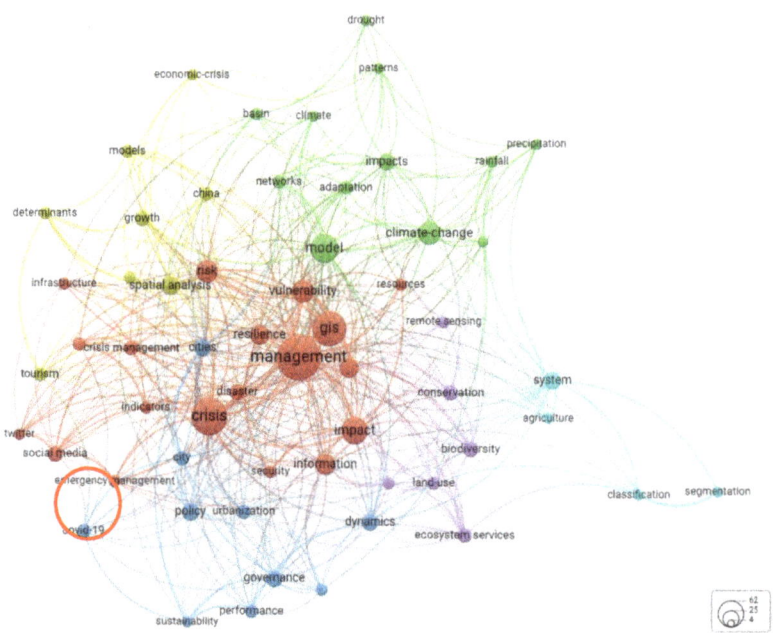

Figure 1. Weighted network visualisation of associations between terms within "crisis management spatial analysis" keyword relations (own study).

The WNV shows a strong presentation of management, crisis, model, and GIS in the body of literature. Also, well-established trends on the possible applications of spatial analysis and SMCA (the analyses take into consideration a group of variable factors and assess their changes over time) were noticeable in broadly understood decision process and decision management with: suitability map [5–9], scenario evaluation method [10–12], resources allocation [13], transportation and vehicle routing [14–18], impact assessment [19–21], location migration and allocation [13,20,22,23], risk management and natural hazards occurrence can be noted [2,24–32]. This state according to [30,33–35] will persist, driven by the new applications of spatial analysis in GIS, and will include crisis management aspects.

More detailed analysis shows the use of the GIS environment [36–38] with recently developed methodologies to support the decision-making process in crisis management at the local level [29,39] and it is emphasized that its essential part was the visualisation of crisis progress, shown with the use of interactive, realistic, large-scale simulations [40].

The results of analyses may be used in several crisis situations like flooding, landslides [24,41] or for vulnerability or risk index estimation of selected areas or infrastructure elements [40,42–44] in order to provide the recommendation for the administrative strategies to minimize the social and economic effects of crisis situations [32,45–47].

According to the authors, the vulnerability index [31], susceptibility models, or susceptibility maps [48,49] should be determined with the use of different methods [50], depending on the area and crisis situation in order to ensure optimal performance and reliable results [51,52]. Reliability of results depends on the accuracy of data which is one of the crucial problems revealed in publications on spatial data next to the techniques for information extraction [24,41,53,54]. Those are followed with conclusions on the use of heterogeneous data sources and remotely sensed data to improve the analysis results, [53,55,56], furthermore, authors show that the potential improvement in the accuracy of GIS-based analysis can be achieved by applying a dedicated approach, for example, neural network [54], integrated uncertainty-sensitivity analysis approach, and attributed model of criteria weights [56].

Pandemic situation publications are considering the causes and potential effects of COVID-19. Researchers show the positive associations between new COVID-19 cases and death cases linked to several factors: public transport usage [15,23,46–60], temperature and humidity [21,61], age, sex, blood group, had influenza [50,62,63], poverty [64], and socio-cultural factors [65]. Furthermore, the juxtaposition of virus transmission acceleration in several countries in relation to the global policy and government responses, human mobility, environmental impact, socioeconomic, lockdown, migration, and vaccination was delivered [20,59,66,67] based on the developed spatiotemporal data matrix of factors and open data sources. The above leads to the determination of the most significant factors, enabling the prediction and modelling of the spatial patterns of virus spread. The researchers commonly use spatial statistic tools such as linear and non-linear regression [50], Bayesian Belief Networks [68], Adaboost algorithm [69], Potential Model [70], Joinpoint analysis [71], machine learning [50,72] in modelling COVID-19 spatial pattern. As a result, it is possible to forecast the COVID spread and to deliver an effective response in cluster containment for crisis situations with intelligent computing [20,62,70,73,74].

Publications considering the effects of the pandemic show the use of socioeconomic data collection on daily new COVID-19 cases to link them to real gross domestic product, unemployment rate, housing prices, export and import, energy system environment [73,75–79].

In the analysed publications on the subject of crisis management, the following problems are considered: the definition of risk, vulnerability, and hazard [80], the analysis of the existing crisis situation, and the management process [2,32,38,65,81–83]. The pivotal role of crisis management is to ensure public safety, in the matter of a pandemic, it is closely related to the capacity of the healthcare system [44,84–86]. Therefore, crisis management has to eliminate the possibility of an overload of the healthcare system, so that the number of new hospitalisations does not exceed the capacity of the healthcare system in a given area, as shown in Figure 2. Therefore, it is necessary to efficiently manage the available forces (medical staff, volunteers, services) and resources (infrastructure, equipment, equipment, and material reserves, restrictions, vaccinations) in time.

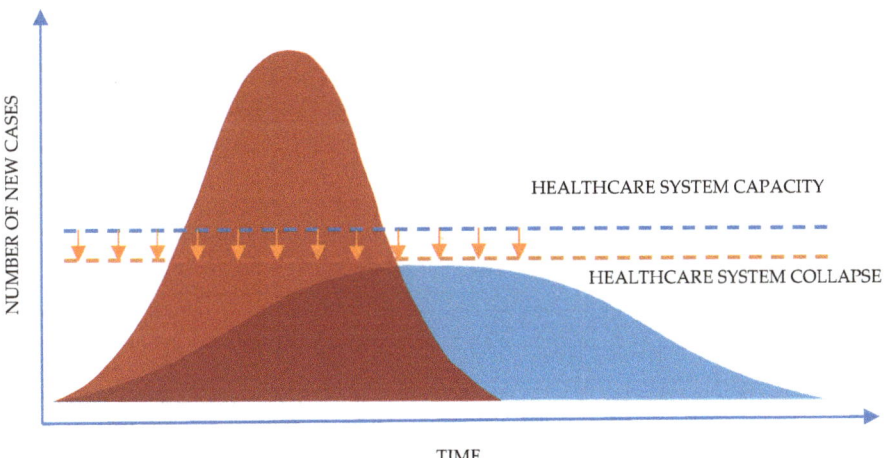

Figure 2. Healthcare system capacity and possible new cases.

Thus, it was assumed that the essential knowledge on the pandemic situation and COVID-19 vulnerability should be considered in a spatiotemporal approach. This determined the aim of our research: to estimate the vulnerability index based on selected criteria along with the determination of its change over time in order to assess the threat caused by COVID-19 in the given area. This will extend the approach presented [31].

Based on a comprehensive analysis of the literature, the aim of this article was to answer the following questions:

- What information can a study of the spatiotemporal vulnerability and risk provide?
- What is the influence of selected criteria on the final value of the COVID-19 vulnerability?
- What direction of changes over time can be observed in the distribution and concentration of vulnerability risk?
- What decisions can be made based on the result of the spatiotemporal vulnerability map?

The novelty of our approach is the use of spatiotemporal multicriteria analysis for COVID-19 situation vulnerability risk assessment in order to support a quick decision-making process. The solution will be valuable to making decisions on implementing preventive actions in the selected area, especially in the initial period of a pandemic by showing the change of vulnerability risk in the selected area in time. Furthermore, the use of basic data in COVID-19 vulnerability estimation plays a pivotal role by addressing the methodology to the countries where more detailed data are not available.

2. Materials and Methods

The spatiotemporal analysis approach applied in this research was based on Spatial Multicriteria Analysis (SMCA) with Analytical Hierarchy Process (AHP) for weights calculation described in. The used methodology is presented in Figure 3. The general concept of SMCA was described in [87,88]. In this article, SMCA allows for the determination of COVID-19 Vulnerability risk—defined as a situation where the risk of exposure to the hazard might be increased [89]. The presented approach allows for the estimation of the COVID-19 Vulnerability risk index (CVI) of the selected area and its characteristics over time. The test field of the solution was Germany.

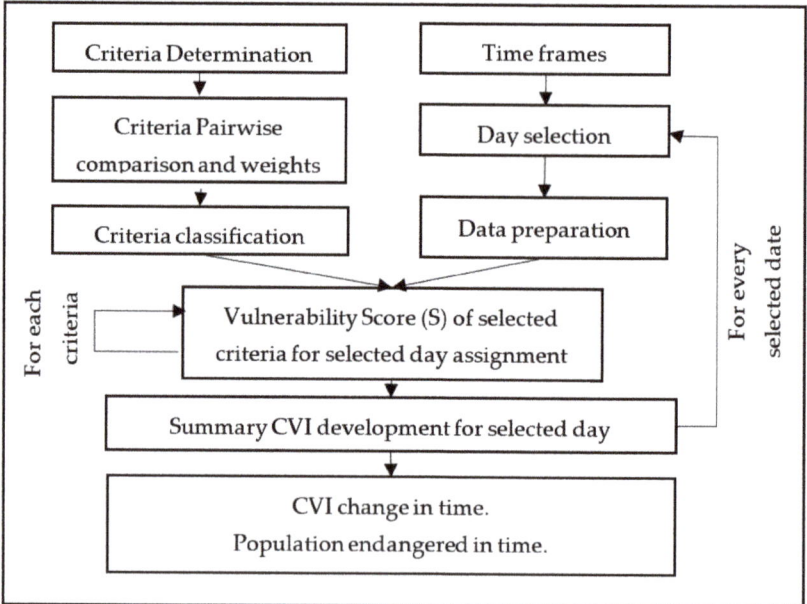

Figure 3. The methodology of spatiotemporal index estimation performed in research (own study).

AHP methodology allows for the importance estimation by calculating the weight of selected criteria by means of pairwise comparisons of each evaluation criterion.

The application of the AHP methodology is based on a value-function type and as such requires an estimation of the value function and criterion weights to determine the summary statistics on the selected area as below [87]:

$$CVI = \sum_{i=1}^{n} W_i \times S_n \quad (1)$$

where CVI is COVID-19 Vulnerability Index, W_i is normalized weight, and S is the Vulnerability Score of the area on the selected layer (n) as value function. Value function and weights are obligatory for estimation. The function values in the paper case study were determined by calculation based on the available dataset. The weights were estimated by pairwise comparisons of each evaluation criteria. This determines the relationship strength between the criteria, that was used to rank selected criteria based to the [90].

In this paper CVI calculations were extended by authors with the spatiotemporal analysis to show CVI change in time as follows:

$$\Delta CVI = CVI_{ti} - CVI_{ti-1} \quad (2)$$

where ΔCVI is the change in time for summary COVID-19 Vulnerability Index for three months' interval.

Furthermore, based on the value of CVI on the selected area the population number endangered with a certain level of vulnerability in time was estimated. This was performed with the use of GIS systems.

The results validation consists of comparing the values of CVI with new cases over time and this is followed with the calculation of the value of the R-squared, to show the proportion of the variance for confirmed COVID-19 cases and CVI index as dependent variables.

Criteria and Weights

Based on the literature review it was assumed that the criteria needed to determine the CVI were basic country demographic statistics listed in Table 1.

Table 1. SMCA criteria and criteria data sources (own study).

Criteria	Criteria Explanation	Data Source	Criteria Type
Cas	Number of COVID cases per 100,000 inhabitants	rki.de	
Serv	Turnover rate for accommodation and food services in relation to the period before the pandemic	destatis.de	
Mb	The estimation of population movement	destatis.de	Dynamic
Hsp	Number of COVID hospitalisations per 100,000 inhabitants	rki.de	
Vacc	Population percentage of two doses vaccinated	rki.de	
Hos	Number of hospitals in the region per 100,000 inhabitants	destatis.de	
Hbed	Total number of hospital beds on region per 100,000 inhabitants	destatis.de	
PDen	Population density per sq. km	destatis.de	Static
Rd	Total length of roads in the region	OSM	
Rs	Total length of railways in the region	OSM	

This simple set of criteria enables the implementation of the COVID-19 vulnerability risk assessment algorithm by all, even less advanced countries if needed. The research was based on several open data sources, such as web services that present demographic statistics: destatis.de [91] and the Robert Koch Institute Site [92], were used. Furthermore, to estimate the information on the transport network, selected data from OpenStreetMap were acquired and analysed. [93]. The case study area was limited to Germany, and the analyses were divided by regions.

The listed criteria presented in Table 1 can be grouped into two categories: dynamic (quickly changing in time) and static (slowly changing in time or static).

The criteria determination process was followed by the pairwise comparison that resulted in the importance determination (in accordance with the AHP methodology). The importance of relations can be found in Table 2. The larger the relative importance values were, the stronger the relation that can be assigned to the pair of criteria.

Table 2. Determination of relative importance based on own study [90].

Relative Importance	Definition	Explanation
1	Equal importance	Two activities contribute equally to objective
3	Weak importance	Experience and judgement slightly favour one activity over another
5	Strong importance	Experience and judgement strongly favour one activity over another
7	Demonstrated importance	One activity is strongly favoured and demonstrated in practice
9	Extreme importance	The evidence favouring one activity over another is of the highest possible order of affirmation
2, 4, 6, 8	Intermediate values	When compromise is needed between two adjacent judgments

The methodology was used to select and compare the criteria. Pairwise comparisons resulted in the estimation of weights that are presented in Table 3. Validation of calculated weights returns Consistency Ratio (CR), which was 0.10; Consistency Index (CI) 0.15. According to the weights listed in the table, the greatest importance can be assigned to the following criteria: Hos, Hbed, Cas, PDen, Hsp.

Table 3. AHP pairwise comparison matrix with calculated weights (own study based the [90]).

	PDen	Serv	Hos	Hbed	Cas	Vacc	Hsp	Mb	Rd	Rs	Criteria Weight
PDen	1.00	6.00	0.25	0.25	0.50	2.00	3.00	4.00	3.00	4.00	0.10
Serv	0.16	1.00	0.11	0.11	0.14	0.25	0.25	0.33	0.50	0.33	0.02
Hos	4.00	9.00	1.00	2.00	3.00	4.00	3.00	8.00	8.00	8.00	0.26
Hbed	4.00	9.00	0.50	1.00	4.00	4.00	6.00	8.00	8.00	8.00	0.25
Cas	2.00	7.00	0.33	0.25	1.00	3.00	3.00	6.00	6.00	6.00	0.14
Vacc	0.50	4.00	0.25	0.25	0.33	1.00	0.25	5.00	4.00	5.00	0.07
Hsp	0.33	4.00	0.33	0.16	0.33	4.00	1.00	4.00	3.00	4.00	0.08
Mb	0.25	3.00	0.13	0.13	0.16	0.20	0.25	1.00	2.00	2.00	0.03
Rd	0.33	2.00	0.13	0.13	0.16	0.25	0.33	0.50	1.00	2.00	0.03
Rs	0.25	3.00	0.13	0.13	0.16	0.20	0.25	0.50	0.50	1.00	0.02

Analysis of results in the static and dynamic groups show that the static criteria affected the CVI estimation twice as strongly as the dynamic criteria (static sum weights: 0.66; dynamic sum weights: 0.34).

To calculate the CVI of the region, the criteria vulnerability score was determined based on the categories in Table 4 (the remaining criteria risk score available in Appendix A). The assigned vulnerability score (VSc) takes values in the range from 2 to 8. The high score represents a high vulnerability in the term of the relevant criterion. For example, density—greater than 2000 people per sq. km—corresponds to the vulnerability value of 8.

Table 4. The selected criteria scores (own study based on [90]).

Criteria/VSc	PDen	Serv	Hos	Hbed	Cas	Vacc
2	<100	<20	>10	>2000	<1	>75
3	100–200	20–40	8–10	1400–2000	1–2	60–75
4	200–300	40–55	6–8	800–1400	2–6	50–60
5	300–500	55–70	4–6	400–800	6–12	30–50
6	500–1000	70–85	2–4	200–400	12–20	15–30
7	1000–2000	85–100	1–2	100–200	20–30	5–15
8	>2000	>100	<1	<100	>30	<5

3. Results and Discussion

3.1. Vulnerability Score Value Analysis for Individual Criteria

For each criterion, the VSc values were estimated. Next, the VSc map was developed as a choropleth map. The example map is presented in Figure 4.

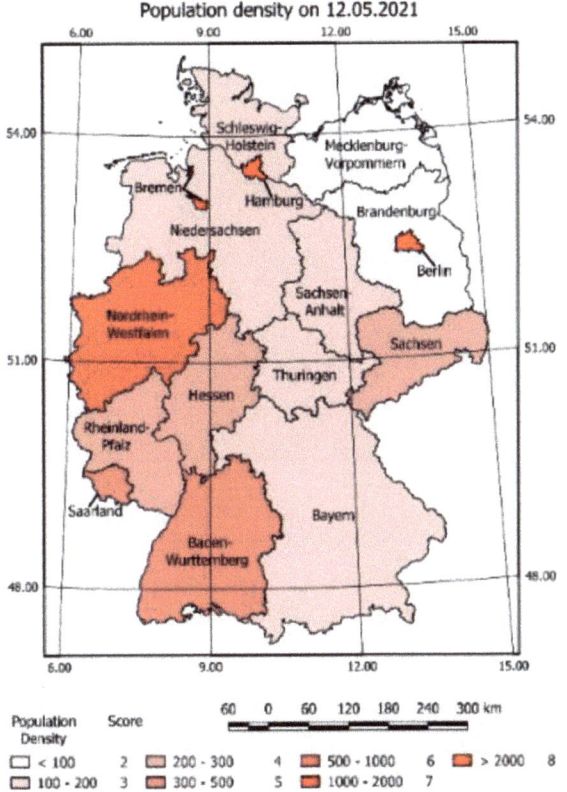

Figure 4. VSc map for population density.

The map shows the information on a selected day (12 May 2021) and gives the representative vulnerability level in accordance with the selected criteria score related to COVID-19 pandemic and its spatial location.

The intensive colours represent large numbers of density and correspond to the high COVID-19 VSc. The light colours represent low populated areas and correspond to a low score of vulnerability for selected criteria. High value can be noticed in Hamburg, Bremen, and Brandenburg. The population density criteria generate vulnerability risk that is constant in time for each region. A similar effect of constant vulnerability can be observed for all static criteria. VSc values of individual criteria can be found in Figures 5 and 6.

All maps present various VSc. The highest score value of criteria in summary for all regions can be assigned to the numbers of hospitalisations and new cases, the lowest to the railway and road density.

Areas marked with the highest score values may generate potential COVID-19 vulnerability risk so the preventive actions should be there considered.

3.2. COVID-19 Vulnerability Index Analysis

The CVI was a result of summaries of the vulnerability values for each criterion multiplied by their weight. The CVI map in Figure 7 presents the various risks classified into five categories from very low to very high. The highest CVI occurs e.g., in the Hamburg, Bremen, Niedersachsen Mecklenburg-Vorpommern, Berlin, Brandenburg. Bayern and Nordrhein-Westfalen were classified as low CVI. The low value of CVI resulted from the summary weighted VSc of criteria.

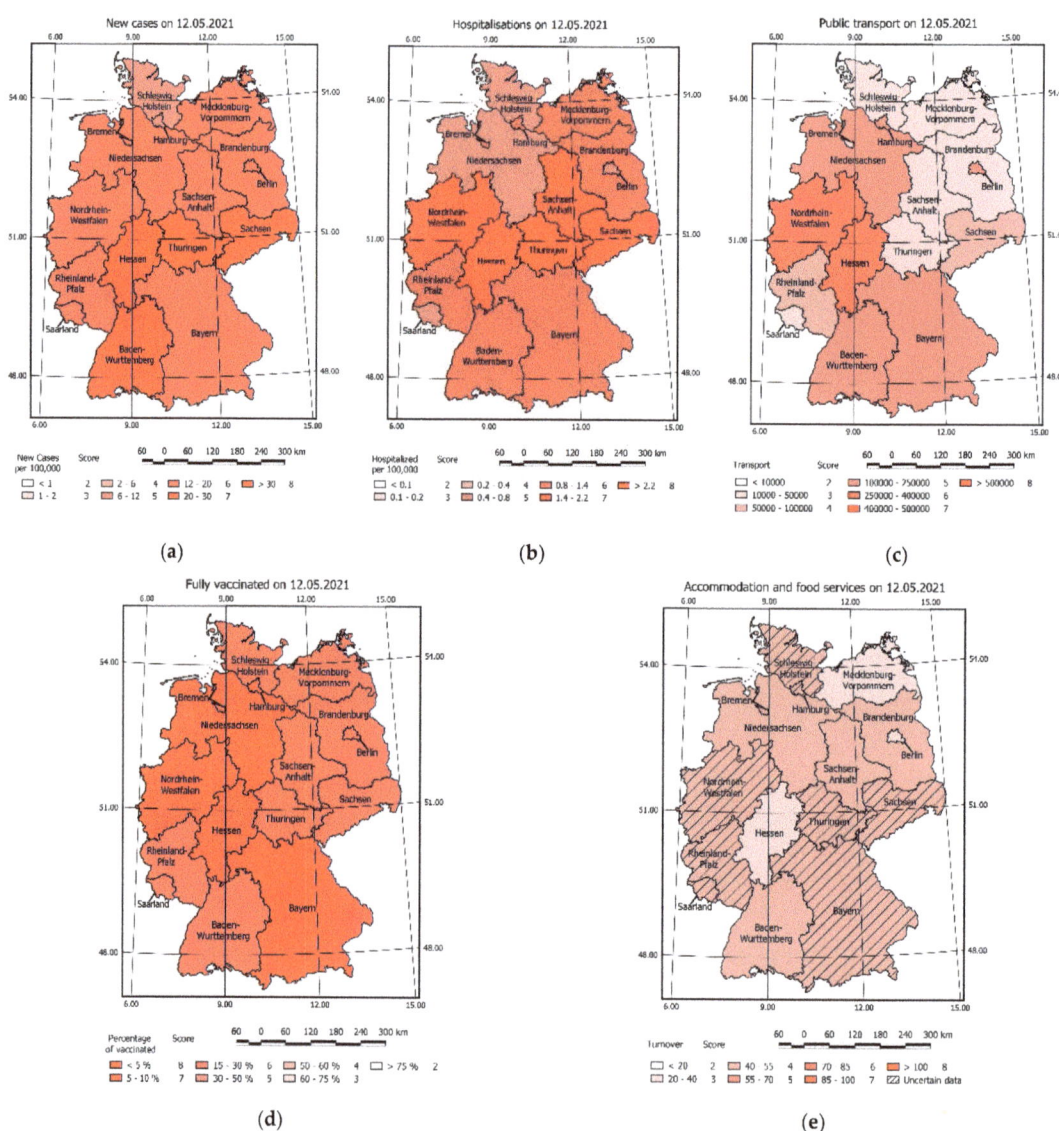

Figure 5. Maps of VSc for selected dynamic criteria on 12 May 2021 (**a**) new cases (**b**) hospitalisations (**c**) public transport (**d**) fully vaccinated (**e**) turnover from food and accommodation services.

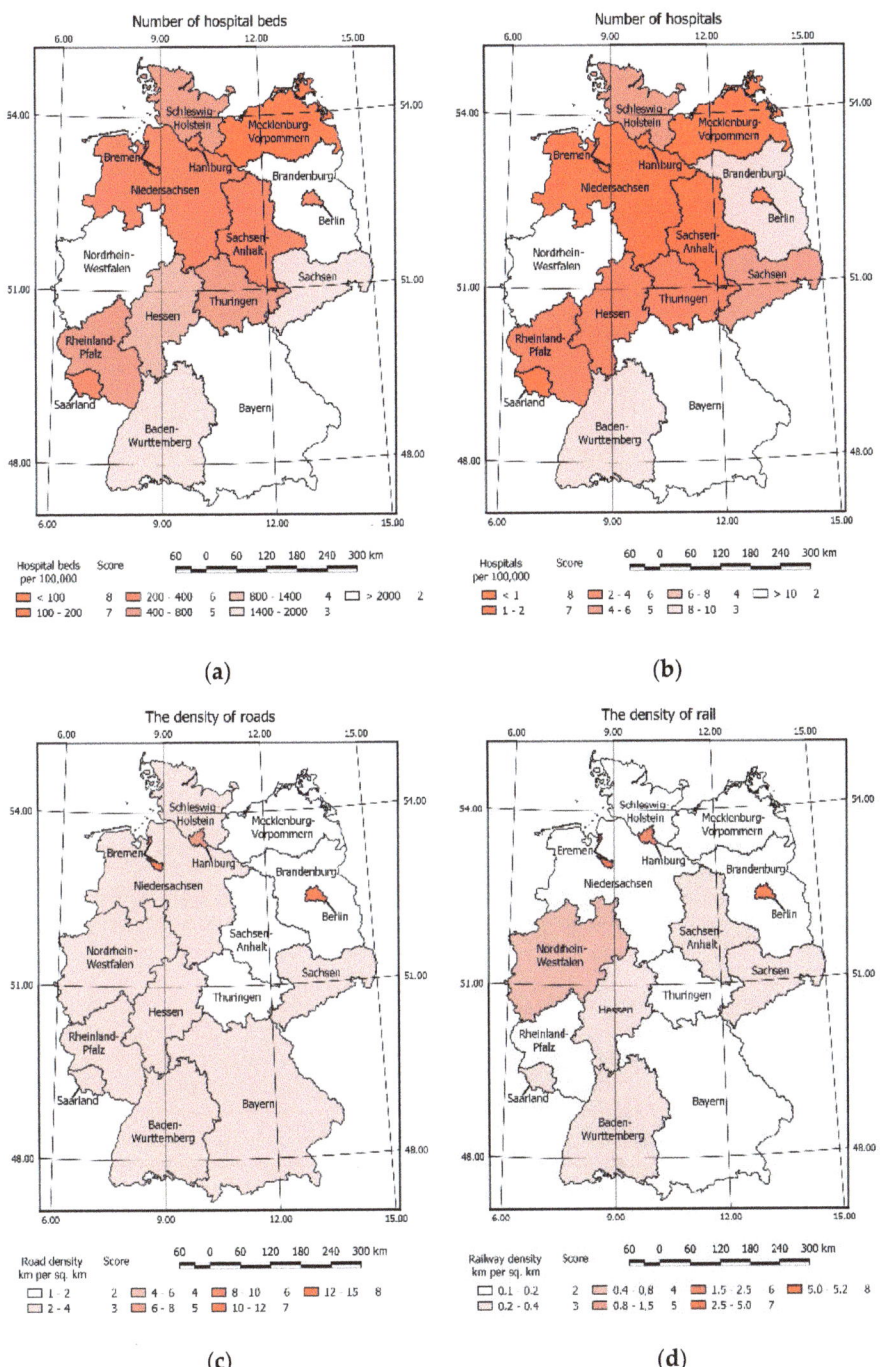

Figure 6. Maps of VSc for selected static criteria on 12 May 2021 (**a**) number of hospital beds (**b**) number of hospitals (**c**) density of roads (**d**) density of railways.

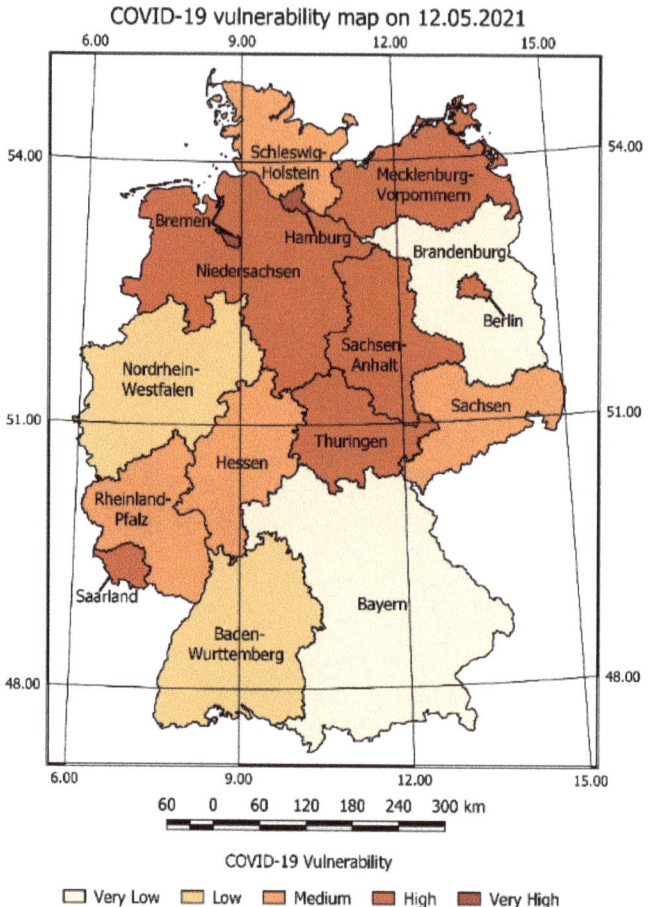

Figure 7. COVID-19 Vulnerability risk map.

Considering the example of Bayern, high VSc values of: new cases, number of hospitals, and number of hospitalisations should result in a high vulnerability risk value; instead the vulnerability of: population density, service turnover, number of vaccinated people, railways, and road lengths caused the occurrence of a low CVI.

The presented CVI analysis may be used in the crisis management process to determine if certain actions (restrictions) have to be taken to prevent further spread of the COVID-19 pandemic. The developed vulnerability risk map allows for measurable assessment of the current situation and determining the risk state of a selected day. The above statements were crucial for research, because the presentation of data on a selected day validates the possibility of the SMCA application in the development of a vulnerability map sequence on selected days and vulnerability change maps over time.

3.3. Criteria Vulnerability Score Analysis in Time

The estimated Vulnerability Score for selected days was presented as a sequence of VSc maps. The example of a selected Vulnerability Score for criteria map on selected days with a three-month interval is shown in Figures 8, 9 and 11. (The number of maps was limited—the remaining maps are provided in Appendix B).

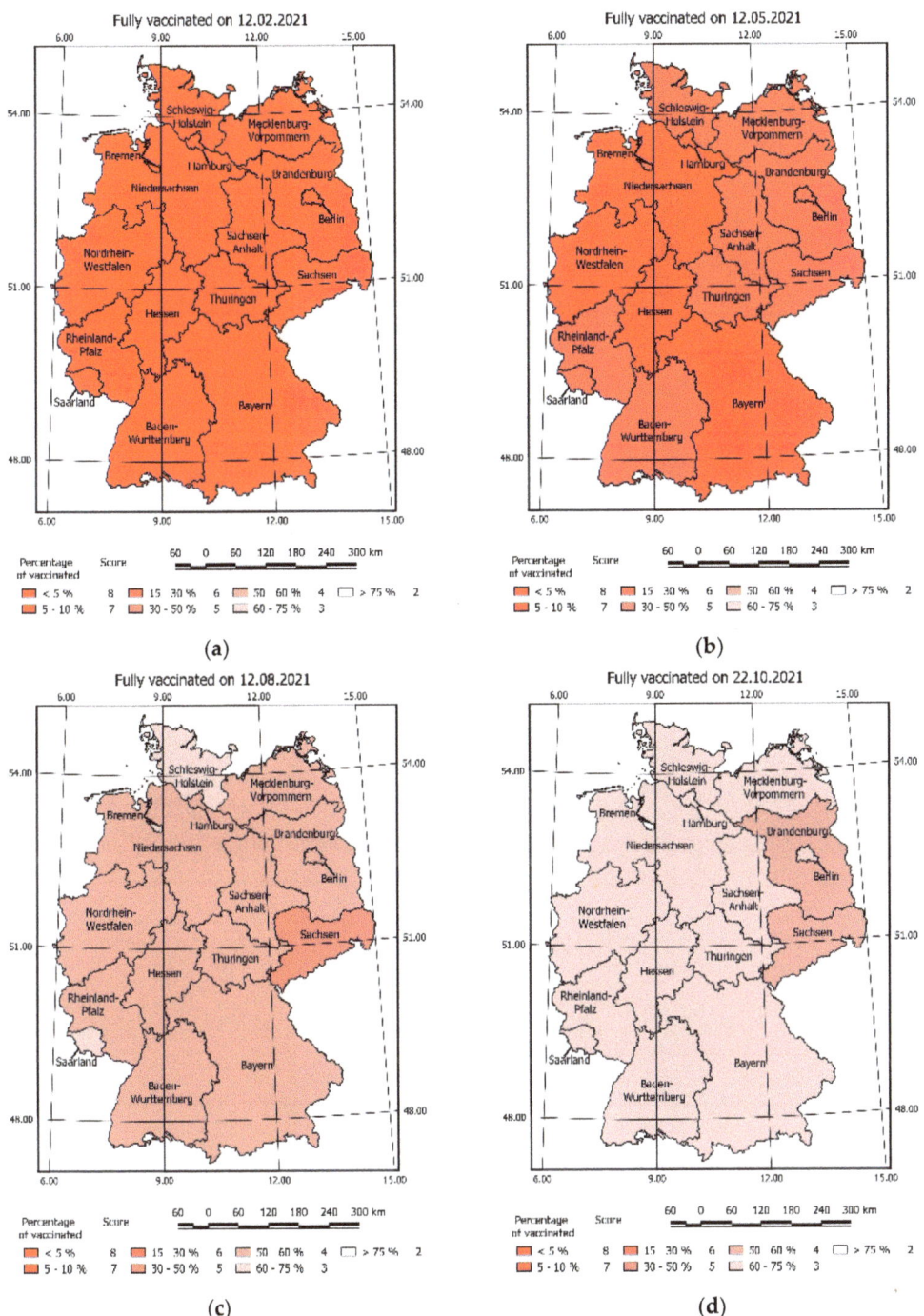

Figure 8. Cumulative COVID-19 Vaccinations on selected days: (**a**) 12 February 2021 (**b**) 12 May 2021 (**c**) 12 August 2021 (**d**) 22 October 2021.

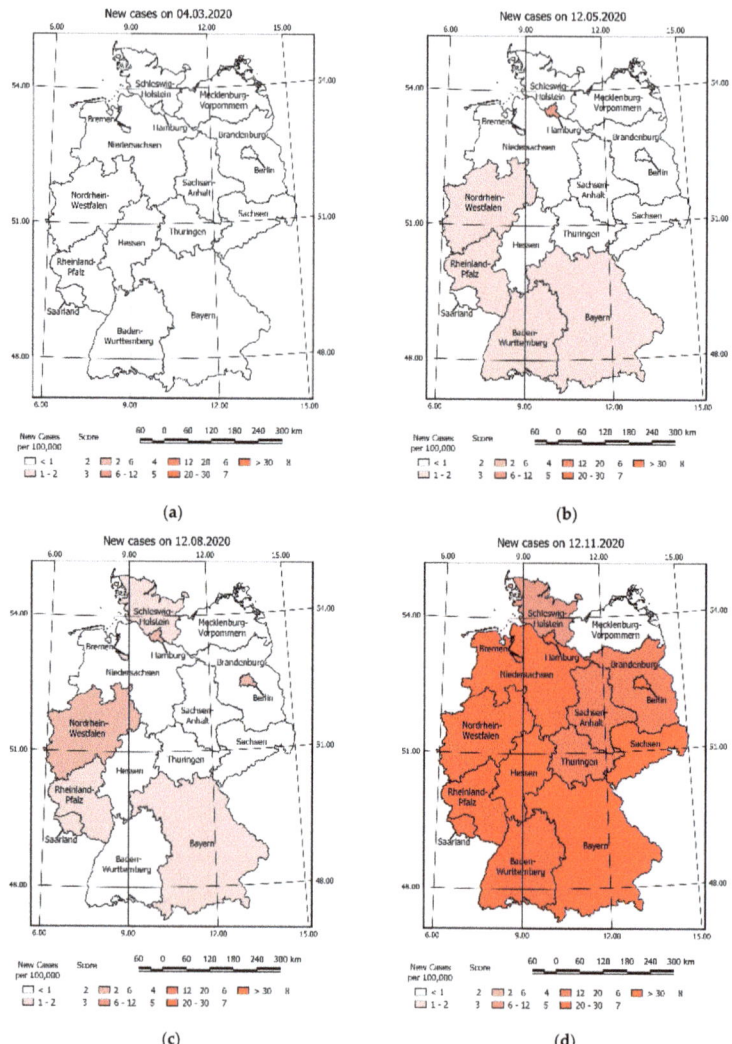

Figure 9. New cases of COVID-19 on selected days: (**a**) 4 March 2020 (**b**) 12 May 2020 (**c**) 12 August 2020 (**d**) 12 November 2020 remaining maps available in Figure A1.

Figure 8 presents the vaccinations vulnerability on selected days. The increase of vaccinated people decreased the risk score. The process of vaccinations began in 2021—all maps before 12 February 2021 present a constant vulnerability risk valued by eight.

Figure 9 shows vulnerability risk resulting in new cases on selected days of the COVID-19 pandemic.

A gradual increase in new cases is noticeable over time. This was confirmed by the chart of new cases according to the data acquired from the Koch Institute (Figure 10).

A juxtaposition of the vaccination vulnerability risk maps and new cases caused by the COVID-19 in corresponding days, explains the fact that at the beginning of 2021 the number of new cases decreased. The noticeable slowing down of the pandemic as a result of reaching 50% vaccination rate of the population in the region visible in Figure 8. Similar observation can be taken on hospitalisations change in time caused by COVID-19 (Figure 11).

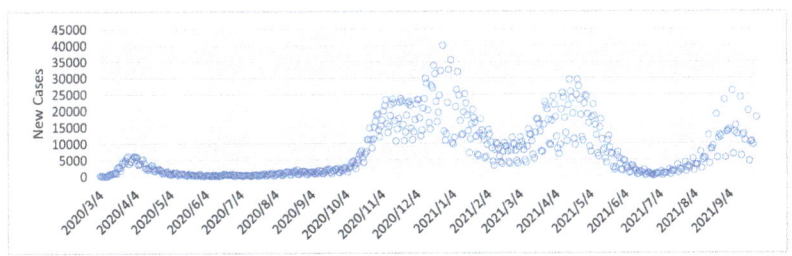

Figure 10. COVID-19 new cases in time chart [93].

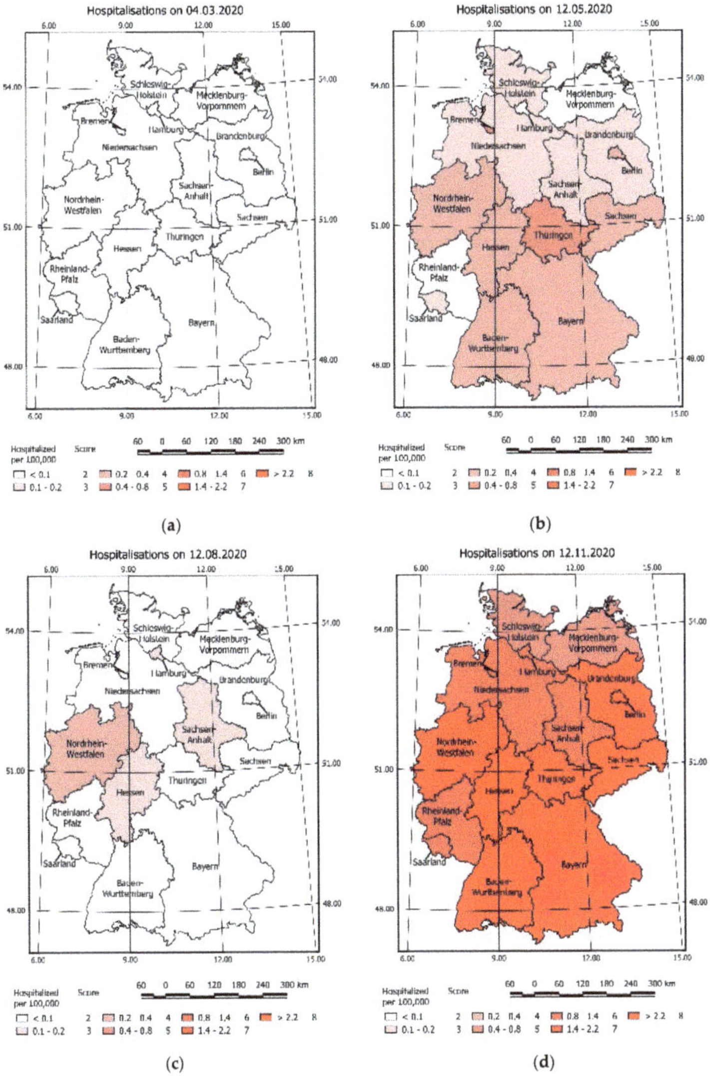

Figure 11. COVID-19 Hospitalisations on selected days: (**a**) 4 March 2020 (**b**) 12 May 2020 (**c**) 12 August 2020 (**d**) 12 November 2020 remaining maps available in Figure A2.

3.4. COVID-19 Vulnerability Index in Time

Based on the Vulnerability Score summaries for selected days, the CVI was calculated. Figure 12 presents the sequence of CVI maps in time. Based on Figure 12a it can be noticed that the federal states: Bremen, Saarland, and Hamburg were classified as high or very high vulnerability risk from the very beginning of the pandemic. This suggests that preventive actions like increasing the number of hospitals beds, preparing field hospitals or restrictions should be considered to ensure public safety in those federal states.

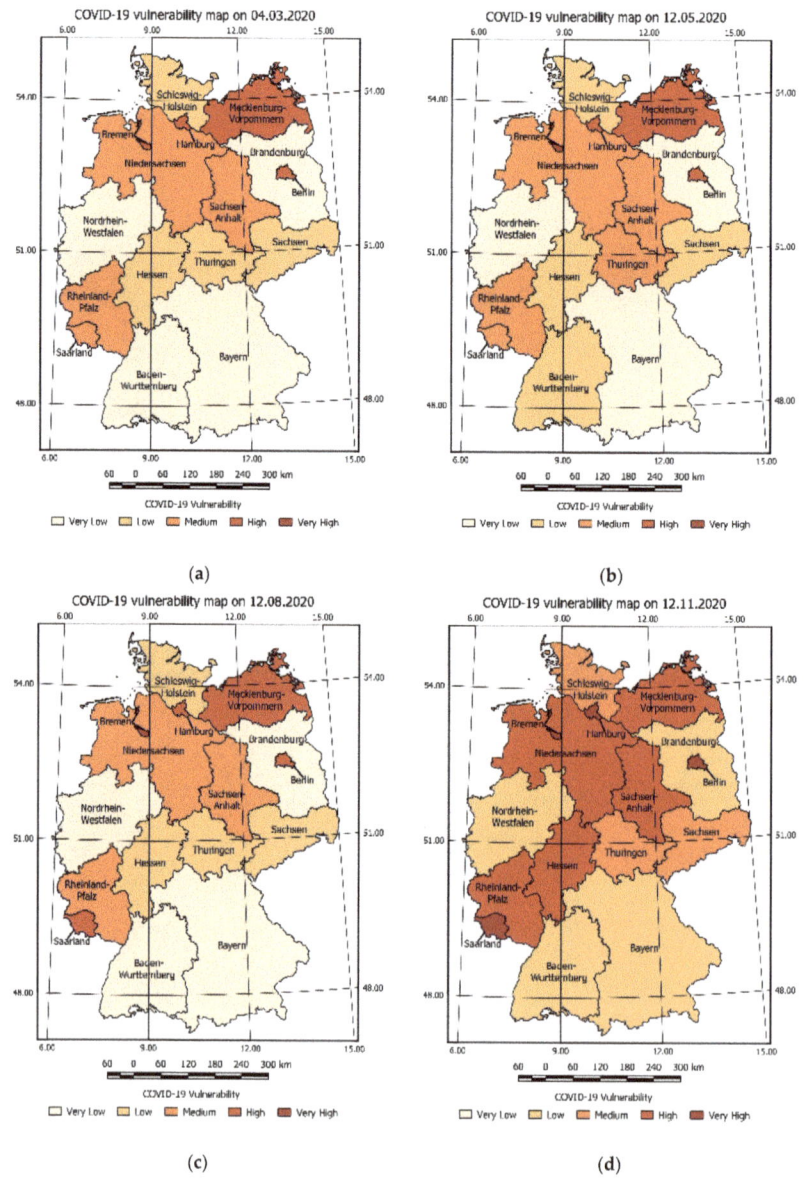

Figure 12. Sequence of CVI estimated in selected days: (**a**) 4 March 2020 (**b**) 12 May 2020 (**c**) 12 August 2020 (**d**) 12 November 2020 remaining maps available in Figure A3.

These recommendations, despite the low number of new cases and hospitalisations, were a result of high vulnerability values assigned to static criteria of the listed federal states. The static and dynamic criteria vulnerabilities of selected countries in time are shown in Figure 13.

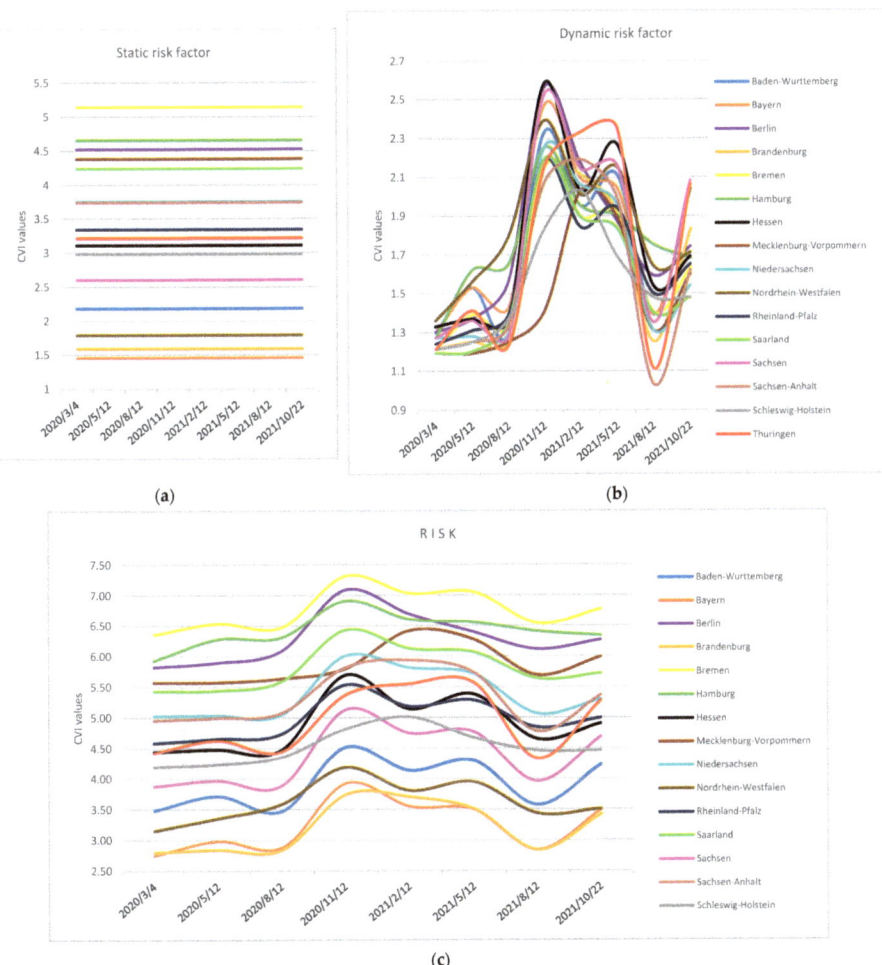

Figure 13. The static (**a**) dynamic (**b**) static and (**c**) summary vulnerability risk for each federal state on selected days.

The high level of static vulnerability increases the overall level of COVID-19 vulnerability as shown in Figure 13a,c. On the other hand, the low level of static vulnerability decreases the final level of COVID-19 vulnerability. In real life scenario, this will correspond to the situation, where the number of hospitals and hospital beds exceeds the number of potential patients.

The analysis in the area of Germany, allows us to estimate the number of people endangered at a certain level of COVID-19 vulnerability in time. Results were presented in Table 5. Pursuant to the above it may be concluded that 22,102,833 population of Germany were at risk of very high COVID-19 vulnerability risk and the number of population endangered changes over time.

Table 5. Number of the German population endangered with a certain level of vulnerability over time.

	4 March 2020	12 May 2020	12 August 2020	12 November 2021	12 February 2021	12 May 2021	12 August 2021	22 October 2021
Very Low	44,717,994	33,610,761	44,717,994	0	13,142,063	15,671,946	44,717,994	33,610,761
Low	15,391,927	24,374,711	15,391,927	44,717,994	31,575,931	29,046,048	9,097,291	14,017,604
Medium	15,273,831	17,398,280	14,288,686	9,097,292	17,366,538	17,366,538	20,583,322	26,770,242
High	7,810,535	7,129,840	8,114,985	22,194,140	13,299,220	18,577,079	6,263,004	8,114,985
Very High	0	680,695	680,695	7,184,861	7,810,535	2,532,676	2,532,676	680,695

The COVID-19 vulnerability risk maps were used to develop the maps shown in Figure 14, One may be easily noticed in which area the pandemic situation has changed.

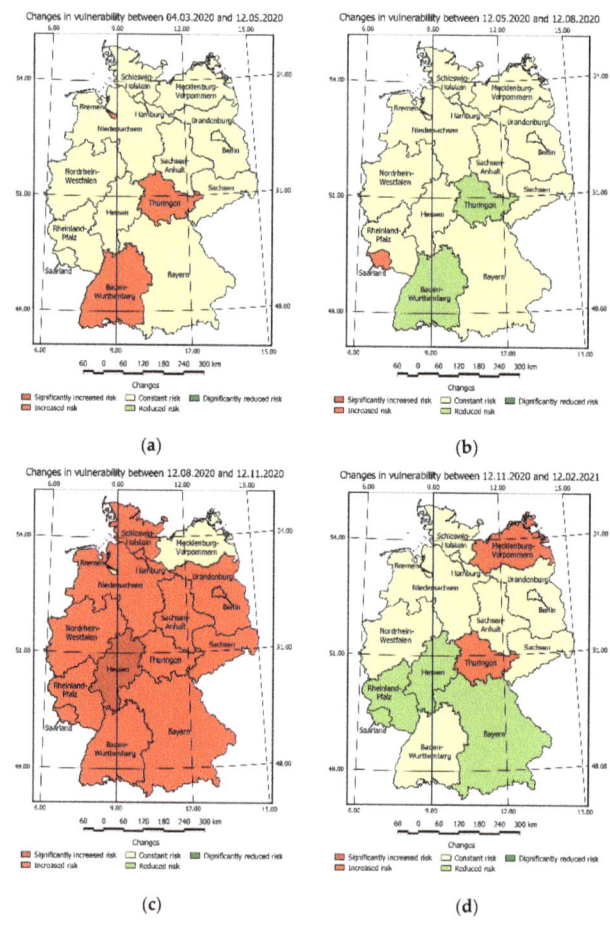

Figure 14. Vulnerability risk changes over time. (a) 4 March 2020–12 May 2020 (b) 12 May 2020–12 August 2020 (c) 12 August 2020–12 November 2020 (d) 12 November 2020–12 February 2021 remaining maps are available in Figure A4.

In this regard, Figure 14c shows the increase in vulnerability caused by post-holiday returns and the re-opening of schools. Figure A4b presents the general decrease in the risk caused by a significant increase in the number of fully vaccinated people. This was followed by another increase in vulnerability Figure A4c.

3.5. Validation

The validation of results was performed in two stages: the first stage was the juxtaposition of CVI and confirmed cases in the time presented. The second stage was the comparison of CVI and COVID-19 active cases. The validation was performed according to the data from Table 6.

Table 6. CVI and new COVID-19 Cases in time for Berlin, Brandenburg, Nordrhein-Westfalen.

		4 March 2020	12 May 2020	12 August 2020	12 November 2020	12 February 2021	12 May 2021	12 August 2021	22 October 2021
Berlin	Cases	7	2	111	1132	485	510	358	713
	CVI	5.52	5.67	5.86	6.34	6.03	5.95	5.67	5.74
Brandenburg	Cases	1	5	8	452	374	397	116	685
	CVI	3.09	3.13	3.21	3.59	3.63	3.43	3.13	3.43
Nordrhein-Westfalen	Cases	115	201	413	4615	1881	3108	1886	2284
	CVI	3.59	3.81	3.82	4.56	4.26	4.32	3.81	3.82

Figure 14 shows the CVI and confirmed cases in selected days on Berlin, Brandenburg, Nordrhein-Westfalen. According to Figure 14 the COVID-19 vulnerability risk in Berlin and Brandenburg, Nordrhein-Westfalen on the first three bars (4 March 2020, 12 May 2020, and 12 August 2020) was growing constantly and this, despite the constant number of new cases, suggests that some actions or preventive steps should be taken in order to reduce the large increase in COVID-19 infections that occurred on the following days: 12 November 2020, 12 February 2021, and 12 May 2021. The above shows that the growing or high value of the COVID-19 vulnerability risk index predicts an upcoming pandemic wave that can be foreseen in a short period of time.

Figure 15 shows the CVI and confirmed cases in selected days on Berlin, Brandenburg, Nordrhein-Westfalen.

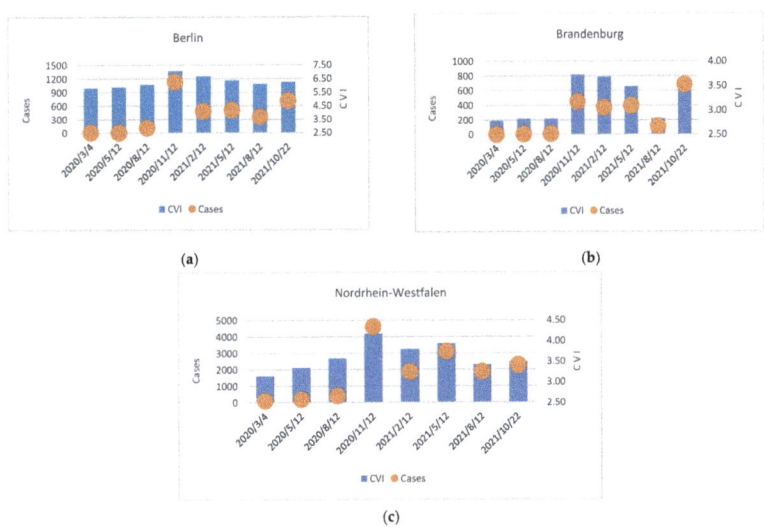

Figure 15. CVI and COVID-19 confirmed cases in (**a**) Berlin, (**b**) Brandenburg and (**c**) Nordrhein-Westfalen.

The chart analysis reveals a positive exponential trend between CVI and the number of confirmed cases with the R^2 value of 0.92 respectively (Figure 16).

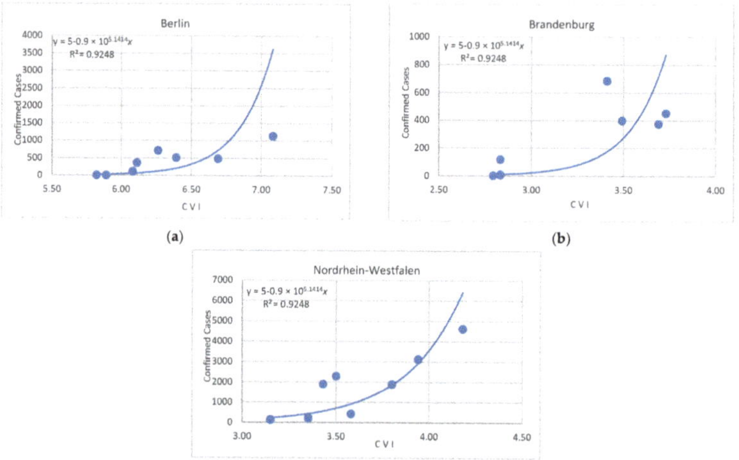

Figure 16. The CVI and new cases relation in the (**a**) Berlin, (**b**) Brandenburg and (**c**) Nordrhein-Westfalen.

The study has the following known limitations:

- Weights summary estimation was based on the AHP method. In this regard, it is essential to pay attention to the problem of criteria selection key and criteria quantity. The increase in criteria quantity would result in a more precise view of the situation in terms of several factors. However, more criteria will cause difficulties in performing analysis due to the lack of available data. If the number of criteria will be decreased—the analysis would be more general, but the data acquisition problem will be less probable.
- Criteria proposed by the authors, and calculated weights create a perspective, focused on health care state image and selected population statistics. This excludes the possibility of insight and of estimating the influence of other factors on pandemic situation. The presented approach and selected criteria include the static criteria groups that allow for early vulnerability risk detection (e.g., in risk of shortage of hospital beds) and furthermore dynamic criteria group for tracking the progress of pandemic in time (new cases).
- The performed analysis was limited to the inference at the strategic level, which results from the limited detailed data access. Obtaining the data in subregions division would allow for more precise identification of pandemic vulnerability risk and would result in appropriate crisis response ensuring public safety. The authors argued that there is quite an immerse gap in the possibilities of conducting spatiotemporal analysis caused to the lack of accurate data. More detailed data are required to prepare recommendations for the selected subregion.

The comparison of the obtained results with the results of works by other authors reveals that those criteria that provide a thematic direction for the analysis results and data are important for the results. As far as the proposed methodology is concerned, data obtained from open data sources were used. What distinguishes the proposed approach from others is the use of both static and dynamic criteria are used, which enable making decisions related to hospital infrastructure and the available resources in the given area. Most studies on COVID-19 involve the modelling of the influence of selected factors, while the proposed approach focuses on modelling the risk connected to the SARS-CoV-2 virus.

4. Conclusions

The outbreak of SARS-CoV-2 caused a pandemic situation and affected the lives of people around the world. For this reason, it became crucial to provide an appropriate crisis response based on research, allowing for the determination of the hazards it implies. The studies on the COVID-19 vulnerability risk index as a result of a weighted summary of the determined individual criteria risk score show the dynamics of threat change in time in the selected area. This allows for tracking the increase of vulnerability risk, caused by the virus spreading and delivering appropriate crisis response.

In terms of the impact of individual criteria on the value of vulnerability risk, it was found that each of the criteria had a different influence on the final value of the CVI coefficient. Furthermore, the division of criteria into static and dynamic ones enabled us to identify factors that were causing a certain level of vulnerability risk to COVID-19 spread even in the early stages of the pandemic. This could help to provide an early reaction, which may prevent the rapid increase of pandemic threat.

The directions of vulnerability risk changes over time were different in each region. However, there is a visible correlation between the CVI change in time and certain, typical events in the annual life cycle e.g., return to school and work from vacation (visible increase) and with such preventive actions as reaching a high level of vaccination (visible decrease), can be noted.

Taking the above into consideration, based on the spatiotemporal vulnerability risk analysis, the decisions on taking actions at an early stage of a pandemic, e.g., relocation of equipment, forces, and resources, are available. Moreover, the conducted analysis illustrates the level of threat better than the number of new cases, which makes it a relevant source of information to identify the areas where restrictions should be introduced.

Furthermore, the performed spatiotemporal analysis allows backward and current modelling of COVID-19 vulnerability risk. The precision of the model of vulnerability risk in the time presented in the case study is low due to the limited number of days taken for the temporal analysis in the article. The increase in time model precision could be obtained as a result of setting smaller time intervals between the COVID-19 vulnerability risk maps. However, this would result in an increased number of maps that would be impossible to be included in the article due to its limited length. Therefore, only the concept and the methodology of the research were presented.

The analysis provided in the case study focused on revealing the COVID-19 vulnerability from the point of view of the healthcare system demonstrated that the spatial data enables the determination of the impact of a crisis situation in the field and, eventually, allows making decisions on an appropriate crisis response. This signifies the role of spatial analysis and spatial data sources in the decision-making process.

According to the authors, future research in this field should be continued and the application of proposed methods with different time data intervals and the results should be assessed to reveal the optimal interval for maps to detect vulnerability change. Moreover, the authors believe that the use of the determined static criteria of vulnerability in combination with the selected pandemic prediction model would extend the perspective to a specific future period of time. This would be a significant potential advantage of the proposed method.

Author Contributions: Conceptualization, M.W. and M.G.; methodology, M.W. and M.G.; software, M.W., M.G. and M.K.; validation, M.W., M.G., K.P. and M.K.; formal analysis, M.W., M.G., K.P. and M.K.; investigation, M.W., M.G. and M.K.; resources, M.W. and M.G.; data curation, M.W., M.G. and K.P.; writing—original draft preparation, M.W., M.G. and M.K.; writing—review and editing, M.W., M.G., K.P. and M.K.; visualization, M.W., M.G. and M.K.; supervision, M.W. All authors have read and agreed to the published version of the manuscript.

Funding: This research was funded by Military University of technology Faculty of Civil Engineering and Geodesy Institute of Geospatial Engineering and Geodesy Statutory Research Founds No. 871/2021.

Acknowledgments: The authors would like to thank Albina Mościcka from MUT Warsaw for comments and supervision while writing this article that greatly improved the research.

Conflicts of Interest: The authors declare no conflict of interest.

Appendix A

Table A1. The remaining criteria scores.

Criteria/Score	Hsp	Mb	Rd	Rs
2	<0.1	<10 K	1–2	0.1–0.2
3	0.1–0.2	10 K–50 K	2–4	0.2–0.4
4	0.2–0.4	50 K–100 K	4–6	0.4–0.8
5	0.4–0.8	100 K–250 K	6–8	0.8–1.5
6	0.8–1.4	250 K–400 K	8–10	1.5–2.5
7	1.4–2.2	400 K–500 K	10–12	2.5–5.0
8	>2.2	>500 K	12–15	5.0–5.2

Appendix B

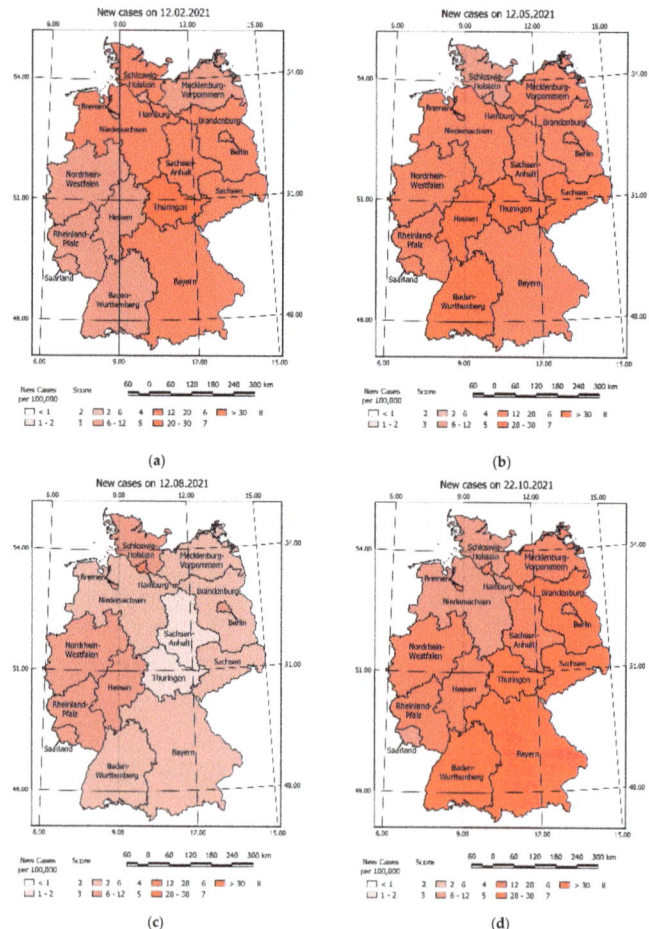

Figure A1. New cases of COVID-19 on selected days: (**a**) 4 March 2020 (**b**) 12 May 2020 (**c**) 12 August 2020 (**d**) 12 November 2020.

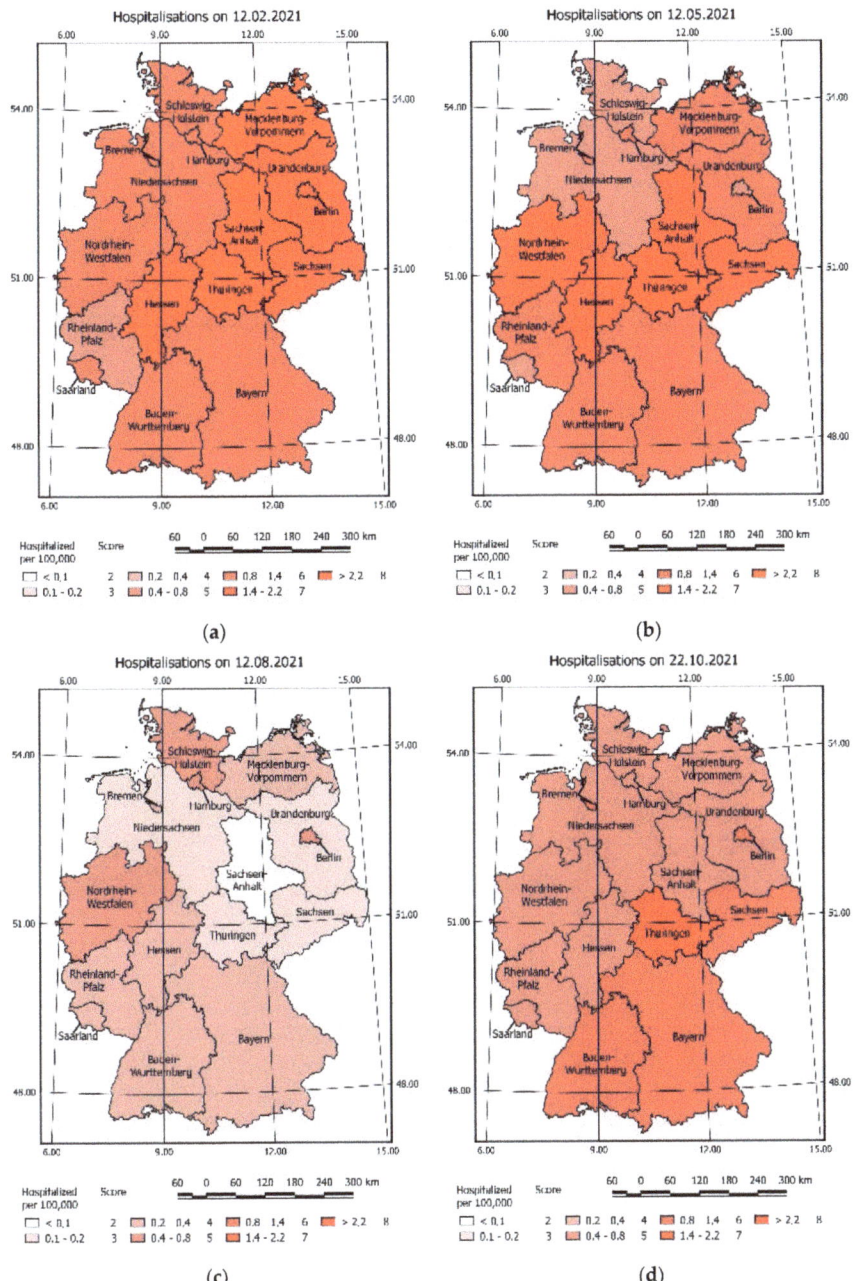

Figure A2. COVID-19 Hospitalisations on selected days: (**a**) 12 February 2021 (**b**) 12 May 2021 (**c**) 12 August 2021, (**d**) 22 October 2021.

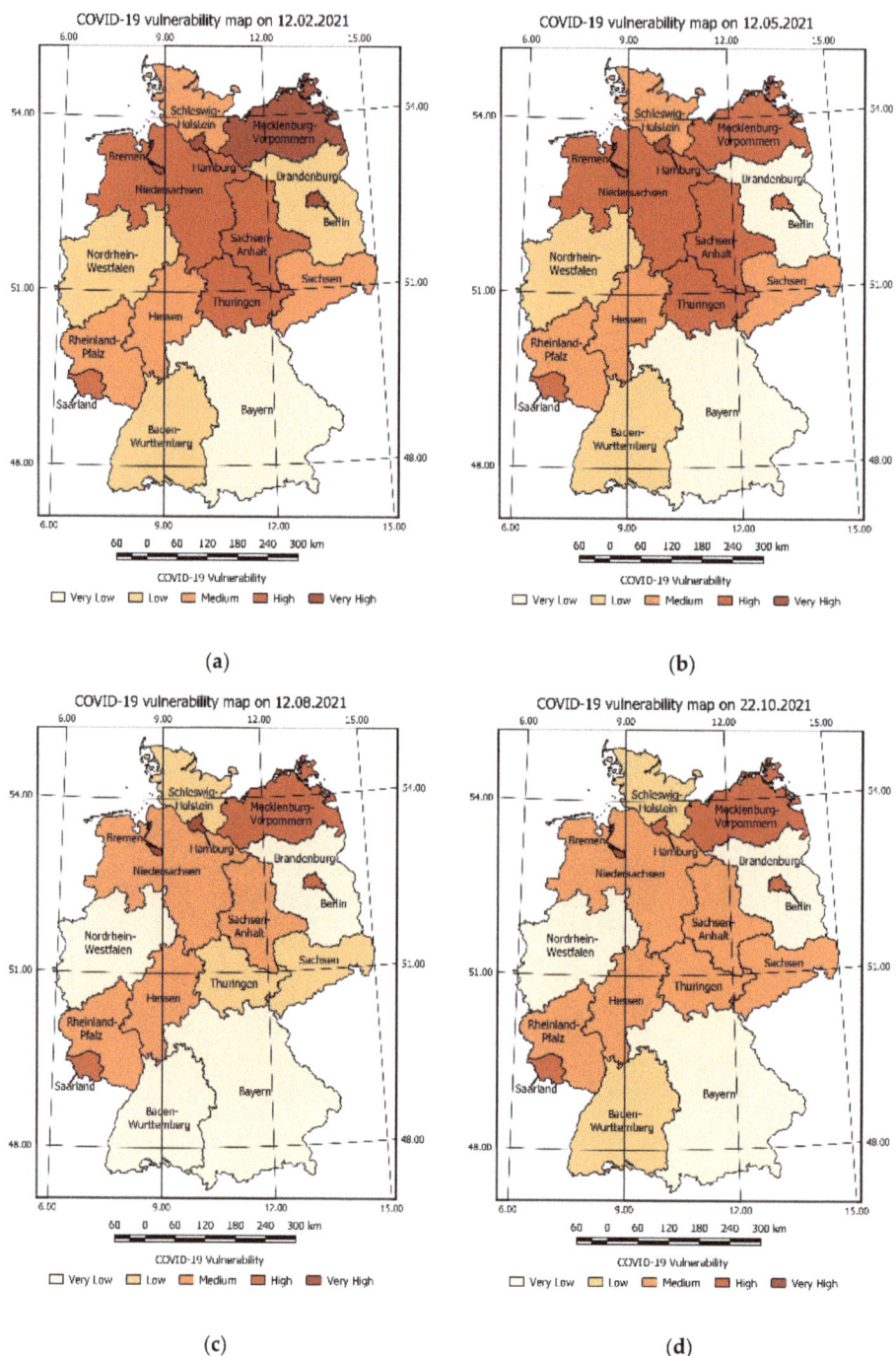

Figure A3. Sequence of CVI estimated in selected days: (**a**) 12 February 2021 (**b**) 12 May 2021 (**c**) 12 August 2021 (**d**) 22 October 2021.

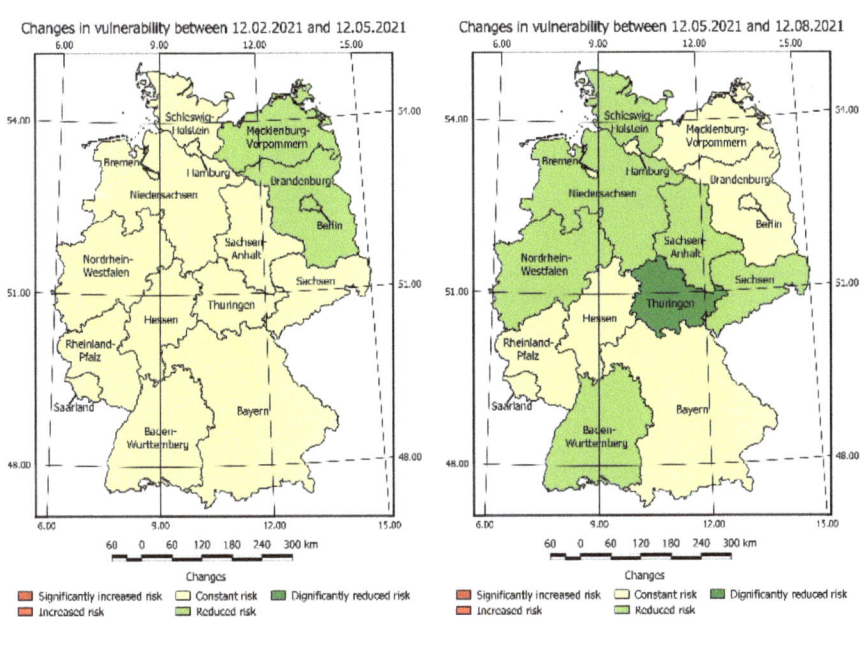

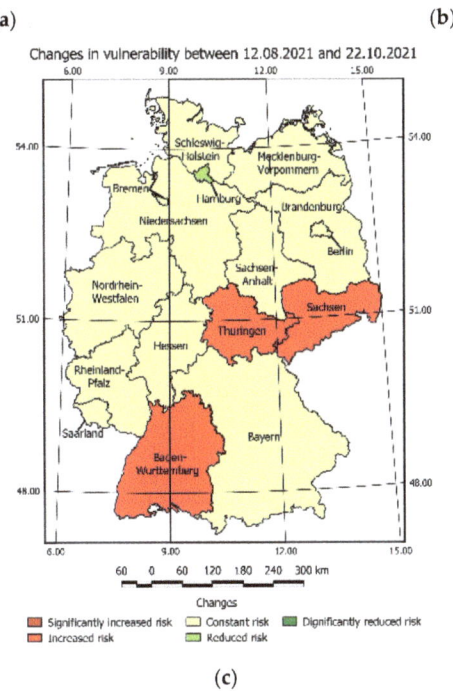

Figure A4. Vulnerability risk change over time. (**a**) 12 February 2021–12 May 2021 (**b**) 12 May 2021–12 August 2021 (**c**) 12 August 2021–22 October 2021.

References

1. Zheng, J. SARS-CoV-2: An Emerging Coronavirus That Causes a Global Threat. *Int. J. Biol. Sci.* **2020**, *16*, 1678–1685. [CrossRef] [PubMed]
2. Wise, T.; Zbozinek, T.D.; Michelini, G.; Hagan, C.C.; Mobbs, D. Changes in Risk Perception and Protective Behavior during the First Week of the COVID-19 Pandemic in the United States. *R. Soc. Open Sci.* **2020**, *7*, 200742. [CrossRef] [PubMed]
3. Al-Khudhairy, D.H.A. Geo-Spatial Information and Technologies in Support of EU Crisis Management. *Int. J. Digit. Earth* **2010**, *3*, 16–30. [CrossRef]
4. Van Eck: VOSviewer Manual: Version 1.6. 5—Google Scholar. Available online: https://scholar.google.com/scholar_lookup?title=VOSviewer+Manual,+Version+1.6.9&author=van+Eck,+N.J.&author=Waltman,+L.&publication_year=2018 (accessed on 19 November 2021).
5. Arabsheibani, R.; Kanani Sadat, Y.; Abedini, A. Land Suitability Assessment for Locating Industrial Parks: A Hybrid Multi Criteria Decision-Making Approach Using Geographical Information System. *Geogr. Res.* **2016**, *54*, 446–460. [CrossRef]
6. Joerin, F.; Thériault, M.; Musy, A. Using GIS and Outranking Multicriteria Analysis for Land-Use Suitability Assessment. *Int. J. Geogr. Inf. Sci.* **2001**, *15*, 153–174. [CrossRef]
7. Bathrellos, G.D.; Skilodimou, H.D.; Chousianitis, K.; Youssef, A.M.; Pradhan, B. Suitability Estimation for Urban Development Using Multi-Hazard Assessment Map. *Sci. Total Environ.* **2017**, *575*, 119–134. [CrossRef]
8. Akpoti, K.; Kabo-bah, A.T.; Zwart, S.J. Review—Agricultural Land Suitability Analysis: State-of-the-Art and Outlooks for Integration of Climate Change Analysis. *Agric. Syst.* **2019**, *173*, 172–208. [CrossRef]
9. Wu, C.; Ding, Y.; Zhou, X.; Lu, G. A Grid Algorithm Suitable for Line and Area Feature Label Placement. *Environ. Earth Sci.* **2016**, *75*, 1368. [CrossRef]
10. Parry, J.T. Terrain Evaluation, Military Purposesterrain Evaluation, Military Purposes. In *Applied Geology*; Finkl, C.W., Ed.; Encyclopedia of Earth Sciences Series; Kluwer Academic Publishers: Dordrecht, The Netherlands, 1984; Volume 3, pp. 570–581, ISBN 978-0-442-22537-7.
11. Sarnowski, Ł.; Podgórski, Z.; Brykała, D. *Planning a Greenway Based on an Evaluation of Visual Landscape Attractiveness*; Biblioteka Uniwersytetu Kazimierza Wielkiego: Bydgoszcz, Poland, 2016.
12. Carver, S.J. Integrating Multi-Criteria Evaluation with Geographical Information Systems. *Int. J. Geogr. Inf. Syst.* **1991**, *5*, 321–339. [CrossRef]
13. Scala, A.; Facchini, A.; Perna, U.; Basosi, R. Portfolio Analysis and Geographical Allocation of Renewable Sources: A Stochastic Approach. *Energy Policy* **2019**, *125*, 154–159. [CrossRef]
14. Kim, T.J.; Choi, K. GIS for Transportation. In *Springer Handbook of Geographic Information*; Kresse, W., Danko, D.M., Eds.; Springer Handbooks; Springer: Berlin/Heidelberg, Germany, 2012; pp. 503–521, ISBN 978-3-540-72680-7.
15. Zhao, S.; Zhuang, Z.; Ran, J.; Lin, J.; Yang, G.; Yang, L.; He, D. The Association between Domestic Train Transportation and Novel Coronavirus (2019-NCoV) Outbreak in China from 2019 to 2020: A Data-Driven Correlational Report. *Travel Med. Infect. Dis.* **2020**, *33*, 101568. [CrossRef] [PubMed]
16. Alexander, D.; Gilbert, R. Infrastructure Assessment Decision Making During a Crisis. *Transp. Res. Rec.* **2009**, *2093*, 93–98. [CrossRef]
17. Ahmed, S.; Ibrahim, R.; Hefny, H. An Efficient Ambulance Routing System for Emergency Cases Based on Dijkstra's Algorithm, AHP, and GIS. *Int. J. Intell. Eng. Syst.* **2018**, *11*, 252–260.
18. Choosumrong, S.; Raghavan, V.; Bozon, N. Multi-Criteria Emergency Route Planning Based on Analytical Hierarchy Process and PgRouting. *Jpn. Soc. Geoinform.* **2012**, *23*, 159–168. [CrossRef]
19. Pelgrum, H. *Spatial Aggregation of Land Surface Characteristics: Impact of Resolution of Remote Sensing Data on Land Surface Modelling*; Wageningen University and Research ProQuest Dissertations Publishing: Wageningen, The Netherlands, 2000.
20. Jithesh, P.K. A Model Based on Cellular Automata for Investigating the Impact of Lockdown, Migration and Vaccination on COVID-19 Dynamics. *Comput. Methods Programs Biomed.* **2021**, *211*, 106402. [CrossRef]
21. Shi, P.; Dong, Y.; Yan, H.; Li, X.; Zhao, C.; Liu, W.; He, M.; Tang, S.; Xi, S. The Impact of Temperature and Absolute Humidity on the Coronavirus Disease 2019 (COVID-19) Outbreak-Evidence from China. *MedRxiv* **2020**. [CrossRef]
22. Pokonieczny, K. Using Artificial Neural Networks to Determine the Location of Wind Farms. Miedzna District Case Study. *J. Water Land Dev.* **2016**, *30*, 101–111. [CrossRef]
23. Chen, Z.-L.; Zhang, Q.; Lu, Y.; Guo, Z.-M.; Zhang, X.; Zhang, W.-J.; Guo, C.; Liao, C.-H.; Li, Q.-L.; Han, X.-H.; et al. Distribution of the COVID-19 Epidemic and Correlation with Population Emigration from Wuhan, China. *Chin. Med. J.* **2020**, *133*, 1044–1050. [CrossRef]
24. French, S.; Argyris, N.; Haywood, S.; Hort, M.; Smith, J. Communicating Geographical Risks in Crisis Management: The Need for Research. *Risk Anal.* **2019**, *39*, 9–16. [CrossRef]
25. Ai, F.; Comfort, L.K.; Dong, Y.; Znati, T. A Dynamic Decision Support System Based on Geographical Information and Mobile Social Networks: A Model for Tsunami Risk Mitigation in Padang, Indonesia. *Saf. Sci.* **2016**, *90*, 62–74. [CrossRef]
26. Ahola, T.; Virrantaus, K.; Krisp, J.M.; Hunter, G.J. A Spatio-temporal Population Model to Support Risk Assessment and Damage Analysis for Decision-making. *Int. J. Geogr. Inf. Sci.* **2007**, *21*, 935–953. [CrossRef]
27. Teodoro, A.C.; Duarte, L. Forest Fire Risk Maps: A GIS Open Source Application—A Case Study in Norwest of Portugal. *Int. J. Geogr. Inf. Sci.* **2013**, *27*, 699–720. [CrossRef]

28. Ejigu, B.A.; Wencheko, E.; Moraga, P.; Giorgi, E. Geostatistical Methods for Modelling Non-Stationary Patterns in Disease Risk. *Spat. Stat.* **2020**, *35*, 100397. [CrossRef]
29. Leone, F.; Colas, A.; Garcin, Y.; Eckert, N.; Jomelli, V.; Gherardi, M. The Snow Avalanches Risk on Alpine Roads Network Assessment of Impacts and Mapping of Accessibility Loss. *Rev. Geogr. Alp.-J. Alp. Res.* **2014**, *102*. [CrossRef]
30. de Brito, M.M.; Evers, M. Multi-Criteria Decision-Making for Flood Risk Management: A Survey of the Current State of the Art. *Nat. Hazards Earth Syst. Sci.* **2016**, *16*, 1019–1033. [CrossRef]
31. Shadeed, S.; Alawna, S. GIS-Based COVID-19 Vulnerability Mapping in the West Bank, Palestine. *Int. J. Disaster Risk Reduct.* **2021**, *64*, 102483. [CrossRef]
32. Doorga, J.R.S.; Magerl, L.; Bunwaree, P.; Zhao, J.; Watkins, S.; Staub, C.G.; Rughooputh, S.D.D.V.; Cunden, T.S.M.; Lollchund, R.; Boojhawon, R. GIS-Based Multi-Criteria Modelling of Flood Risk Susceptibility in Port Louis, Mauritius: Towards Resilient Flood Management. *Int. J. Disaster Risk Reduct.* **2022**, *67*, 102683. [CrossRef]
33. Geneletti, D.; Scolozzi, R.; Adem Esmail, B. Assessing Ecosystem Services and Biodiversity Tradeoffs across Agricultural Landscapes in a Mountain Region. *Int. J. Biodivers. Sci. Ecosyst. Serv. Manag.* **2018**, *14*, 188–208. [CrossRef]
34. Gonzalez, A.; Enríquez-de-Salamanca, Á. Spatial Multi-Criteria Analysis in Environmental Assessment: A Review and Reflection on Benefits and Limitations. *J. Environ. Assess. Policy Manag.* **2018**, *20*, 1840001. [CrossRef]
35. Argyris, N.; Ferretti, V.; French, S.; Guikema, S.; Montibeller, G. Advances in Spatial Risk Analysis. *Risk Anal.* **2019**, *39*, 1–8. [CrossRef]
36. Majlingova, A.; Buzalka, J. Crisis Management Based on GIS—Case Study. In Proceedings of the Fire Protection, Safety and Security 2017, Zvolen, Slovakia, 3–5 May 2017; Majlingova, A., VelKova, V., Eds.; pp. 340–350.
37. Becker, T.; Konig, G. Generalized Cartographic and Simultaneous Representation of Utility Networks for Decision-Support Systems and Crisis Management in Urban Environments. In Proceedings of the International Geoinformation Conference, Kuala Lumpur, Malaysia, 28–30 October 2015; Rahman, A., Isikdag, U., Castro, F., Eds.; Volume II–2, pp. 19–28.
38. Reeves, J.J.; Hollandsworth, H.M.; Torriani, F.J.; Taplitz, R.; Abeles, S.; Tai-Seale, M.; Millen, M.; Clay, B.J.; Longhurst, C.A. Rapid Response to COVID-19: Health Informatics Support for Outbreak Management in an Academic Health System. *J. Am. Med. Inf. Assoc.* **2020**, *27*, 853–859. [CrossRef] [PubMed]
39. Ernst, V.; Ostrovskii, M. *Intelligent Cartographic Presentations for Emergency Situations*; Loffler, J., Klann, M., Eds.; Springer: Berlin/Heidelberg, Germany, 2007; Volume 4458, pp. 77–84.
40. Kehl, C.; de Haan, G. *Interactive Simulation and Visualisation of Realistic Flooding Scenarios*; Zlatanova, S., Dilo, A., Peters, R., Scholten, H., Eds.; Springer: Berlin/Heidelberg, Germany, 2013; pp. 79–93.
41. Dilo, A.; Zlatanova, S. Spatiotemporal Data Modeling for Disaster Management in The Netherlands. In Proceedings of the Joint ISCRAM-CHINA and GI4DM Conference, Harbin, China, 4 August 2008.
42. The Use of Subjective-Objective Weights in GIS-Based Multi-Criteria Decision Analysis for Flood Hazard Assessment: A Case Study in Mazandaran, Iran-Web of Science Core Collection. Available online: https://www-1webofscience-1com-100003exr00f6.han.wat.edu.pl/wos/woscc/full-record/WOS:000617914700020 (accessed on 7 November 2021).
43. Chen, W.; Zhang, S.; Li, R.; Shahabi, H. Performance Evaluation of the GIS-Based Data Mining Techniques of Best-First Decision Tree, Random Forest, and Naive Bayes Tree for Landslide Susceptibility Modeling. *Sci. Total Environ.* **2018**, *644*, 1006–1018. [CrossRef] [PubMed]
44. Bezerra, É.C.D.; dos Santos, P.S.; Lisbinski, F.C.; Dias, L.C. Análise espacial das condições de enfrentamento à COVID-19: Uma proposta de Índice da Infraestrutura da Saúde do Brasil. *Ciênc. Saúde Coletiva* **2020**, *25*, 4957–4967. [CrossRef] [PubMed]
45. Water Crisis Analysis Using GIS; Case Study: Nishabur Plain, Iran. Available online: https://scialert.net/fulltext/?doi=ajps.2007.884.891 (accessed on 9 December 2021).
46. Budzynski, M.; Luczkiewicz, A.; Szmaglinski, J. Assessing the Risk in Urban Public Transport for Epidemiologic Factors. *Energies* **2021**, *14*, 4513. [CrossRef]
47. Davidovsky, A. *System Analysis and Forecasting of the Relationship between Economic Factors and the Epidemic Process COVID-19 to Optimize International Transport Communications in the Context of a Pandemic*; Atlantis Press: Amsterdam, The Netherlands, 2020; pp. 473–479.
48. Kim, J.-C.; Lee, S.; Jung, H.-S.; Lee, S. Landslide Susceptibility Mapping Using Random Forest and Boosted Tree Models in Pyeong-Chang, Korea. *Geocarto Int.* **2018**, *33*, 1000–1015. [CrossRef]
49. Pourghasemi, H.R.; Gayen, A.; Edalat, M.; Zarafshar, M.; Tiefenbacher, J.P. Is Multi-Hazard Mapping Effective in Assessing Natural Hazards and Integrated Watershed Management? *Geosci. Front.* **2020**, *11*, 1203–1217. [CrossRef]
50. Pourghasemi, H.R.; Pouyan, S.; Heidari, B.; Farajzadeh, Z.; Fallah Shamsi, S.R.; Babaei, S.; Khosravi, R.; Etemadi, M.; Ghanbarian, G.; Farhadi, A.; et al. Spatial Modeling, Risk Mapping, Change Detection, and Outbreak Trend Analysis of Coronavirus (COVID-19) in Iran (Days between February 19 and June 14, 2020). *Int. J. Infect. Dis.* **2020**, *98*, 90–108. [CrossRef]
51. Feizizadeh, B.; Blaschke, T. GIS-Multicriteria Decision Analysis for Landslide Susceptibility Mapping: Comparing Three Methods for the Urmia Lake Basin, Iran. *Nat. Hazards* **2013**, *65*, 2105–2128. [CrossRef]
52. Pham, B.T.; Bui, D.T.; Pourghasemi, H.R.; Indra, P.; Dholakia, M.B. Landslide Susceptibility Assessment in the Uttarakhand Area (India) Using GIS: A Comparison Study of Prediction Capability of naïve Bayes, Multilayer Perceptron Neural Networks, and Functional Trees Methods. *Theor. Appl. Climatol.* **2017**, *128*, 255–273. [CrossRef]

53. Mohamed, S.; El-Raey, M. Vulnerability Assessment for Flash Floods Using GIS Spatial Modeling and Remotely Sensed Data in El-Arish City, North Sinai, Egypt. *Nat. Hazards* **2020**, *102*, 707–728. [CrossRef]
54. Jena, R.; Pradhan, B.; Al-Amri, A.; Lee, C.W.; Park, H.-J. Earthquake Probability Assessment for the Indian Subcontinent Using Deep Learning. *Sensor* **2020**, *20*, 4369. [CrossRef] [PubMed]
55. Web-Based Geospatial Multiple Criteria Decision Analysis Using Open Software and Standards-Web of Science Core Collection. Available online: https://www-1webofscience-1com-100003exr00f6.han.wat.edu.pl/wos/woscc/full-record/WOS:000374902300010 (accessed on 7 November 2021).
56. Feizizadeh, B.; Jankowski, P.; Blaschke, T. A GIS Based Spatially-Explicit Sensitivity and Uncertainty Analysis Approach for Multi-Criteria Decision Analysis. *Comput. Geosci.* **2014**, *64*, 81–95. [CrossRef] [PubMed]
57. Warren, M.S.; Skillman, S.W. Mobility Changes in Response to COVID-19. *arXiv* **2020**, arXiv:2003.14228.
58. Yang, C.; Sha, D.; Liu, Q.; Li, Y.; Lan, H.; Guan, W.W.; Hu, T.; Li, Z.; Zhang, Z.; Thompson, J.H.; et al. Taking the Pulse of COVID-19: A Spatiotemporal Perspective. *Int. J. Digit. Earth* **2020**, *13*, 1186–1211. [CrossRef]
59. Zheng: Spatial Transmission of COVID-19 via Public . . . —Google Scholar. Available online: https://scholar.google.com/scholar_lookup?title=Spatial+transmission+of+COVID-19+via+public+and+private+transportation+in+China&author=Zheng,+R.&author=Xu,+Y.&author=Wang,+W.&author=Ning,+G.&author=Bi,+Y.&publication_year=2020&journal=Travel+Med.+Infect.+Dis.&volume=34&pages=101626&doi=10.1016/j.tmaid.2020.101626 (accessed on 27 November 2021).
60. Ma, Y.; Zhao, Y.; Liu, J.; He, X.; Wang, B.; Fu, S.; Yan, J.; Niu, J.; Zhou, J.; Luo, B. Effects of Temperature Variation and Humidity on the Death of COVID-19 in Wuhan, China. *Sci. Total Environ.* **2020**, *724*, 138226. [CrossRef] [PubMed]
61. Shakhovska, N.; Izonin, I.; Melnykova, N. The Hierarchical Classifier for COVID-19 Resistance Evaluation. *Data* **2021**, *6*, 6. [CrossRef]
62. Liu, Q.; Liu, W.; Sha, D.; Kumar, S.; Chang, E.; Arora, V.; Lan, H.; Li, Y.; Wang, Z.; Zhang, Y.; et al. An Environmental Data Collection for COVID-19 Pandemic Research. *Data* **2020**, *5*, 68. [CrossRef]
63. Ferreira, M.C. Spatial Association between the Incidence Rate of COVID-19 and Poverty in the São Paulo Municipality, Brazil. *Geospat. Health* **2020**, *15*. [CrossRef]
64. Dryhurst, S.; Schneider, C.R.; Kerr, J.; Freeman, A.L.J.; Recchia, G.; van der Bles, A.M.; Spiegelhalter, D.; van der Linden, S. Risk Perceptions of COVID-19 around the World. *J. Risk Res.* **2020**, *23*, 994–1006. [CrossRef]
65. Carcione, J.M.; Santos, J.E.; Bagaini, C.; Ba, J. A Simulation of a COVID-19 Epidemic Based on a Deterministic SEIR Model. *Front. Public Health* **2020**, *8*, 230. [CrossRef]
66. Chen: Transmission Dynamics of a Two-City SIR Epidemic . . . —Google Scholar. Available online: https://scholar.google.com/scholar_lookup?title=Transmission+dynamics+of+a+two-city+SIR+epidemic+model+with+transport-related+infections&author=Chen,+Y.&author=Yan,+M.&author=Xiang,+Z.&publication_year=2014&journal=J.+Appl.+Math.&volume=2014&doi=10.1155/2014/764278 (accessed on 27 November 2021).
67. Pagano, A.; Pluchinotta, I.; Giordano, R.; Petrangeli, A.; Fratino, U.; Vurro, M. Dealing with Uncertainty in Decision-Making for Drinking Water Supply Systems Exposed to Extreme Events. *Water Resour. Manag.* **2018**, *32*, 2131–2145. [CrossRef]
68. Epidemic Analysis of COVID-19 in Italy Based on Spatiotemporal Geographic Information and Google Trends-Niu-2021- Transboundary and Emerging Diseases—Wiley Online Library. Available online: https://onlinelibrary.wiley.com/doi/10.1111/tbed.13902 (accessed on 19 November 2021).
69. Mościcka, A.; Araszkiewicz, A.; Wabiński, J.; Kuźma, M.; Kiliszek, D. Modeling of Various Spatial Patterns of SARS-CoV-2: The Case of Germany. *J. Clin. Med.* **2021**, *10*, 1409. [CrossRef] [PubMed]
70. Wang, Y.; Liu, Y.; Struthers, J.; Lian, M. Spatiotemporal Characteristics of the COVID-19 Epidemic in the United States. *Clin. Infect. Dis.* **2021**, *72*, 643–651. [CrossRef] [PubMed]
71. Javidan, N.; Kavian, A.; Pourghasemi, H.R.; Conoscenti, C.; Jafarian, Z.; Rodrigo-Comino, J. Evaluation of Multi-Hazard Map Produced Using MaxEnt Machine Learning Technique. *Sci. Rep.* **2021**, *11*, 6496. [CrossRef]
72. Sha, D.; Malarvizhi, A.S.; Liu, Q.; Tian, Y.; Zhou, Y.; Ruan, S.; Dong, R.; Carte, K.; Lan, H.; Wang, Z.; et al. A State-Level Socioeconomic Data Collection of the United States for COVID-19 Research. *Data* **2020**, *5*, 118. [CrossRef]
73. Swapnarekha, H.; Behera, H.S.; Nayak, J.; Naik, B. Role of Intelligent Computing in COVID-19 Prognosis: A State-of-the-Art Review. *Chaos Solitons Fractals* **2020**, *138*, 109947. [CrossRef]
74. Zhang, Z.; Cheshmehzangi, A.; Ardakani, S.P. A Data-Driven Clustering Analysis for the Impact of COVID-19 on the Electricity Consumption Pattern of Zhejiang Province, China. *Energies* **2021**, *14*, 8187. [CrossRef]
75. Nagaj, R.; Žuromskaitė, B. Tourism in the Era of COVID-19 and Its Impact on the Environment. *Energies* **2021**, *14*, 2000. [CrossRef]
76. Navon, A.; Machlev, R.; Carmon, D.; Onile, A.E.; Belikov, J.; Levron, Y. Effects of the COVID-19 Pandemic on Energy Systems and Electric Power Grids—A Review of the Challenges Ahead. *Energies* **2021**, *14*, 1056. [CrossRef]
77. Polikarpov, I.; Al-Yamani, F.; Petrov, P.; Saburova, M.; Mihalkov, V.; Al-Enezi, A. Phytoplankton Bloom Detection during the COVID-19 Lockdown with Remote Sensing Data: Using Copernicus Sentinel-3 for North-Western Arabian/Persian Gulf Case Study. *Mar. Pollut. Bull.* **2021**, *171*, 112734. [CrossRef]
78. Nayak, J.; Mishra, M.; Naik, B.; Swapnarekha, H.; Cengiz, K.; Shanmuganathan, V. An Impact Study of COVID-19 on Six Different Industries: Automobile, Energy and Power, Agriculture, Education, Travel and Tourism and Consumer Electronics. *Expert Syst.* **2022**, *39*, e12677. [CrossRef] [PubMed]

79. Chretien: Influenza Forecasting in Human Populations: ... —Google Scholar. Available online: https://scholar.google.com/scholar_lookup?title=Influenza%20forecasting%20in%20human%20populations%3A%20a%20scoping%20review&publication_year=2014&author=J.P.%20Chretien&author=D.%20George&author=J.%20Shaman&author=R.A.%20Chitale&author=F.E.%20McKenzie (accessed on 27 December 2021).
80. Collins, A.; Florin, M.-V.; Renn, O. COVID-19 Risk Governance: Drivers, Responses and Lessons to Be Learned. *J. Risk Res.* **2020**, *23*, 1073–1082. [CrossRef]
81. Board: A World at Risk—Google Scholar. Available online: https://scholar.google.com/scholar_lookup?hl=en&publication_year=2019&author=Global+Preparedness+Monitoring+Board&title=A+World+at+Risk%3A+Annual+Report+on+Global+Preparedness+for+Health+Emergencies. (accessed on 19 November 2021).
82. Alharbi, R. A GIS-Based Decision Support System for Reducing Air Ambulance Response Times: A Case Study on Public Schools in Jeddah City. *J. Geogr. Inf. Syst.* **2015**, *07*, 384. [CrossRef]
83. Chopra, V.; Toner, E.; Waldhorn, R.; Washer, L. How Should US Hospitals Prepare for Coronavirus Disease 2019 (COVID-19)? *Ann. Intern. Med.* **2020**, *172*, 621–622. [CrossRef]
84. Swerdlow, D.L.; Finelli, L. Preparation for Possible Sustained Transmission of 2019 Novel Coronavirus: Lessons From Previous Epidemics. *JAMA-J. Am. Med. Assoc.* **2020**, *323*, 1129–1130. [CrossRef]
85. Liu, Q.; Luo, D.; Haase, J.E.; Guo, Q.; Wang, X.Q.; Liu, S.; Xia, L.; Liu, Z.; Yang, J.; Yang, B.X. The Experiences of Health-Care Providers during the COVID-19 Crisis in China: A Qualitative Study. *Lancet Glob. Health* **2020**, *8*, E790–E798. [CrossRef]
86. Malczewski, J. GIS-based Multicriteria Decision Analysis: A Survey of the Literature. *Int. J. Geogr. Inf. Sci.* **2006**, *20*, 703–726. [CrossRef]
87. Malczewski, J.; Jankowski, P. Emerging Trends and Research Frontiers in Spatial Multicriteria Analysis. *Int. J. Geogr. Inf. Sci.* **2020**, *34*, 1257–1282. [CrossRef]
88. Flanagan, B.E.; Hallisey, E.J.; Adams, E.; Lavery, A. Measuring Community Vulnerability to Natural and Anthropogenic Hazards: The Centers for Disease Control and Prevention's Social Vulnerability Index. *J. Environ. Health* **2018**, *80*, 34–36.
89. Saaty, T.L. *The Analytic Hierarchy Process: Planning, Priority Setting, Resource Allocation*; RWS: Chalfont Saint Peter, UK, 1990; ISBN 978-0-9620317-2-4.
90. Corona-Pandemie Führt zu Übersterblichkeit in Deutschland. Available online: https://www.destatis.de/DE/Presse/Pressemitteilungen/2021/12/PD21_563_12.html (accessed on 1 February 2022).
91. RKI-COVID-19-COVID-19. Available online: https://www.rki.de/EN/Content/infections/epidemiology/outbreaks/COVID-19/COVID19.html (accessed on 1 February 2022).
92. OpenStreetMap. Available online: https://www.openstreetmap.org/ (accessed on 1 February 2022).
93. COVID-19-Trends in Deutschland Im Überblick. Available online: https://www.rki.de/DE/Content/InfAZ/N/Neuartiges_Coronavirus/Situationsberichte/COVID-19-Trends/COVID-19-Trends.html?__blob=publicationFile#/home (accessed on 25 November 2021).

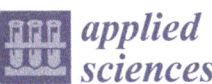

Article

Survey of BERT-Base Models for Scientific Text Classification: COVID-19 Case Study

Mayara Khadhraoui [1,2,*], Hatem Bellaaj [2], Mehdi Ben Ammar [3,4], Habib Hamam [4,5,6,7] and Mohamed Jmaiel [2]

1. National Engineering School of Sfax (ENIS), University of Sfax, Sfax 3038, Tunisia
2. ReDCAD Laboratory, Department of Computer Engineering and Applied Mathematics, University of Sfax, Sfax 3029, Tunisia; hatem.bellaaj@redcad.org (H.B.); mohamed.jmaiel@redcad.org (M.J.)
3. Solutions Galore Inc., Moncton, NB E1C 5Y1, Canada; mehdi.benammar@gmail.com
4. Faculty of Engineering, Université de Moncton, Moncton, NB E1A 3E9, Canada; habib.hamam@umoncton.ca
5. International Institute of Technology and Management, Commune d'Akanda, Libreville BP 1989, Gabon
6. Spectrum of Knowledge Production & Skills Development, Sfax 3027, Tunisia
7. Department of Electrical and Electronic Engineering Science, School of Electrical Engineering, University of Johannesburg, Johannesburg 2006, South Africa
* Correspondence: khadhraouimayara@gmail.com

Abstract: On 30 January 2020, the World Health Organization announced a new coronavirus, which later turned out to be very dangerous. Since that date, COVID-19 has spread to become a pandemic that has now affected practically all regions in the world. Since then, many researchers in medicine have contributed to fighting COVID-19. In this context and given the great growth of scientific publications related to this global pandemic, manual text and data retrieval has become a challenging task. To remedy this challenge, we are proposing CovBERT, a pre-trained language model based on the BERT model to automate the literature review process. CovBERT relies on prior training on a large corpus of scientific publications in the biomedical domain and related to COVID-19 to increase its performance on the literature review task. We evaluate CovBERT on the classification of short text based on our scientific dataset of biomedical articles on COVID-19 entitled COV-Dat-20. We demonstrate statistically significant improvements by using BERT.

Keywords: BERT; COVID-19; scientific text classification; transfer learning; scientific publications; deep learning

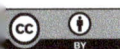

1. Introduction

Since December 2019 and possibly before, the world has faced one of the most serious dangers in its history: the new coronavirus pandemic [1]. By the end of February 2022, the world had recorded an affected population of more than 430 million people and around 6 million deaths [2]. The entire world is on high alert to find a radical solution to this pandemic and to minimize the cases of death.

1.1. Context

We collaborated with epidemiologists to help medical researchers accelerate research on COVID-19. The researchers appreciated having relevant data exposed and classified. Research laboratories in epidemiology constantly need to collect relevant and pertinent data to be able to analyze an epidemic (or pandemic), predict the evolution of contamination in the population in question, determine the shape of the virus, discover its genome sequencing, produce a vaccine, develop a drug, conceive a screening method or implement a medical device dedicated to the epidemic (intensive care, etc.). We are aware of the time and effort put in by medical researchers to develop their epidemiological studies. The manual pre-screening by researchers of all the information available on the web, in specialized datasets and other research, can be overwhelming as well as time and energy consuming. Search engines provide an astronomical amount of information; many are unclassified and irrelevant to the researcher's query. Therefore, we aimed at providing epidemiology researchers with a configurable open-source platform for automatic pertinent data retrieval and classification from scientific abstracts and full papers on COVID-19 by using various search engines, in particular PubMed, Google Scholar, Science Direct, etc. To achieve our goal, we advanced Deep Learning (DL) techniques to classify unclassified biomedical abstracts. In the context of scientific research, DL, part of the large field of artificial intelligence, allows machines to learn and perform decisions in an automatic way. Given the heterogeneity of the data available in the scientific field, the search for information seems to be a difficult task and can generate difficulties for researchers. For our work, we were interested in the literature review component in the field of epidemiological research, which represents a challenging task. Particular attention was given to this major challenge. To overcome it, DL techniques and algorithms were investigated and adapted to our context of text classification related to fighting COVID-19. In this context, we exploited algorithms to facilitate the learning process based on sourced data in order to better manipulate target data. The main approach is called transfer learning, which enables information and knowledge from a past task in order to improve the next task [3,4]. Transfer learning is based on a recent approach called "Universal Embeddings", which is essentially pre-trained embeddings obtained from the training models of DL on a large corpus. In fact, "Universal Embeddings" enables using the pre-trained embeddings in various NLP tasks, including scenarios with constraints such as heterogeneity of unlabeled data.

The aim of this article is twofold:

1. First, to produce an appropriate dataset for training. Our research is oriented to multiclass classification rather than to multilabel classification. When we began our research in January 2020, we could not find any datasets on COVID-19 with short text that is classified according to categories. For this reason, we were required to build a new dataset on COVID-19 by using the PubMed search engine, and it was validated by experts from Community and Preventive Medicine at the Faculty of Medicine, Department of Epidemiology. The validation process took over 6 months. We advance a method to build the required dataset and address our needs.

   The proposed dataset, entitled Cov-Dat-20, contains 4304 papers distributed in an equitable manner according to four categories, namely: COVID-19, Virology, Public Health and Mental Health.

2. Based on the literature, we considered concerns and issues that can now be addressed through natural language processing (NLP) based on different pre-trained language models including Glove [5], ELMo [6], OpenAI GPT model [7] and Bidirectional Encoder Representations from Transformers (abbreviated as BERT) [8]. Compared to the cited models, BERT provides better results for many use cases and without necessarily requiring a large amount of labelled data thanks to a "pre-training" phase without labels, allowing it to acquire a more detailed knowledge of the language. In addition, the BERT model uses a specific manner to handle several limits such as the reduced size of input text and the lack of vocabulary as was our case when we deal with the summary of scientific articles. Bearing in mind the several benefits of BERT, we propose the CovBERT model to help medical research epidemiologists fight against COVID-19. We have released the CovBERT model as a new resource to enhance the performance of NLP tasks in the scientific domain. Our proposed model is a pre-trained language model based on BERT and trained on our large corpus of scientific text, Cov-Dat-20. After training, we fine-tuned the CovBERT model with a specific subject related to COVID-19. Finally, we evaluated the CovBERT model on different numerously studied text classification datasets.

1.2. Traditional ML versus DL Models

Since 2005, the outlook of artificial intelligence has changed dramatically with machine learning (ML) and the emergence of DL, which draws inspiration from neuroscience. In fact, traditional learning, or ML, as part of artificial intelligence is using techniques (such as DL) which allow machines to learn from their experiences in order to improve the way they perform their tasks. In traditional learning, the learning process is based on several steps:

- Feed an algorithm with data;
- Use this data to train a model;
- Test and deploy the model;
- Use the deployed model to perform an automated predictive task.

DL is one of the main ML and artificial intelligence technologies that are based on neural networks. The learning process is qualified as deep because the structure of artificial neural networks consists of several input, output and hidden layers. Each layer contains units that turn the input data into information that the next layer can use for a specific predictive task. Based on this structure, a machine can learn through its own data processing.

The remainder of the paper is organized in four sections in addition to the introduction. The present introduction includes a first subsection illustrating the context of our work. Traditional versus DL models are then discussed in a separate subsection. Section 2 is devoted to presenting related works. In Section 3, we will provide our methodology. Section 4 discusses the presented experimental results. In Section 5, we will have our concluding remarks and include our strategies for future research.

2. Related Works

This section is devoted to past and current research in biomedical text classification [9,10]. Text classification is a fundamental task of natural language processing (NLP), with the aim of assigning a text to one or more categories. The applications of text classification include sentiment analysis [11], question classification [12] and topic classification [13], the latter of which we are interested in for this work. We investigated several proposed approaches related to text-classification tasks based on deep neural networks and pre-trained language models.

Today, deep neural networks have several techniques and models that prove/demonstrate new state-of-the-art results on fully examined text-classification datasets. There are some models, such as convolutional neural networks (CNN) [14], recurrent neural networks (RNN) [15] and artificial neural networks (ANN) [16], as well as some more complex networks such as C-LSTM [17], CNN-LSTM [18] and DRNN [19].

Nevertheless, DL models mention additive advantages over traditional ML models based on the backpropagation algorithm. In fact, related to [20], the backpropagation algorithm is an optimization algorithm that adjusts the parameters of a network of multi-layer neurons to match inputs and outputs referenced in a learning dataset. According to reference [21], the usage of DL for text classification requires entering the text into a deep network to obtain the text representation then entering it into the Softmax() function and obtaining the probability of each category. Yao et al. [22] proposed an improvement of distributed document representations by adding descriptions of medical concepts for the classification task of the clinical files for the benefit of traditional Chinese medicine. The active learning technique [23] was applied in the clinical domain, which exploits untagged corpora to enhance the clinical text-classification process. An ordinary approach is to first map the narrative text to concepts of different knowledge sources such as the Unified Medical Language System (UMLS), then train the classifiers on document representations that include the unique concept identifiers of the UMLS—Concept Unique Identifiers (CUIs)—as functionalities [24]. In [25], the authors are interested in the acute kidney injury (AKI) prediction based on DL models. They used knowledge-guided CNNs to merge word features with UMLS CUI features. They used pre-trained word embeddings and CUI embeddings of clinical notes as the input.

Nevertheless, the neural networks proved their effectiveness until the advent of the transfer learning approach. In 2018, that main approach appeared and proved its effectiveness. It consists of training a complete model to perform a task with many data.

Then, the pre-trained model can be used to complete other tasks, building on previous learning. This is called transfer learning.

By definition, a pre-trained model is a recorded network that has already been trained on a large dataset. Generally, we use them on large-scale text-classification tasks. A pre-trained model is ready to be used as is, or, based on the transfer learning technique, the model can become personalized for a given task. The intuition behind transfer learning for text classification is that if a model is trained on a sufficiently large and general dataset, that model will effectively serve as a generic model. The model is efficient at taking advantage of the data learned without the necessity of starting from scratch by training a large model on a large dataset.

In general, NLP projects rely on pre-trained word embedding on large volumes of unlabeled data by means of algorithms such as word2vec [26] and GloVe [5]. They aim at initializing the first layer of a neural network. Then, the obtained model is trained on specific data for a particular task. That said, many current models for supervised NLP tasks are pre-trained as models in language modeling (which is an unsupervised task) and then fine-tuned (which is a supervised task) with tagged task-specific data. Recent advances in ULMFiT [27], ELMo [6], OpenAI Transformer [28] and BERT [8] present a quintessential shift, in paradigmatic terms, from the simple initialization of the first layer of models to pre-training the entire model with hierarchical representations to improve the natural language processing process, including text classification. All these approaches enable pre-training an unsupervised language model on a large dataset such as Wikipedia and then fine-tuning these pre-trained models on specific tasks.

Instead of associating a static embedding vector with each word, pre-trained models build richer representations that consider the semantic and syntactic context of each word.

Related to [27], ULMFiT (Universal Language Model Fine-Tuning) is a recent generic method used to build efficient text-classification systems, setting a new state of the art on several benchmarks in NLP tasks. The present method has proven its efficiency in terms of not requiring a huge amount of data to train the model.

In addition, ELMo (Embeddings from Language Models) examines the entire sentence before assigning and embedding each word it contains instead of using a fixed embedding for each word [6]. It uses a bidirectional LSTM trained on a particular task to be able to create these embeddings. ELMo can be trained on a massive dataset. ELMo is trained to reveal the next word in each sentence. This is convenient because of the large amount of textual data.

In [7], the authors present the OpenAI GPT, short for Generative Pre-Training Transformer, which is a multi-layered unidirectional transformer decoder. The proposed model was trained on a huge corpus and aims to perform various NLP tasks based on precise adjustments. To start, the transformer language model was trained in an unsupervised manner. The training process is based on a few thousand books from the Google Books corpus. From there, the pre-trained model will be adapted to the supervised target task.

In the same context, recently, the BERT model has achieved state-of-the-art results in a broad range of NLP tasks [8]. It is a variation of transfer learning. The main operating mode of BERT corresponds to a transfer by fine-tuning that is like the one used by ULMFiT. Furthermore, BERT can also be used in the transfer mode by extracting features like ELMo. The BERT model uses transformer architecture, which is a recent and powerful alternative to RNNs to achieve deep bidirectional pre-training. In addition, the use of two new tasks for pre-training, one at the word level and the other at the sentence level, defines the main innovation of BERT.

In our work, we revolve around the classification of scientific text in the biomedical field, and we intersect with the summary of the scientific article. The main challenge encountered is a reduced size of text and the lack of vocabulary. Based on BERT's advantages, the main model is instantiated in different general and specialized domains (biomedical and scientific domains, for example). In fact, BERT's contextualization introduces different advantages related to the performance of the model, the learning time, the learning cost, the quantity of data requested for the learning, the length of the input text, etc. In our context, we looked at BERT-base models in three different fields: multiple domains (the general case), the scientific domain (the scientific articles) and the biomedical domain (the COVID-19 case study) presented in Table 1.

Table 1. A comparative study of pre-trained Bert-base models.

Models	Summary	NLP Tasks	Datasets	Learning Type	Mono/Multi-Class	Accuracy Model/Bert	Domain
BoostingBERT	The model integrates multi-class boosting into the BERT model. The boosting technique is demonstrated to be able to be used to enhance the performance of BERT, instead of other techniques such as bagging or stacking. Based on the experimental results, BoostingBERT outperforms the bagging BERT constantly. Two approaches are compared, making use of the base transformer classifier in the BoostingBERT model: weights privacy vs. weights sharing, and the former one constantly outperforms the latter one.	Multiple NLP tasks	GLUE dataset	Ensemble learning	Multi-class	82.93%/80.72% with CoLa dataset 93.35/92.55 with SST-2 dataset	Multi-domain
EduBERT	The use of pre-trained models has proven a great advance in learning analytics. They apply the BERT approach to the three LAK tasks previously explored on the MOOC forum data: detection of confusion, urgent intervention by teachers and classification of sentimentality. The experimental results have proven an improvement in performance beyond the state of the art.	Sentiment analysis (SA), named entity recognition (NER) and question answering (QA)	Stanford MOOCPosts dataset	Supervised/unsupervised	Not mentioned	89.78%/89.47%	Multi-domain
ALBERT	ALBERT introduces two optimizations to reduce model size: a factorization of the embedding layer and parameter sharing across the hidden layers of the network. The result of combining these two approaches results in a baseline model with only 12M parameters, compared to BERT's 108M, with an accuracy of 80.1% on several NLP benchmarks compared with BERT's 82.3% average.	Question answering	GLUE SQuAD RACE	Supervised/unsupervised	Not mentioned	88.7%/85.2%	Multi-domain
FinBERT	FinBERT is a language model based on BERT for financial NLP tasks. FinBERT is evaluated on two financial sentiment analysis datasets. The authors achieve the state of the art on FiQA sentiment scoring and Financial PhraseBank. They implement two other pre-trained language models, ULMFit and ELMo, for financial sentiment analysis to compare with FinBERT. Experiments are conducted to investigate the effects of further pre-training on the financial corpus, training strategies to prevent catastrophic forgetting and fine-tuning only a small subset of model layers for decreasing training time without a significant drop in performance.	Sentiment analysis and text classification	Financial sentiment analysis datasets	Supervised/unsupervised	Not Mentioned	86%	Scientific domain
SciBERT	The authors release SCIBERT, a pre-trained language model based on BERT to address the scientific data. SCIBERT leverages unsupervised pre-training on a large multi-domain corpus of scientific publications to improve performance on downstream scientific NLP tasks. SCIBERT largely outperforms BERT and previous state-of-the-art models in a variety of biomedical text-mining tasks including sequence tagging, sentence classification and dependency parsing, with datasets from a variety of scientific domains. SCIBERT makes improvements over BERT.	Named entity recognition (NER), PICO extraction (PICO), text classification (CLS), relation classification (REL), dependency parsing (DEP)	Corpus of scientific text	Supervised/unsupervised	Not mentioned	99.01%/88.85%	Scientific domain

Table 1. Cont.

Models	Summary	NLP Tasks	Datasets	Learning Type	Mono/Multi-Class	Accuracy Model/Bert	Domain
KnowBert	KnowBert represents a general method to embed multiple knowledge bases (KBs) into large-scale models. The proposed model aims to enhance scientific data representations with structured, human-curated knowledge. For each KB, the retrieval of the relevant entity is based on an integrated entity linker; then, the contextual word representations are updated via a form of word-to-entity attention. After integrating WordNet and a subset of Wikipedia into BERT, KnowBert demonstrates improved perplexity, ability to recall facts as measured in a probing task and downstream performance on relationship extraction, entity typing and word sense disambiguation. KnowBert's runtime is comparable to BERT's, and it scales to large KBs.	Relation extraction, entity typing, word sense disambiguation	Wikipedia	Supervised/unsupervised	Not mentioned	89.01%/89%	Scientific domain
ClinicalBert	The authors are exploring and releasing BERT models for clinical text: one for generic clinical text and another for discharge summaries specifically. The main approach demonstrates that using a domain-specific model enhances performance improvements on three common clinical NLP tasks compared with nonspecific embeddings. These domain-specific models are not as performant on two clinical de-identification tasks, and the authors argue that this is a natural consequence of the differences between de-identified source text and synthetically non-de-identified task text.	Readmission prediction, diagnosis predictions, mortality risk estimation	MIMIC-III dataset	Supervised/unsupervised	Not mentioned	80.8%/77.6%	Biomedical domain
BlueBERT	The proposed approach is a BERT-base model pre-trained on PubMed abstracts and MIMIC-III clinical notes. Based on the BERT model, BlueBERT is specialized by an extra linear layer on top of the existing model to transform the output into 10 classes, one for each ICD-9 code. The authors implemented the BCEWithLogits loss for multi-class classification. Related to the BERT model's architecture, BlueBERT introduces three small architectural variations: (1) adding three linear layers with ReLU non-linearity instead of just one linear layer, (2) freezing the BlueBERT weights from the first variant so that only the linear layer weights would be tuned and (3) adding a dropout layer after the BERT layer from the second variant.	Text classification	PubMed abstracts and MIMIC-III datasets	Supervised/unsupervised	Multi-class	89.2%/86.9%	Biomedical domain
BioBERT	The BioBERT (Bidirectional Encoder Representations from Transformers for Biomedical Text Mining) model is a domain-specific language representation model pre-trained on large-scale biomedical corpora. Based on experimental results, BioBERT largely outperforms BERT and previous state-of-the-art models in a variety of biomedical text-mining tasks when pre-trained on biomedical corpora. BioBERT outperforms on the following three representative biomedical text-mining tasks: biomedical named entity recognition, biomedical relation extraction and biomedical question answering. The analysis results show that pre-training BERT on biomedical corpora helps it to understand complex biomedical texts.	NER Biomedical relation extraction Bio question answering	PubMed abstracts/4,5B PMC full papers/13,5B	Supervised/unsupervised	Not mentioned	89.04%/88.30%	Biomedical Domain

3. Methodology

We are interested in offering relevant information when searching available media (search engines, datasets). In this context, text classification [29–31], defined as the process of associating a category with a text of various length based on the information it contains, is an important element of information-retrieval systems. We face text-classification challenges and accuracy issues. For each new entry, the main challenge consists of determining the category to which this entry belongs. The text annotation process is time-consuming and is generally performed manually because of the language complexity. Therefore, the automation of this process has become a priority for the scientific community to be efficient. For our work, we aim to collaborate with epidemiologists to help medical research fight COVID-19. Our main goal is to not only classify scientific texts but to predict unseen data based on the pre-trained model.

3.1. COV-Dat-20 Dataset Creation

We propose a dataset containing data on COVID-19 extracted from summaries of PubMed. It is made up of 4304 articles distributed in an equitable manner according to four categories, namely: COVID-19, Virology, Public Health and Mental Health.

For the methodology, amongst the articles that were proposed by PubMed, some could have been classified under more than one category. For our work, our research is oriented to the multiclass classification type rather than to multilabel classification. In this case, our experts in the Department of Epidemiology recommended that we classify the articles based on the highest percentage proposed by PubMed.

The Cov-Dat-20 dataset is elaborated based on advanced SQL queries from PubMed. For example, we present an advanced SQL query in PubMed: ((("public health" [MeSH Major Topic]) OR "preventive medicine" [MeSH Major Topic])) AND "COVID-19" [Supplementary Concept]; (health knowledge, attitudes, practice [MeSH Terms]) AND COVID-19 [Supplementary Concept]; (((COVID-19 [Title/Abstract]) OR COVID-19 [Supplementary Concept])) AND (((epidemiological assessment [Title/Abstract]) OR public health interventions [Title/Abstract]) OR epidemiology [Title/Abstract]).

Figure 1 presents the scientific paper distribution in the dataset according to the categories mentioned above.

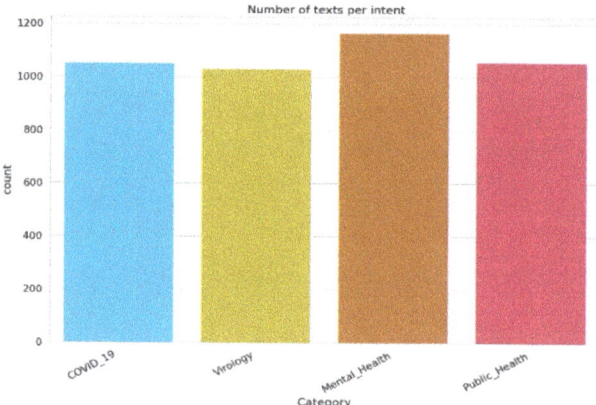

Figure 1. Data repartition in the Cov-Dat-20 dataset.

For more details, 4304 rows and 3 columns, 1,013,901 words, 43,123 unique words and 4304 sentences characterize the Cov-Dat-20 dataset.

Table 2 presents the label encoding related to our dataset. In our work, we were interested in the multi-class concept in the classification process. For each category, we offer a selective and detailed list of keywords.

Table 2. Label encoding.

Category	Description
COVID-19	It is interested in scientific papers of probable treatment and the different symptoms related to COVID-19.
Virology	It deals with scientific papers about the study of viruses, genome sequencing, etc.
Public Health	It focuses on scientific papers about the study, prevention, control, in particular through vaccination, and epidemiological data against COVID-19.
Mental Health	It spotlights several scientific papers about the impact of COVID-19 on mental health.

- COVID-19: focus on the (1) COVID-19 treatment and (2) COVID-19 symptoms: (1) treatment, chloroquine, hydroxychloroquine, interferon beta-1a, remdesivir, lopinavir/ritonavir; (2) fever, headache, cough, chills, shortness of breath or difficulty breathing, muscle pain, repeated shaking with chills, new loss of taste or smell;
- Virology: genome sequencing, phylogenetic analysis, SARS-CoV-2, MERS-CoV, nomenclature, virus composition, virus layers;
- Public Health: COVID-19, interventions, awareness, behavior, behavioral change, coronavirus, pandemic, public health protection, public health measures;
- Mental Health: COVID-19, mental health disorders, SARS-CoV-2, neural taxonomies, personalized medicine, precision psychiatry, social connection, mental health, psychiatry.

The Cov-Dat-20 is available on https://www.kaggle.com/mayarakh/Cov-Dat-20 accessed on 6 March 2022.

3.2. Data Pre-Processing

Raw data needs to be transformed into an understandable format. To do this, we opted for applying data pre-processing techniques to build a DL classifier. In fact, data pre-processing techniques eliminate characteristics of less important data and improve accuracy.

For our case, we used a common preprocessing approach that can integrate with various NLP (natural language processing) tasks using NLTK (Natural Language Toolkit) [32]. Before tackling the learning process, the text in the dataset goes through some stages, namely, the elimination of punctuation, putting all the text in lower case, tokenization, cleaning and lemmatization.

- Lowercasing is a widespread approach to reduce all the text to lower case for simplicity.
- Tokenization: text pre-processing step, which involves splitting the text into tokens (words, sentences, etc.)
- Cleaning is a form of pre-processing to filter out useless data such as punctuation removal and stop-word removal (a stop word is a commonly used word in text and stop-word removal is a form pre-processing to filter out useless data).
- Lemmatization is an alternative approach to stemming for removing inflection.

At the end of this step, data are ready to move to the step of decomposing the dataset into a part for "Learning" and a part reserved for the "Test" phase. We chose to carry out this decomposition by reserving 80% for the training set and 20% for testing.

3.3. Exploration of the BERT Model

As mentioned before, we focused on the scientific-text-classification task. In the same context, Google's BERT [8], having received deep bidirectional training using the transformer, gave state-of-the-art results for many NLP tasks, more precisely, in the text-classification task. In addition, our decision to explore the BERT model is justified by its several advantages compared to similar models. BERT aims at improving the understanding of users' requests in order to provide more relevant results, especially for requests formulated in a natural way.

3.3.1. BERT-Base Characteristics

BERT is a neural network that can treat a wide variety of NLP (natural language processing) tasks [8]. To do so, the learning phase is broken down into two phases. First, we proceed with the pre-training phase, which is very time and computation consuming. Once this phase is performed, a network is created that has a certain general understanding of the language. Then, the second phase is called the adjustment phase, which trains the network on a specific task. Moreover, BERT uses a part of the transformer network architecture. The advantage of this architecture is that it treats the relationships between distant words better than recurrent networks (LSTM/GRU) [33]. On the other hand, the network cannot process sequences of any length but has a finite input dimension to learn in a reasonable time. At the scale of this work, we use the basic model of BERT-base with fixed characteristics: 12-layer, 768-hidden, 12-heads, 110 M parameters.

3.3.2. BERT-Base Operation

The Bert model is a bidirectional model. Unlike its predecessors, which were unidirectional and so read the text in a particular direction (e.g., left to right), the main model of BERT goes through the entire text in both directions simultaneously, which presents the property of "bidirectionality". Technically speaking, BERT consists of multiple layers forming a "Transformer", which learns contextual relationships between the different words composing the text. The transformers aim at analyzing the words of a complex query to relate them in order to comprehend the semantics of the sentence and to better understand its overall meaning. TPU Clouds are integrated circuits that accelerate the workload of transformers to make them faster and more efficient.

The BERT architecture in our proposal is illustrated in Figure 2. We took the case of the category Virology and an input text composed of two sentences: "The COVID-19 genome is decrypted. The virus composition is ...". The algorithm will go in both directions, from sentence 1 to sentence 2 until the end of the text (Abstract, full article, ...) but also from sentence 2 to sentence 1 until the beginning of the text as depicted in Figure 2.

The core of the architecture is mainly decomposed into two components. It uses an encoder to read the input text and thus generates a vector representation of the words. In addition, BERT uses a specific decoder to perform the expected prediction task.

BERT-base offers a vocabulary of 30,522 words. The vocabulary is built in a way that is based on the tokenization process. Indeed, the main process consists in dividing the input text into a list of words, called tokens, that are available in the constructed vocabulary. To process words that are out-vocabulary, BERT-base uses a technique, called BPE-based WordPiece tokenization. Regarding non-vocabulary words, this approach proposes to divide them into sub-words. Each word is then represented by a group of sub-words. For each sub-word, BERT-base provides contextual representations. Therefore, the context of the word is merely the combination of the sub-words' contexts. In this work, we adopted the BERT idea to epidemiology by optimizing the word keys and subkeys.

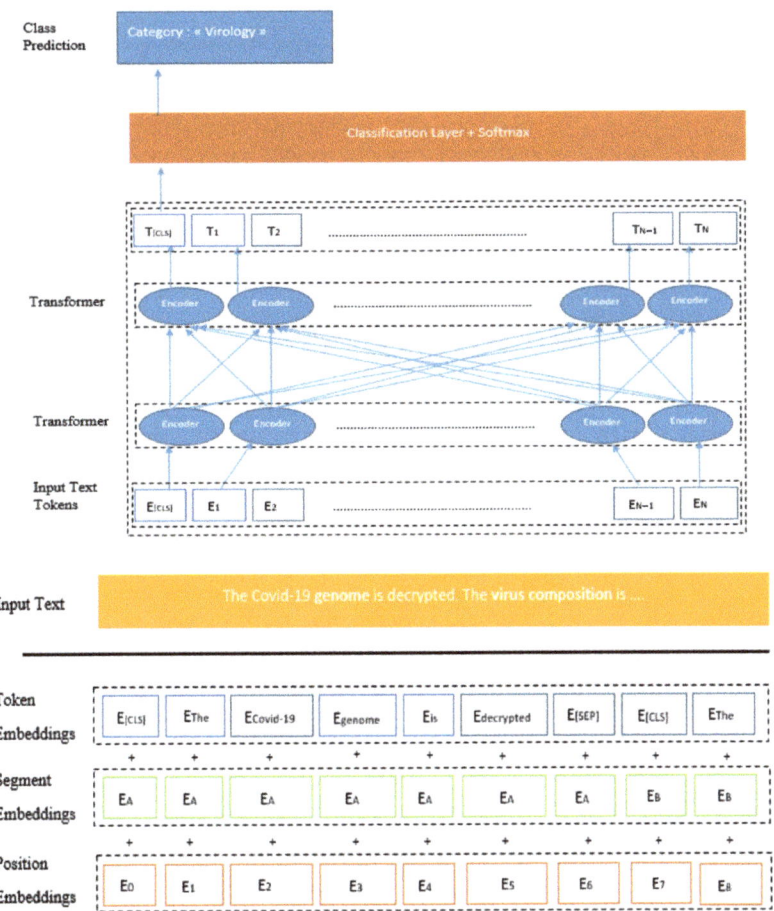

Figure 2. BERT-base fine-tuning model architecture: COVID-19 case study.

3.3.3. Contextual Embeddings in Biomedical and Scientific Domains

Considering the literature, the word-embedding technique shows its effectiveness in traditional word-level vector representations [25] GloVe [5] and fastText [34]. However, this technique faces some limitations by expressing all possible meanings of a word as a single vector representation. In addition, it cannot disambiguate the word senses based on the surrounding context. To overcome these limitations, ELMo and BERT present efficient solutions by providing contextualized word representations. For example, ELMo creates a context-sensitive embedding for each word in each sentence by pre-training it on a large text corpus as a language model. Compared to ELMo, BERT goes deeper and involves much more parameters for contextualized word representations. It can be fine-tuned to accomplish a specific task in several domains such as the biomedical domain. In this context, we present BioBERT and ClinicalBERT models. In [35], BioBERT is a BERT-base model finetuned over a corpus of biomedical research articles from PubMed. BioBERT focused on several NLP tasks presented in Table 2. In the same context, we present the ClinicalBERT model [36]. The main model is based on BERT and then pre-trained on clinical notes from the MIMICIII dataset. In addition, several works utilize the BERT-base model and then perform fine-tuning in scientific domains, such as SciBERT [37]. SciBERT is concerned with named entity recognition, relation extraction and text classification as pointed out in Table 2. Furthermore, we used the BERT model pre-trained in the English language to classify scientific papers from PubMed, and we aim to fine-tune it in the field of COVID-19 for biomedical- and scientific-text-classification tasks.

In Table 3, we produce a comparative study of BERT and its variants in terms of NLP tasks. The dataset and the main size, the special domain, the several hyper parameters, the length period and the different methods used are presented in Table 3.

Table 3. Comparative study of BERT variations.

Model	NLP Tasks	Dataset /Size	Characteristics	Hyperparameters	Learning Period	Methods
BioBERT [35]	NER Biomedical relation extraction Bio question answering	PubMed Abstracts/4,5B PMC Full Papers/13,5B	Biomedical domain	Sentence length: 128–512 tokens	23 days 8 NVIDIA V100 (32GB) GPUs	Word piece tokenization Pre-training BERT on biomedical corpora: Naver Smart ML Fine-tuning BioBERT
ClinicalBERT [36]	Readmission prediction Diagnosis predictions Mortality risk estimation	MIMIC-III	Clinical domain	Sequence length: 128–512 tokens	Amazon Web Services using a single K80 GPU	Subword embeddings Self-attention mechanism
SciBERT [37]	NER Text classification Relation classification Dependency parsing	Semantic Scolar/1.14M	Scientific domain	Sentence length: 128–512 tokens	5 days + 2 days TPU v3 with 8 cores	Finetuning BERT: Frozen BERT embeddings Contextualize word embeddings
KnowBERT [38]	Relation extraction Entity typing Word sense disambiguation	Wikipedia	Knowledge domain	-	-	Mention-span representations Retrieval of relevant entity embeddings Recontextualization of entity span embeddings

3.3.4. Self-Attention Mechanism

This section is devoted to detailing the self-attention mechanism. In fact, the functioning of our cerebral cortex freely inspires the attention mechanism. For example, when analyzing an image to describe it, our attention is instinctively focused on a few areas containing important information without looking at every part of the image equally. This mechanism, therefore, resembles a means of saving processing resources in the face of complex data for analysis. Similarly, when an interpreter translates a text from a source language into a target language, it focuses, based on several experiences, on which words in a source sentence are associated with a certain term in the translated sentence. This attention mechanism is now an integral part of most modern semantic analysis solutions [39]. The attention mechanism is formulated as follows:

$$\text{Attention}(Q, K, V) = \text{softmax}\left(\frac{QK^T}{\sqrt{d_k}}\right)V \tag{1}$$

where the parameters Q, K and V stand for three vectors, which are query, key and value, generated through input embedding, and d_k designates the size of key vectors. K^T stands for transposed vector of K. For example, let us consider that we have four queries, which means:

$$Q = \begin{bmatrix} q_1 \\ q_2 \\ q_3 \\ q_4 \end{bmatrix}, \text{ and three keys } (d_k = 3), \text{ that is} = \begin{bmatrix} k_1 \\ k_2 \\ k_3 \end{bmatrix}, \text{ then}$$

$$\frac{QK^T}{\sqrt{d_k}} = \begin{bmatrix} q_1 \\ q_2 \\ q_3 \\ q_4 \end{bmatrix} \cdot \begin{bmatrix} k_1 & k_2 & k_3 \end{bmatrix} = \frac{1}{\sqrt{d_k}} \begin{bmatrix} q_1 \cdot k_1 & q_1 \cdot k_2 & q_1 \cdot k_3 \\ q_2 \cdot k_1 & q_2 \cdot k_2 & q_2 \cdot k_3 \\ q_3 \cdot k_1 & q_3 \cdot k_2 & q_3 \cdot k_3 \\ q_4 \cdot k_1 & q_4 \cdot k_2 & q_4 \cdot k_3 \end{bmatrix} \quad (2)$$

where, for example, $q_3 \cdot k_2$ means the second key, k_2, applied on the third query, q_3. Then, the maximum of the matrix is calculated according to the function Softmax(), also called soft argmax or normalized exponential function.

4. Pre-Training BERT-Base on COV-Dat-20

To demonstrate the pertinence of Cov-Dat-20 for language model pre-training, we trained BERT-base on 4304 abstracts on several topics such as COVID-19 treatment, COVID-19 symptoms, virology, public health and mental health. Therefore, CovBERT is a BERT-base model trained on multiple domains of scientific abstracts. In fact, we chose to focus on abstracts only from the complete scientific papers. Our choice is justified by a comparative study [40] between the experimental results of a scientific-text-classification approach based on (1) the full article and (2) the abstract only. Based on the experimental results, we observed that the abstract classification approach is more efficient than the full article approach in terms of learning time, the model size and complexity.

Furthermore, the tokenization step is essential in the BERT fine-tuning phase. To feed our text into BERT, we divided it into tokens, and then these tokens were mapped to their index in the tokenizer vocabulary. Related to BERT-base model, the maximum sentence length is 512 tokens. Applying pre-trained BERT requires us to use the tokenizer provided by the model. In fact, the BERT-base generates a specific vocabulary of a fixed size. Added to that, BERT's tokenizer uses a specific manner to handle out-of-vocabulary words.

4.1. Importing Libraires

In order to adjust the BERT-base model to our needs, we imported several necessary libraries related to the text-classification task, such as tensorflow, pandas, numpy, transformers, etc.

4.2. Needed Parameters for Training

In order to obtain a high performance of our model, we followed the pre-training hyper-parameters used in BERT [8]. For fine-tuning, most hyper-parameters are the same as pre-training, except for batch size, learning rate and number of training epochs.

- Max Length: 64;
- Batch size: 32;
- Learning rate (Adam): 2e-5;
- Number of epochs: 4;
- Seed val.: 42.

4.3. Model Characteristics

In order to be suitable to our classification task, we modified the pre-trained BERT model and we trained it on our dataset. The CovBERT model has several layers and output types designed to accommodate our specific NLP task.

4.4. Evaluation Metrics

In the main subsection, we present several indicators measuring the quality of the model. To measure the performance of this classifier, we introduce four types of elements classified for the desired class, namely, TP, FP, TN and FN:

- TP: the positive class correctly predicted by the models;
- FP: the positive class incorrectly predicted by the models;
- TN: the false class correctly predicted by the models;
- FN: the false class incorrectly predicted by the models.

In what follows, we present the evaluation metrics adopted to measure the performance of the different DL models used. Indeed, our assessment is based on four different measures, including: *Accuracy, Precision, Recall, F1-Score*. The evaluation metrics are defined as follows:

$$Accuracy = \frac{TP + TN}{TP + TN + FP + FN} \quad (3)$$

$$Precision = \frac{TP}{TP + FP} \quad (4)$$

$$Recall = \frac{TP}{TP + FN} \quad (5)$$

$$F1Score = 2 * \frac{Precision * Recall}{Precision + Recall} \quad (6)$$

We tackled the text-classification task based on the BERT-base model after exploring DL and experimenting with its limitations. Let us begin by describing our experiments. We started with the automatic collection of scientific papers related to COVID-19 from PubMed. We then created our dataset made up of 4304 scientific papers distributed in an equitable way on four different categories: COVID-19, Virology, Public Health and Mental Health. In order to validate the data classification process in our dataset, we contacted epidemiologists to carry out this task. Based on the manual verification, we concluded that some papers were misclassified. Based on our previous experiments and considering some related works, we opted for performing the scientific paper classification with the PubMed engine. We converged towards a DL solution to tackle the pandemic of COVID-19. We named our model CovBERT.

To adapt the existing pre-trained BERT model to our needs, we applied some modifications, and we trained it on our dataset Cov-Dat-20. We then explored the modified BERT-base model with the graphics processing unit (GPU) to obtain a better performance in terms of learning cost. In addition, we fixed the training hyper-parameters such as the max. length, the batch size, the learning rate, the epoch's number, and the seed val. We monitored the validation loss and kept the best model on the validation set.

Figure 3 presents the CovBERT accuracy with four epochs. We notice, with CovBERT, an accuracy of 94% at epoch four. Beyond four epochs, we risk falling into overfitting.

```
begin training using onecycle policy with max lr of 2e-05...
Epoch 1/4
373/373 [==============================] - 143s 382ms/step - loss: 0.7852 - accuracy: 0.6732
Epoch 2/4
373/373 [==============================] - 142s 380ms/step - loss: 0.3422 - accuracy: 0.8644
Epoch 3/4
373/373 [==============================] - 142s 381ms/step - loss: 0.2780 - accuracy: 0.8912
Epoch 4/4
373/373 [==============================] - 142s 380ms/step - loss: 0.1630 - accuracy: 0.9418
<tensorflow.python.keras.callbacks.History at 0x7feb0a3c4748>
```

Figure 3. CovBERT model accuracy.

The related confusion matrix of the proposed model is presented in Figure 4. We noticed that the high precision was maintained for the Public Health category with 94%. It was also maintained for the Mental Health and the Virology categories with 79% being the least precision value.

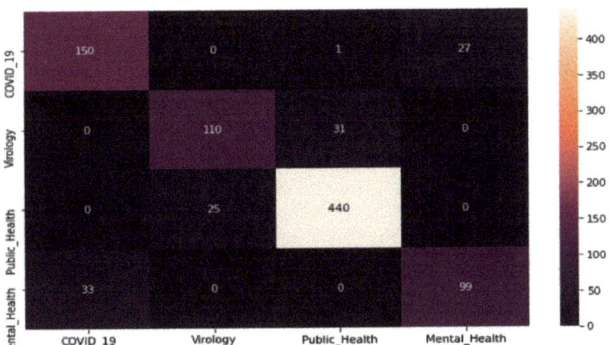

Figure 4. Model confusion matrix of our proposed CovBERT model.

The error related to the training set (training loss) of the proposed dataset is shown in Figure 5. The training loss value starts with 0.8. Then, it gradually falls until 0.2 in the third epoch. Figure 6 shows the accuracy evolution over time. We noticed that the accuracy increases over time from 84% in epoch 1 to 94% in epoch 4. We concluded that, from one epoch to another, the model acquired more knowledge and proved its effectiveness.

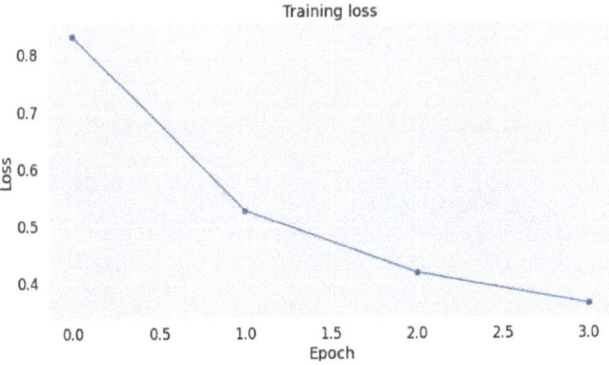

Figure 5. Training loss of our proposed CovBERT model.

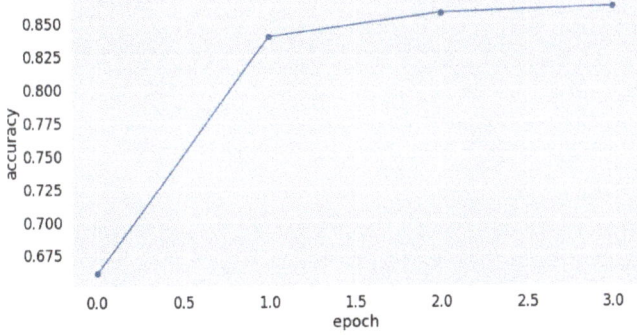

Figure 6. CovBERT model accuracy evolution over time with 4 epochs.

In summary, we proved the high performance of the modified BERT model. We noticed that this training model is better suited for the specific NLP task compared to other DL training models such as CNN and BiLSTM. Among the advantages of the modified BERT model, we noticed that it is easy to implement. The pre-trained modified BERT model weights already encode a large quantity of information on the English language. The fine-tuning step is based on a much smaller dataset for a specific task. Furthermore, we noticed that using the modified BERT model is more efficient in terms of cost and learning time, as well as in terms of model complexity and size.

5. Discussion

In this section, we present, in Table 4, BERT's variants, the relative domains and natural language processing (NLP) tasks. Then, we discuss the main results of our comparative study. Indeed, we used Huggingface's models in our approach resumed in Table 5.

Table 4. BERT's variants, relative domain and NLP tasks.

Models	Domain	NLP Tasks
roberta-base	Multi-Domain	1. Named Entity Recognition 2. Sequence Classification 3. Question Answering
albert-base-v1	Multi-Domain	1. Sequence Classification 2. Question Answering
allenai/scibert_scivocab_uncased	Scientific Domain	1. Named Entity Recognition (NER) 2. PICO Extraction 3. Text Classification 4. Relation Classification (REL) 5. Dependency Parsing (DEP)
allenai/scibert_scivocab_cased	Scientific Domain	1. Named Entity Recognition (NER) 2. PICO Extraction 3. Text Classification 4. Relation Classification (REL) 5. Dependency Parsing (DEP)
emilyalsentzer/Bio_ClinicalBERT	Biomedical Domain	1 Biomedical Named Entity Recognition 2. Biomedical Relation Extraction 3. Biomedical Question Answering
dmis-lab/biobert-base-cased-v1.1	Biomedical Domain	1. Biomedical Named Entity Recognition 2. Biomedical Relation Extraction 3. Biomedical Question Answering
monologg/biobert_v1.1_pubmed	Biomedical Domain	1. Biomedical Named Entity Recognition 2. Biomedical Relation Extraction 3. Biomedical Question Answering
dmis-lab/biobert-v1.1	Biomedical Domain	1. Biomedical Named Entity Recognition 2. Biomedical Relation Extraction 3. Biomedical Question Answering
gsarti/biobert-nli	Biomedical Domain	1. Biomedical Named Entity Recognition 2. Biomedical Relation Extraction 3. Biomedical Question Answering
CovBERT	Biomedical and Scientific Domains	1. Text Classification

Table 5. Comparative study of BERT, its variants and our proposed CovBERT model.

Models	Accuracy	Average Loss	Recall	Precision	F1 Metric
roberta-base	83%	29%	51%	68%	57%
albert-base-v1	84%	39%	41%	56%	47%
allenai/scibert_scivocab_uncased	84%	33%	70%	71%	69%
allenai/scibert_scivocab_cased	84%	30%	74%	74%	73%
emilyalsentzer/Bio_ClinicalBERT	87%	25%	83%	82%	82%
dmis-lab/biobert-base-cased-v1.1	87%	14%	68%	68%	66%
monologg/biobert_v1.1_pubmed	87%	17%	77%	79%	76%
dmis-lab/biobert-v1.1	88%	19%	68%	68%	66%
gsarti/biobert-nli	89%	19%	66%	71%	65%
CovBERT	**94%**	**18%**	**88%**	**86%**	**86%**

Based on the Tables 4 and 5, we conclude that BERT-base models that are instantiated in the biomedical domain perform better in terms of accuracy than models that are instantiated in other domains.

Table 5 presents a comparative study of the initial BERT [8] and its variants such as SciBERT [37], BioBERT [35] and CovBERT. We noticed that the BERT model has proven its effectiveness in 11 NLP tasks. The BERT model is fine-tuned in several domains such as the scientific domain, SciBERT, for five NLP tasks, namely, NER, PICO extraction, text classification, relation classification and dependency parsing. In addition, BioBERT is another BERT variant for the biomedical domain. BioBERT focuses on the recognition of biomedical named entities, on biomedical relation extraction, as well as on biomedical question answering. Furthermore, we presented our proposed model, titled CovBERT, trained on PubMed abstracts in the scientific and biomedical domains.

Based on the comparative study, we concluded that BERT-base multi-domain models, such as ALBERT and Roberta, are less relevant than domain-specific models, with 84% and 83% accuracy, respectively. In addition, models pre-trained on biomedical domains are more accurate than models in the scientific domain with 89% accuracy. In addition, models in the biomedical field (specific field) are more relevant than pre-trained models in scientific domain (several fields). From there comes the effectiveness of our model, which concentrates the biomedical and scientific fields. We were able to show an accuracy improvement in the text-classification NLP task from 84% (SciBERT) in the scientific domain to 94% in the biomedical and scientific domains (CovBERT).

6. Conclusions

In this context of COVID-19, we advanced a new BERT-base pre-training model, referred to as CovBERT. The BERT model largely outperforms previous state-of-the-art models in a variety of NLP tasks. Furthermore, our choice is justified by the effectiveness of BERT to handle a lack of vocabulary, considering that, in our context, we deal with short texts (the summary of scientific articles). To assess the performance of our proposed model, we created a novel dataset, Cov-Dat-20, in the context of COVID-19, which contains several scientific papers collected from PubMed and classified into different categories according to COVID-19. Based on our experience, the CovBERT model outperforms the BERT-base model on text-classification tasks. The main approach is promising and presents an efficient increase based on the accuracy, precision, recall and F1 metrics. In future work, we intend to extend this study by enriching our dataset and developing our model in order to improve classification and prediction performance and to compare the new results to the present ones. Based on our promising results, we are inspired and aim to adapt our techniques to other subjects.

Author Contributions: Conceptualization: M.K. and M.B.A.; methodology, M.K., M.B.A., H.H., H.B. and M.J.; writing—original draft preparation, M.K.; writing—review and editing, M.K., M.B.A., H.H.,

H.B. and M.J.; supervision, M.J. and H.B. All authors have read and agreed to the published version of the manuscript.

Funding: This research received no external funding.

Institutional Review Board Statement: Not applicable.

Informed Consent Statement: Not applicable.

Data Availability Statement: Not applicable.

Acknowledgments: The authors would like to thank Jihene Maatoug and Sihem Ben Fradj, members of the Epidemiology Department of CHU Farhat Hached, in Sousse, for their valuable cooperation and revision of our dataset. The authors also thank the Natural Sciences and Engineering Research Council of Canada (NSERC) and New Brunswick Innovation Foundation (NBIF) for their financial support of the global project. These granting agencies did not contribute to the design of the study or the collection, analysis and interpretation of the data.

Conflicts of Interest: The authors declare no conflict of interest.

References

1. Zu, Z.; Jiang, M.; Xu, P.; Chen, W.; Ni, Q.; Lu, G.; Zhang, L. Coronavirus disease 2019 (COVID-19): A perspective from china. *Radiology* **2020**, *296*, E15–E25. [CrossRef] [PubMed]
2. Worldometers for COVID-19. Available online: https://www.worldometers.info/ (accessed on 30 January 2020).
3. Pan, S.; Yang, Q. A survey on transfer learning. Knowledge and Data Engineering. *IEEE Trans.* **2010**, 1345–1359.
4. Yousaf, A.; Asif, R.M.; Shakir, M.; Rehman, A.U.; Alassery, F.; Hamam, H.; Cheikhrouhou, O. A Novel Machine Learning-Based Price Forecasting for Energy Management Systems. *Sustainability* **2021**, *13*, 12693. [CrossRef]
5. Pennington, J.; Socher, R.; Manning, C. Glove: Global vectors for word representation. In Proceedings of the Empiricial Methods in Natural Language Processing (EMNLP), Doha, Qatar, 25–29 October 2014; Volume 12, pp. 1532–1543.
6. Peters, M.; Neumann, M.; Iyyer, M.; Gardner, M.; Clark, C.; Lee, K.; Zettlemoyer, L. Deep contextualized word representations. In Proceedings of the 2018 Conference of the North American Chapter of the Association for Computational Linguistics: Human Language Technologies, New Orleans, LA, USA, 1–6 June 2018; pp. 2227–2237.
7. Alt, C.; Hübner, M.; Hennig, L. Fine-tuning pre-trained transformer language models to distantly supervised relation extraction. In Proceedings of the 57th Annual Meeting of the Association for Computational Linguistics, Florence, Italy, 28 July–2 August 2019; pp. 1388–1398. [CrossRef]
8. Devlin, J.; Chang, M.W.; Lee, K.; Toutanova, K. Bert: Pre-training of deep bidirectional transformers for language understanding. In Proceedings of the 2019 Conference of the North American Chapter of the Association for Computational Linguistics: Human Language Technologies, Minneapolis, MN, USA, 2–7 June 2019; pp. 4171–4186.
9. Mirónczuk, M.; Protasiewicz, J. A recent overview of the state-of-the-art elements of text classification. *Expert Syst. Appl.* **2018**, *106*, 36–54. [CrossRef]
10. Holzinger, A.; Kieseberg, P.; Weippl, E.; Tjoa, A.M. Current Advances, Trends and Challenges of Machine Learning and Knowledge Extraction: From Machine Learning to Explainable AI. In Proceedings of the International Cross-Domain Conference CD-MAKE 2018, Hamburg, Germany, 27–30 August 2018; pp. 1–8.
11. Maas, A.; Daly, R.; Pham, P.; Huang, D.; Ng, A.; Potts, C. Learning word vectors for sentiment analysis. In Proceedings of the 49th Annual Meeting of the Association for Computational Linguistics: Human Language Technologies, Portland, OR, USA, 19–24 June 2011; pp. 142–150. [CrossRef]
12. Zhang, D. Question classification using support vector machines. In Proceedings of the 26th Annual International ACM SIGIR Conference on Research and Development in Information Retrieval, Toronto, ON, Canada, 28 July–1 August 2003; pp. 26–32. [CrossRef]
13. Wang, S.; Manning, C. Baselines and bigrams: Simple, good sentiment and topic classification. In Proceedings of the 50th Annual Meeting of the Association for Computational Linguistics: Short Papers, Jeju Island, Korea, 8–14 July 2012; Association for Computational Linguistics: Stroudsburg, PA, USA, 2012; pp. 90–94. [CrossRef]
14. Wang, X.; Yin, S.; Shafiq, M.; Laghari, A.A.; Karim, S.; Cheikhrouhou, O.; Alhakami, W.; Hamam, H. A New V-Net Convolutional Neural Network Based on Four-Dimensional Hyperchaotic System for Medical Image Encryption. *Secur. Commun. Netw.* **2022**, *2022*, 4260804. [CrossRef]
15. Chung, J.; Gulcehre, C.; Cho, K.; Bengio, Y. Empirical evaluation of gated recurrent neural networks on sequence modelling. IPS 2014 Workshop on Deep Learning. *arXiv* **2014**, arXiv:1412.3555.
16. Al-Shayea, Q. Artificial neural networks in medical diagnosis. *J. Appl. Biomed.* **2013**, *11*, 150–154. [CrossRef]
17. Shi, M.; Wang, K.; Li, C. A C-LSTM with Word Embedding Model for News Text Classification. In Proceedings of the IEEE/ACIS 18th International Conference on Computer and Information Science (ICIS), Beijing, China, 17–19 June 2019; pp. 253–257.
18. Xiao, Y.; Cho, K. Efficient character-level document classification by combining convolution and recurrent layers. *arXiv* **2016**, arXiv:1602.00367.

19. Wang, B. Disconnected recurrent neural networks for text categorization. In Proceedings of the 56th Annual Meeting of the Association for Computational Linguistics, Melbourne, Australia, 15–20 July 2018; pp. 2311–2320. [CrossRef]
20. Wang, X.; Lu, H.; Wei, X.; Wei, G.; Behbahani, S.S.; Iseley, T.T. Application of artificial neural network in tunnel engineering: A systematic review. *IEEE Access* **2020**, *8*, 119527–119543. [CrossRef]
21. Zheng, S.; Yang, M. A New Method of Improving BERT for Text Classification. In Proceedings of the Intelligence Science and Big Data Engineering. Big Data and Machine Learning, Nanjing, China, 17–20 October 2019; pp. 442–452. [CrossRef]
22. Yao, L.; Zhang, Y.; Wei, B.; Li, Z.; Huang, X. Traditional chinese medicine clinical records classification using knowledge-powered document embedding. In Proceedings of the 2016 IEEE International Conference on Bioinformatics and Biomedicine (BIBM), Shenzhen, China, 15–18 December 2016. [CrossRef]
23. Figueroa, R.; Zeng-Treitler, Q.; Ngo, L.; Goryachev, S.; Wiechmann, E. Active learning for clinical text classification: Is it better than random sampling? *J. Am. Med. Inform. Assoc.: JAMIA* **2012**, *19*, 809–816. [CrossRef]
24. Garla, V.; Brandt, C. Knowledge-based biomedical word sense disambiguation: An evaluation and application to clinical document classification. *J. Am. Med. Inform. Assoc.* **2012**, *20*, 882–886. [CrossRef] [PubMed]
25. Yao, L.; Mao, C.; Luo, Y. Clinical text classification with rule-based features and knowledge-guided convolutional neural networks. *BMC Med. Inform. Decis. Mak.* **2018**, *19*, 70–71. [CrossRef]
26. Asgari-Chenaghlu, M. Word Vector Representation, Word2vec, Glove, and Many More Explained. Ph.D. Thesis, University of Tabriz, Tabriz, Iran, 2017. [CrossRef]
27. Howard, J.; Ruder, S. Universal language model fine-tuning for text classification. In Proceedings of the 56th Annual Meeting of the Association for Computational Linguistics, Melbourne, Australia, 15–20 July 2018; pp. 328–339. [CrossRef]
28. Radford, A.; Karthik, N.; Tim, S.; Ilya, S. Improving Language Understanding by Generative Pre-Training. 2018. Available online: https://s3-us-west-2.amazonaws.com/openai-assets/research-covers/language-unsupervised/language_understanding_paper.pdf (accessed on 1 October 2021).
29. Salton, G.; Buckley, C. Term-weighting approaches in automatic text retrieval. *Inform. Process. Man.* **1988**, *24*, 513–523. [CrossRef]
30. Joulin, A.; Grave, E.; Bojanowski, P.; Mikolov, T. Bag of tricks for efficient text classification. In Proceedings of the 15th Conference of the European Chapter of the Association for Computational Linguistics, Valencia, Spain, 3–7 April 2017; pp. 427–431. [CrossRef]
31. Sokolova, M.; Lapalme, G. A systematic analysis of performance measures for classification tasks. *Inf. Process. Manag.* **2009**, *45*, 427–437. [CrossRef]
32. Bird, S. NLTK: The natural language toolkit. In Proceedings of the COLING/ACL on Interactive Presentation Sessions Association for Computational Linguistics 2006, Sydney, Australia, 17–18 July 2006; pp. 69–72.
33. Yu, Y.; Si, X.; Hu, C.; Zhang, J. A review of recurrent neural networks: Lstm cells and network architectures. *Neural Comput.* **2019**, *31*, 1–36. [CrossRef] [PubMed]
34. Xu, J.; Du, Q. A deep investigation into fasttext. In Proceedings of the IEEE 21st International Conference on High Performance Computing and Communications, Zhangjiajie, China, 10–12 August 2019; pp. 1714–1719. [CrossRef]
35. Lee, J.; Yoon, W.; Kim, S.; Kim, D.; Kim, S.; So CKang, J. Biobert: A pre-trained biomedical language representation model for biomedical text mining. *Bioinformatics* **2019**, *36*, 1234–1240. [CrossRef] [PubMed]
36. Huang, K.; Altosaar, J.; Ranganath, R. Clinicalbert: Modeling clinical notes and predicting hospital readmission. *arXiv* **2019**, arXiv:1904.05342.
37. Beltagy, I.; Cohan, A.; Lo, K. Scibert: Pretrained contextualized embeddings for scientific text. In Proceedings of the 2019 Conference on Empirical Methods in Natural Language Processing and the 9th International Joint Conference on Natural Language Processing (EMNLP-IJCNLP) 2019, HongKong, China, 3–7 November 2019.
38. Matthew, E.P.; Mark, N.; Robert, L.; Roy, S.; Vidur, J.; Sameer, S.; Noah, A.S. Knowledge Enhanced Contextual Word Representations. In Proceedings of the 2019 Conference on Empirical Methods in Natural Language Processing and the 9th International Joint Conference on Natural Language Processing (EMNLP-IJCNLP), HongKong, China, 3–7 November 2019; pp. 43–54. [CrossRef]
39. Ashish, V.; Noam, S.; Niki, P.; Jakob, U.; Llion, J.; Aidan, N.G.; Lukasz, K.; Illia, P. Attention is all you need. In Proceedings of the 31st Conference on Neural Information Processing Systems (NIPS 2017), Long Beach, CA, USA, 4–9 December 2017; pp. 6000–6010.
40. Khadhraoui, M.; Bellaaj, H.; Ben Ammar, M.; Hamam, H.; Jmaiel, M. Machine Learning Classification Models with SPD/ED Dataset: Comparative Study of Abstract Versus Full Article Approach. In Proceedings of the ICOST 2020, Hammamet, Tunisia, 24–26 June 2020; pp. 24–26. [CrossRef]

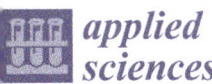

Article

Design of a Wearable Healthcare Emergency Detection Device for Elder Persons

Flora Amato, Walter Balzano and Giovanni Cozzolino *

Department of Electrical Engineering and Information Technology, University of Naples Federico II, 80125 Napoli, Italy; flora.amato@unina.it (F.A.); walter.balzano@unina.it (W.B.)
* Correspondence: giovanni.cozzolino@unina.it

Abstract: Improving quality of life in geriatric patients is related to constant physical activity and fall prevention. In this paper, we propose a wearable system that takes advantage of sensors embedded in a smart device to collect data for movement identification (running, walking, falling and daily activities) of an elderly user in real-time. To provide high efficiency in fall detection, the sensor's readings are analysed using a neural network. If a fall is detected, an alert is sent though a smartphone connected via Bluetooth. We conducted an experimental session using an Arduino Nano 33 BLE Sense board in inside and outside environments. The results of the experiment have shown that the system is extremely portable and provides high success rates in fall detection in terms of accuracy and loss.

Keywords: neural networks; e-health; Arduino; wearable; machine learning

Citation: Amato, F.; Balzano, W.; Cozzolino, G. Design of a Wearable Healthcare Emergency Detection Device for Elder Persons. *Appl. Sci.* **2022**, *12*, 2345. https://doi.org/10.3390/app12052345

Academic Editors: Stefano Silvestri and Francesco Gargiulo

Received: 20 November 2021
Accepted: 18 February 2022
Published: 23 February 2022

Publisher's Note: MDPI stays neutral with regard to jurisdictional claims in published maps and institutional affiliations.

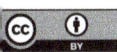

Copyright: © 2022 by the authors. Licensee MDPI, Basel, Switzerland. This article is an open access article distributed under the terms and conditions of the Creative Commons Attribution (CC BY) license (https:// creativecommons.org/licenses/by/ 4.0/).

1. Introduction

Among the leading causes of severe harm and death in the elderly, there is the problem of falls at home. Lack of balance, sudden lurching and confusion after getting out of bed cause much mortality and bedriddenness. The effect is greatest in patients with dementia, who often receive harm that limits their mobility, forcing them to spend the rest of their lives bedridden or in assisted living residences.

According to the best statistics available, in Italy, people over 65 years of age fall at least once during the year. Of these, 43% fall more than once, and of these falls, over 60% occur at home. A large portion of those who fall are seniors with dementia. The bedroom accounts for as many as 25% of total falls. In the United States, falls are the leading cause of unintentional death and the 7th leading cause of death in persons aged ≥65 years. In 2018, there were 32,522 fall-related deaths of people ≥65 and only 4933 fall-related deaths of people younger than 65; thus, 85% of fall-related deaths occur in the 13% of the population who are ≥65 [1].

How a person falls will dictate the types of injuries that may result. For example, falling forward or backwards, striking the hand first as an unconditional reflex, usually causes a wrist fracture. Instead, a rupture of the hip is characteristic of falls to one side or the other. When an older adult suddenly gets out of bed, their or her body needs time to restore balance and cope with the new situation.

The main problem is not the fall and the fracture, but its consequences. In fact, in the elderly, pathologies such as osteoporosis and other physiological changes related to ageing cause slower healing, additional discomfort and effects from the psychological point of view. Many elderly patients are reluctant to report falling because they view falling as part of the ageing process or fear being restricted in their activities or hospitalised.

Falls can impair the independence of older adults and cause a range of personal and socioeconomic consequences. In fact, falls were responsible for more than 3 million emergency department visits by older persons. Medical expenditures for nonfatal fall injuries were approximately $50 billion in 2019 and are sure to increase [2]. However, clinicians often underestimate the damage from a fall unless the patient has an obvious injury, as history and objective examination usually do not include detailed assessments.

Anyone who lives with, helps or works with seniors, particularly those with illnesses, knows how difficult it is to get them to listen to and follow the suggestions and directions they are given. Therefore, we designed a wearable emergency recognition device for elder persons with the aim of detecting dangerous events, such as falls, in order to trigger assistance. In our case study, we used patients with metabolic disorders, who are more likely to be prone to falls.

The paper is organised as follows. Section 2 reports a discussion of related works on the fall detection topic. In Section 3, we describe our fall detection system and its constituent components. In Section 4, the experimental results and evaluation are presented. Lastly, conclusions and future work are described in Section 5.

2. Related Works

At present, several solutions have been proposed for elderly fall detection. Such solutions are categorised into three main types according to the sensor-technology used: non-wearable systems (NWS), wearable systems (WS) and fusion or hybrid systems (FS).

In particular, NWS systems [3–5] use vision-based sensors strategically distributed in the home of the elder. They have been proven powerful and robust at detecting falls; however, these systems have high costs, can be obviously be effective only in indoor environments and could generate privacy issues for the elders or the people that assist them.

To overcome these limitations, WS systems were proposed. They typically use inertial sensors, such as an accelerometer or gyroscope, usually attached to the elder for motion detection. Accelerometers are being increasingly used in WS systems because they offer advantages: low power consumption; affordability; lightness; ease of use; small size; the potential to be mounted on various body parts; and most importantly, extreme portability. Therefore, in some representative papers [6–8] a 3-axis accelerometer with the threshold-based algorithm was used. In these papers, the authors detected falls when the acceleration from a 3-axis accelerometer exceeded the threshold. One of the essential advantages of using the threshold-based method is that it is less complex and less computationally intensive than the other methods. However, finding suitable thresholds to detect all types of falls without mislabelling activities of daily living (ADL) has proven to be a complex problem.

A similar approach uses a smartphone's built-in accelerometer to monitor the movement data of an elderly person continuously. In [9], the collected data were used to test three different learning classifiers offline: decision trees, k-nearest-neighbours (KNN) and naive Bayes. The results show that the decision-trees-based algorithm had the best performance, with more equilibrated sensitivity and specificity values compared with the other algorithms. Nevertheless, due to smartphones' relatively high energy consumption, this system could only be active for a short period.

Recently, WS systems based on machine learning (ML) approaches have been proposed [10–14] to address these limitations and improve the accuracy of fall detection. One study [15] used a nonlinear support vector machine to extract features and gain meaning from body data captured by an accelerometer attached to a smart textile. Two feature extractions were required to identify the peak to detect the fall direction, requiring more processing than a single extraction algorithm. The authors of [16] detected and predicted falls using a method based on the hidden Markov model (HMM), which involved gathering time series from the movements obtained by a three-axis accelerometer placed on the upper body. The test results show a perfect success rate of drop detection (100% sensitivity and 100% specificity). However, they used data samples from adolescents' simulated activities to train and adjust the HMM and the system's thresholds.

3. Fall Detection System

Our methodology foresees developing a wearable system for detecting falls of older people, which takes advantage of low-power smart devices' capabilities and a neural network for movement detection recognition. In this work, we have followed an ML approach by using a neural network for fall detection, but we differ from related works in the system's design.

While other related works exploit multiple sensors that collect movements and send data to a device that analyse them, in this work, we used a single device for activity monitoring and recognition through a neural network deployed on an Arduino nano 33 BLE Sense board. The board has a small size of 45 × 18 mm, which makes it suitable for prototype wearables, and is equipped with several integrated sensors to measure environmental variables. In Figure 1, one can see the board's main components and input/output interfaces. This choice brings versatility and portability advantages, since the other related works' solutions are constrained to indoor environments that rely on non-portable infrastructures or require multiple sensors to be worn on the body.

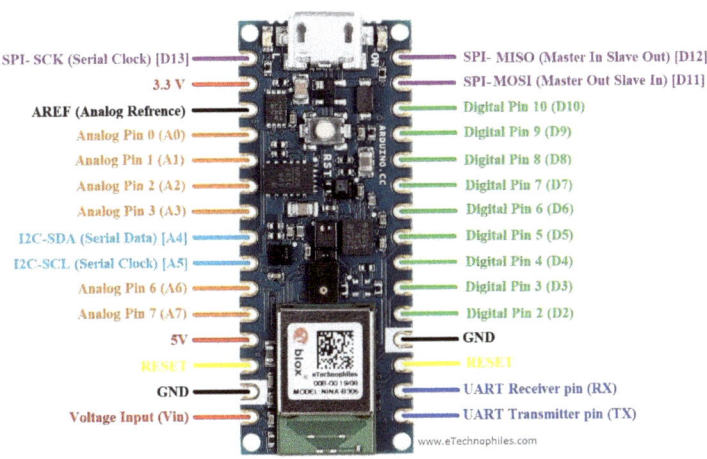

Figure 1. Arduino 33 Nano BLE Sense pinout.

Another innovation of our work is that the monitoring board interacts with a smartphone to collect and manage events. The board can communicate with the smartphone through a Bluetooth Low Energy (BLE) module: when it detects a fall, it sends a notification to the smartphone. To avoid false alarms, a mobile application on the smartphone manages the notifications, asking to the user if there is an emergency. If no response is provided within 60 s, the smartphone forwards an alert by calling a healthcare professional and sending information about the location of the older person. Furthermore, the detected events are stored on the smartphone—one the one hand to give more accurate information to healthcare professionals and on the other hand to provide an efficient way to enhance the neural network's training, together with feedback provided in response to detected events.

3.1. Datasets

The analysis of the recent related literature showed that current studies tend to prefer the use of already existing public repositories containing falls and ADLs, although no particular dataset can be considered a globally accepted benchmarking tool. For neural network training, we used two different datasets.

The first dataset chosen for recognition of falls and daily activities (ADL) [17] includes 11 activities and three trials for each of them. For the dataset collection, 17 different subjects performed six different activities of daily living (walking, standing, lifting an object, sitting and lying down) and five different types of falls (falling forward using hands, falling forward using knees, falling backwards, falling sitting, and falling sideways). Data were collected with a multi-modal approach using wearable sensors, ambient sensors and vision devices. For data consistency, we selected a single subject and chose to refer only to the data acquired by inertial sensors placed on the right wrist. For each type of activity (excluding walking), we selected five samples for a total of 50 samples for falls and daily activities, respectively.

We used Power BI to eliminate redundant data and measurements unrelated to the right wrist or related to the three axes of acceleration and gyroscope. Therefore, the resulting dataset was trimmed to be used in the training of the neural network that we show in detail in the dedicated section.

The *Run or Walk* dataset [18] contains running and walking data collected from iOS devices. Initially, the dataset consisted of a single file representing 88,588 data samples collected by the device's accelerometer and gyroscope during an interval of 10 s and at a frequency of approximately 5.4/s. For each row, there is an activity type represented by "activity" column which acts as label and a "wrist" column which represents the wrist whereupon the device was placed to collect samples. Specifically, each row of the dataset contained:

- acceleration_x;
- acceleration_y;
- acceleration_z;
- gyro_x;
- gyro_y;
- gyro_z;
- label "0" for walking;
- label "1" for running;
- label "0" for the left wrist;
- label "1" for the right wrist.

The original dataset also contained the columns columns "date", "time" and "username", which for obvious reasons, have been eliminated by PowerBI. Moreover, we chose to consider the measurements made only on the right wrist (for consistency with data collected for the others activities). Then, we collected 50 samples for walking and 50 for running. Angular velocity values were transformed from rad/s to deg/s to align them with the fall/adl dataset values. Therefore, all values contained in the gyro axes columns were multiplied by 57.2958°/rad.

3.2. Data Pre-Processing

When data are transmitted to the designed neural network, the size of each input datum should be the same as the number of input layer variables (in our model, the input layer size is 300). However, since the duration of each action, including falling, is different, we needed to make the sizes of the data the same. Based on this, all data were unified to have 50 values.

We split complete dataset into four lists of gestures, namely, "adl", "fall", "walk" and "run"; we had 50 samples for each gesture. For each of these files we had to normalise input data between 0 and 1 in order to create tensors. Each row contained normalised input data, coming from acceleration and angular velocity values, and the output represented by an eye matrix encoding the expected activity value. Data pre-processing reported in the following Listing 1.

Listing 1. Dataset parsing and pre-processing.

```python
# Set a fixed random seed value, for reproducibility, this will allow us to
    get the same random numbers each time the notebook is run
SEED = 1337
np.random.seed(SEED)
tf.random.set_seed(SEED)

# the list of gestures that data is available for
GESTURES = ["adl", "fall", "walk", "run",]
NUM_GESTURES = len(GESTURES)
SAMPLES_PER_GESTURE = 50

# create a one-hot encoded matrix that is used in the output
ONE_HOT_ENCODED_GESTURES = np.eye(NUM_GESTURES)

inputs = []
outputs = []

# read each csv file and push an input and output
for gesture_index in range(NUM_GESTURES):
  gesture = GESTURES[gesture_index]
  print(f"Processing index {gesture_index} for gesture '{gesture}'.")

  output = ONE_HOT_ENCODED_GESTURES[gesture_index]

  df = pd.read_csv("/content/" + gesture + ".csv")

  # calculate the number of gesture recordings in the file
  num_recordings = int(df.shape[0] / SAMPLES_PER_GESTURE)

  print(f"\tThere are {num_recordings} recordings of the {gesture} gesture.")

  for i in range(num_recordings):
    tensor = []
    for j in range(SAMPLES_PER_GESTURE):
      index = i * SAMPLES_PER_GESTURE + j
      # normalize the input data, between 0 and 1:
      tensor += [
          (df['aX'][index] + 4) / 8,
          (df['aY'][index] + 4) / 8,
          (df['aZ'][index] + 4) / 8,
          (df['gX'][index] + 1000) / 2000,
          (df['gY'][index] + 1000) / 2000,
          (df['gZ'][index] + 1000) / 2000
      ]

    inputs.append(tensor)
    outputs.append(output)

# convert the list to numpy array
inputs = np.array(inputs)
outputs = np.array(outputs)

print("Data set parsing and preparation complete.")
```

3.3. Training, Testing and Validation Datasets

For model training we randomly split input and output pairs into a training set (60%), a testing set (20%) and a validation set (20%), as reported in the following Listing 2.

Listing 2. Dataset randomisation and splitting.

```python
# Randomise the order of the inputs, so they can be evenly distributed for
    training, testing, and validation
num_inputs = len(inputs)
randomise = np.arange(num_inputs)
np.random.shuffle(randomize)

# Swap the consecutive indexes (0, 1, 2, etc) with the randomised indexes
inputs = inputs[randomise]
outputs = outputs[randomise]

# Split the recordings (group of samples) into three sets: training, testing
    and validation
TRAIN_SPLIT = int(0.6 * num_inputs)
TEST_SPLIT = int(0.2 * num_inputs + TRAIN_SPLIT)

inputs_train, inputs_test, inputs_validate = np.split(inputs, [TRAIN_SPLIT,
    TEST_SPLIT])
outputs_train, outputs_test, outputs_validate = np.split(outputs, [
    TRAIN_SPLIT, TEST_SPLIT])

print("Data set randomisation and splitting complete.")
```

3.4. Model Training

In this work, we used Google TensorFlow for neural network configuration and learning, since it makes neural network implementation convenient, because it provides functions used for machine learning, including activation functions and an initialisation function.

To exploit the advantages of neural networks while keeping a simple model, able to be deployed on the Arduino board, we designed a sequential neural network model for ADL recognition consisting of:

- A dense layer with 50 neurons and a *sigmoid* activation function;
- A dense level with 25 neurons and a *sigmoid* activation function;
- A final level with four neurons and an activation function *softmax*.

The following Listing 3 shows the implemented model:

Listing 3. Neural network model definition and training.

```python
# build the model and train it
model = tf.keras.Sequential()
model.add(tf.keras.layers.Dense(50, activation='ReLU'))
model.add(tf.keras.layers.Dense(25, activation='ReLU'))
# softmax is used, because we only expect one gesture to occur per input
model.add(tf.keras.layers.Dense(NUM_GESTURES, activation='softmax'))
model.compile(optimizer='adam', loss='mse', metrics=['accuracy'])
history = model.fit(inputs_train, outputs_train, epochs=80, batch_size=1,
    validation_data=(inputs_validate, outputs_validate))
```

Since the sample size of the experiment was 50, and we had three components for acceleration and angular velocity per sample (x, y and z; gx, gy and gz), the number of variables in the input layer was set to 50×6. In the hidden layers, a ReLU function was used as the activation function, for performance reasons.

The output layer consists of four neurons—[0, 1]—for the "adl", "fall", "walk" and "run" activities. In the output stage, the activation function is *softmax*, so the sum of the output probabilities has to be 1. In our case, having four different classes, we obtained a probability for each of them. The predicted movement is the one with the highest probability.

3.5. Model Deployment

The model was built and trained using the TensorFlow and Keras libraries. The obtained model was converted to a Tensor Flow Lite version, as reported in Listing 4, suitable to be loaded into the Arduino IDE and then flashed into the board. Thus we built a classifier that prints a prediction on a serial monitor and sends emergency notifications through Bluetooth messages to a smartphone.

Listing 4. Neural Network conversion into Tensorflow Lite model.

```
# Convert the model to the TensorFlow Lite format without quantization
converter = tf.lite.TFLiteConverter.from_keras_model(model)
tflite_model = converter.convert()

# Save the model to disk
open("model.tflite", "wb").write(tflite_model)

import os
basic_model_size = os.path.getsize("model.tflite")
print("Model is %d bytes" % basic_model_size)
```

The classifier implemented for the Arduino board predicts four possible motions (as illustrated above). The detection of a movement is signalled by turning on the RGB LED of the board, as shown in Figure 2, according to the following scheme:

- Red LED, when a fall is detected;
- Blue LED, for running;
- Green LED, for walking;
- LED off, for actions of daily life (ADL).

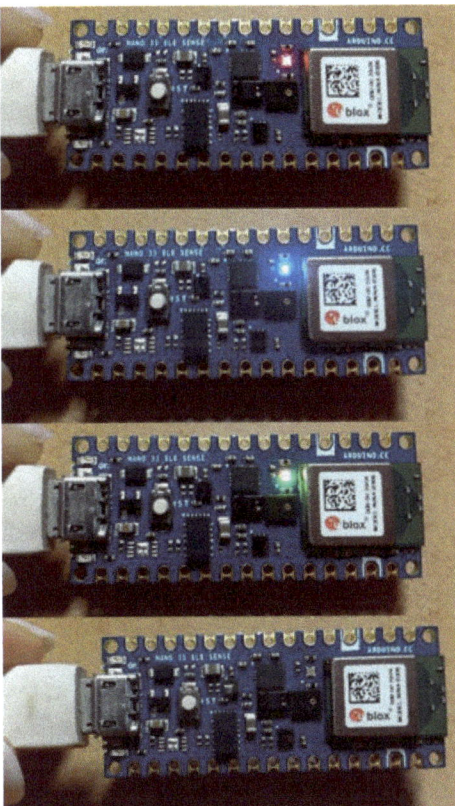

Figure 2. From the top: falling, running, walking and standing detection.

4. Results

How to evaluate fall detection systems (FDSs) in realistic conditions is still an unresolved experimental problem. The main users of FDSs are supposed to be the elderly. The current public databases containing actual falls experienced by older adults are certainly scarce. In our scenario of monitoring older persons' activities (generally people with limited mobility), falls could be identified as movements that clearly deviate from the detected patterns of the samples in the training set. Anyway, in the absence of measurement repositories with a significant number of actual falls, experiments were conducted to obtain the acceleration values of falls. We excluded older people from falls simulations because they could have resulted in severe injuries to such subjects.

For fall simulations, we prepared an experimental environment consisting of a floor mat capable of absorbing one's fall on which we put an unstable platform. The subject, to which the smart device was attached on the right wrist by a strip string, was asked to stand on the unstable platform. By slightly moving the platform, the subject's fall was induced.

The model for motion detection (ADL, fall, walk, run) was trained for 80 epochs, obtaining the results shown in Figure 3.

The parameters shown are:

- *loss*, defined as the root mean square error between the actual value and the predicted value during training;
- *accuracy*, as the percentage of correct predictions, compared to the total predictions during training;
- *val_loss*, loss on the validation data;
- *val_accuracy*, accuracy on the validation data.

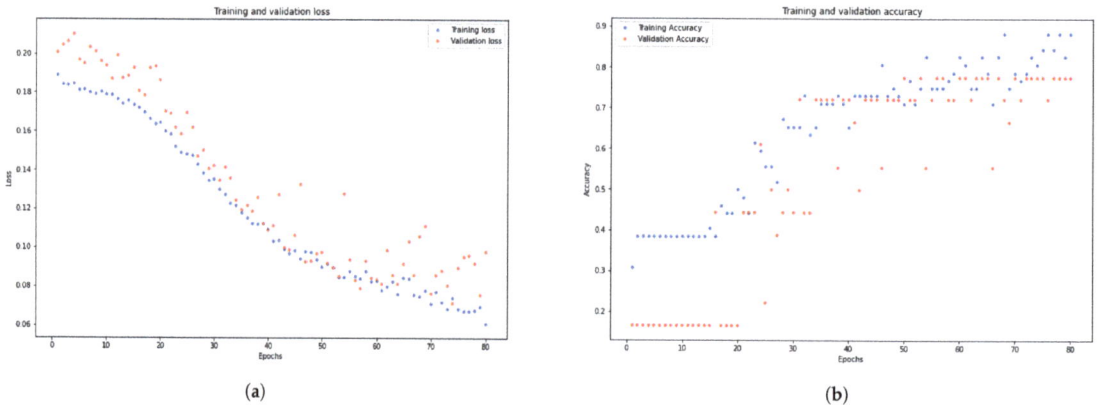

Figure 3. Training of the movement detection model: (**a**) *loss* and *val_loss* functions for the movement classifier. (**b**) *accuracy* and *val_accuracy* functions for the movement classifier.

Figure 3a shows the loss and *val_loss* obtained for the motion classifier. On the validation data, the loss function was 0.10. Figure 3b shows the accuracy and *val_accuracy* obtained for the motion classifier. On the validation data, the accuracy did not get beyond 78%.

For a real-world validation session, we tested an elderly person performing ADLs and walking, since they are safe experiments. These data are more representative of the posture, walking speed and other factors typical of older people.

The subject performed ADLs wearing the device for a week and provided feedback on the alert notifications prompted by the smartphone. The subject also performed a prefixed set of activities at the end of each day to compare the results. We estimated network classification performance at the beginning and the end of the experiment by evaluating samples of data collected during test set of activities performed on day 1 and day 7. We reported the results in Figure 4.

Figure 4a shows the confusion matrix obtained by the model during day 1. The recognition of fall, walk and run activities were good (all five running activities were recognised, along with the four walking activities and the two falling activities). However, in the case of the ADLs, due to their variability, only one was recognised adequately, and the remainder were predicted to be falls. Figure 4b shows the model's confusion matrix obtained during day 7, after tuning the network with feedback provided by the subject through the smartphone. Fall, walk and run recognition were still good; and in ADLs recognition, 50% of events were correctly recognised.

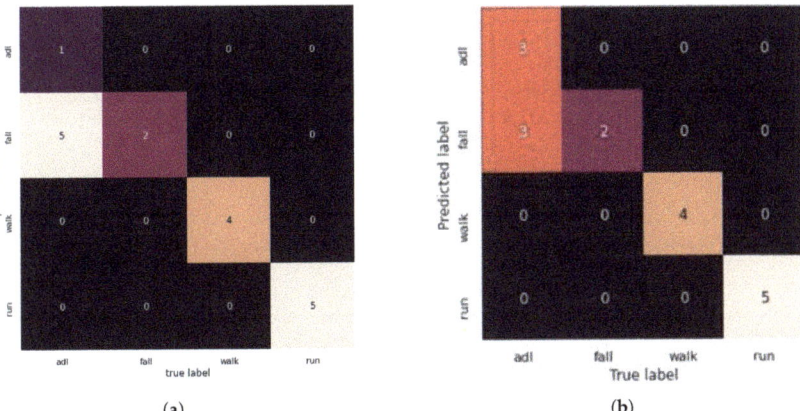

Figure 4. Model's confusion matrix. (**a**) Confusion matrix for the movement detection classifier on 1. (**b**) Confusion matrix for the movement detection classifier on day 7.

5. Conclusions

In this work we have presented a system for fall detection for elderly people. The system exploits a smart sensor board on which we use a neural network trained to recognise and monitor the activity of the patient. The board interacts with a smartphone application, connected through Bluetooth with the board, which is responsible for getting user feedback to supposed fall events and forwarding emergency calls if necessary.

In previous fall detection studies, falls have recognised using acceleration sensors on the waist or the chest, and the recognition rate has been over 95%. However, when an acceleration sensor on the wrist was used, the recognition rate was about 75%. The artificial neural network proposed in this work was able to recognise activities with 78% accuracy using the acceleration of the wrist. This is a relatively small improvement compared to the conventional fall detection mechanism, which is due to the simple neural network model that was designed to suit the limited computational capabilities of such devices.

However, with wrist-band type devices, we can cut down the system costs (we may use existing smart-watches or bands) and provide comfort to the user. Moreover the proposed system is portable, usable in outdoor environments and upgradeable through the firmware. Furthermore, the system analyses sensor data with an embedded computational unit (CU), not having the need for streaming data to an external CU, thereby preventing draining of the battery of the connected smartphone. The latter is only responsible for obtaining feedback from the user and forwarding emergency notifications.

In future developments we will provide the ability to classify more activities, so that the living patterns of older persons can be better recognised. Furthermore, we could also integrate speech recognition features to recognise help requests, including those not related to falls [19,20]. Moreover, we foresee the need to apply security and privacy techniques in order to process the data acquired by the sensors [21,22].

Author Contributions: Conceptualization, F.A., W.B. and G.C.; methodology, F.A., W.B. and G.C.; software, F.A., W.B. and G.C.; validation, F.A., W.B. and G.C.; formal analysis, F.A., W.B. and G.C.; data curation, F.A., W.B. and G.C.; writing—original draft preparation, F.A., W.B. and G.C.; writing—review and editing, F.A., W.B. and G.C. All authors have read and agreed to the published version of the manuscript.

Funding: This research received no external funding.

Institutional Review Board Statement: Not applicable.

Informed Consent Statement: Informed consent was obtained from all subjects involved in the study.

Data Availability Statement: https://sites.google.com/up.edu.mx/har-up/, https://www.kaggle.com/vmalyi/run-or-walk (accessed on 18 November 2021).

Conflicts of Interest: The authors declare no conflict of interest.

References

1. Older Adult Falls. Available online: https://injuryfacts.nsc.org/home-and-community/safety-topics/older-adult-falls/ (accessed on 28 November 2021).
2. Older Adult Fall Prevention. Available online: https://www.cdc.gov/falls/ (accessed on 28 November 2021).
3. Harrou, F.; Zerrouki, N.; Sun, Y.; Houacine, A. Vision-based fall detection system for improving safety of elderly people. *IEEE Instrum. Meas. Mag.* **2017**, *20*, 49–55. [CrossRef]
4. Solbach, M.D.; Tsotsos, J.K. Vision-based fallen person detection for the elderly. In Proceedings of the IEEE International Conference on Computer Vision Workshops, Venice, Italy, 22–29 October 2017; pp. 1433–1442.
5. De Miguel, K.; Brunete, A.; Hernando, M.; Gambao, E. Home camera-based fall detection system for the elderly. *Sensors* **2017**, *17*, 2864. [CrossRef] [PubMed]
6. Dias, P.V.G.; Costa, E.D.M.; Tcheou, M.P.; Lovisolo, L. Fall detection monitoring system with position detection for elderly at indoor environments under supervision. In Proceedings of the 2016 8th IEEE Latin-American Conference on Communications (LATINCOM), Medellin, Colombia, 16–18 November 2016; pp. 1–6.
7. Phu, P.T.; Hai, N.T.; Tam, N.T. A threshold algorithm in a fall alert system for elderly people. In Proceedings of the 5th International Conference on Biomedical Engineering in Vietnam, Ho Chi Minh City, Vietnam, 16–18 June 2015; Springer: Berlin/Heidelberg, Germany, 2015; pp. 347–350.
8. Santiago, J.; Cotto, E.; Jaimes, L.G.; Vergara-Laurens, I. Fall detection system for the elderly. In Proceedings of the 2017 IEEE 7th Annual Computing and Communication Workshop and Conference (CCWC), Las Vegas, NV, USA, 9–11 January 2017; pp. 1–4.
9. Aguiar, B.; Rocha, T.; Silva, J.; Sousa, I. Accelerometer-based fall detection for smartphones. In Proceedings of the 2014 IEEE International Symposium on Medical Measurements and Applications (MeMeA), Lisbon, Portugal, 11–12 June 2014; pp. 1–6.
10. Pannurat, N.; Thiemjarus, S.; Nantajeewarawat, E. Automatic fall monitoring: A review. *Sensors* **2014**, *14*, 12900–12936. [CrossRef] [PubMed]
11. Hwang, J.Y.; Kang, J.; Jang, Y.W.; Kim, H.C. Development of novel algorithm and real-time monitoring ambulatory system using Bluetooth module for fall detection in the elderly. In Proceedings of the 26th Annual International Conference of the IEEE Engineering in Medicine and Biology Society, San Francisco, CA, USA, 1–5 September 2004; Volume 1, pp. 2204–2207.
12. Noury, N.; Hervé, T.; Rialle, V.; Virone, G.; Mercier, E.; Morey, G.; Moro, A.; Porcheron, T. Monitoring behavior in home using a smart fall sensor and position sensors. In Proceedings of the 1st Annual International IEEE-EMBS Special Topic Conference on Microtechnologies in Medicine and Biology. Proceedings (Cat. No. 00EX451), Lyon, France, 12–14 October 2000; pp. 607–610.
13. Hussain, F.; Ehatisham-ul Haq, M.; Azam, M.A.; Khalid, A. Elderly assistance using wearable sensors by detecting fall and recognizing fall patterns. In Proceedings of the 2018 ACM International Joint Conference and 2018 International Symposium on Pervasive and Ubiquitous Computing and Wearable Computers, Singapore, 8–12 October 2018; pp. 770–777.
14. Gharghan, S.K.; Mohammed, S.L.; Al-Naji, A.; Abu-AlShaeer, M.J.; Jawad, H.M.; Jawad, A.M.; Chahl, J. Accurate fall detection and localization for elderly people based on neural network and energy-efficient wireless sensor network. *Energies* **2018**, *11*, 2866. [CrossRef]
15. Mezghani, N.; Ouakrim, Y.; Islam, M.R.; Yared, R.; Abdulrazak, B. Context aware adaptable approach for fall detection bases on smart textile. In Proceedings of the 2017 IEEE EMBS International Conference on Biomedical & Health Informatics (BHI), Orlando, FL, USA, 16–19 February 2017; pp. 473–476.
16. Tong, L.; Song, Q.; Ge, Y.; Liu, M. HMM-based human fall detection and prediction method using tri-axial accelerometer. *IEEE Sens. J.* **2013**, *13*, 1849–1856. [CrossRef]
17. Martínez-Villaseñor, L.; Ponce, H.; Brieva, J.; Moya-Albor, E.; Núñez-Martínez, J.; Peñafort-Asturiano, C. UP-fall detection dataset: A multimodal approach. *Sensors* **2019**, *19*, 1988. [CrossRef] [PubMed]
18. Run or Walk—A Dataset Containing Labeled Sensor Data from Accelerometer and Gyroscope. Available online: https://www.kaggle.com/vmalyi/run-or-walk (accessed on 18 November 2021).

19. Silvestri, S.; Gargiulo, F.; Ciampi, M.; De Pietro, G. Exploit multilingual language model at scale for ICD-10 clinical text classification. In Proceedings of the 2020 IEEE Symposium on Computers and Communications (ISCC), Rennes, France, 7–10 July 2020; pp. 1–7.
20. Ciampi, M.; De Pietro, G.; Masciari, E.; Silvestri, S. Some lessons learned using health data literature for smart information retrieval. In Proceedings of the 35th Annual ACM Symposium on Applied Computing, Brno, Czech Republic, 30 March–3 April 2020; pp. 931–934.
21. Amato, F.; Casola, V.; Cozzolino, G.; De Benedictis, A.; Mazzocca, N.; Moscato, F. A Security and Privacy Validation Methodology for e-Health Systems. *ACM Trans. Multimedia Comput. Commun. Appl.* **2021**, *17*, 1–22. [CrossRef]
22. Amato, F.; Castiglione, A.; Cozzolino, G.; Narducci, F. A semantic-based methodology for digital forensics analysis. *J. Parallel Distribut. Comput.* **2020**, *138*, 172–177. [CrossRef]

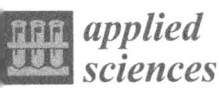

Article

Reducing the Heart Failure Burden in Romania by Predicting Congestive Heart Failure Using Artificial Intelligence: Proof of Concept

Maria-Alexandra Pană [1], Ștefan-Sebastian Busnatu [1,*], Liviu-Ionut Serbanoiu [1], Electra Vasilescu [2], Nirvana Popescu [2], Cătălina Andrei [1] and Crina-Julieta Sinescu [1]

[1] Department of Cardiology, University of Medicine and Pharmacy "Carol Davila", Emergency Hospital "Bagdasar-Arseni", 050474 Bucharest, Romania; maria.alexandra.pana@drd.umfcd.ro (M.-A.P.); liviu-ionut.serbanoiu@rez.umfcd.ro (L.-I.S.); catalina.andrei@umfcd.ro (C.A.); crina.sinescu@umfcd.ro (C.-J.S.)
[2] Computer Science Department, Politehnica University of Bucharest, 060042 Bucharest, Romania; electra.vasilescu@gmail.com (E.V.); nirvana.popescu@cs.pub.ro (N.P.)
* Correspondence: stefan.busnatu@umfcd.ro; Tel.: +40-732154643

Citation: Pană, M.-A.; Busnatu, Ș.-S.; Serbanoiu, L.-I.; Vasilescu, E.; Popescu, N.; Andrei, C.; Sinescu, C.-J. Reducing the Heart Failure Burden in Romania by Predicting Congestive Heart Failure Using Artificial Intelligence: Proof of Concept. *Appl. Sci.* **2021**, *11*, 11728. https://doi.org/10.3390/app112411728

Academic Editors: Stefano Silvestri and Francesco Gargiulo

Received: 25 October 2021
Accepted: 8 December 2021
Published: 10 December 2021

Publisher's Note: MDPI stays neutral with regard to jurisdictional claims in published maps and institutional affiliations.

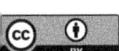

Copyright: © 2021 by the authors. Licensee MDPI, Basel, Switzerland. This article is an open access article distributed under the terms and conditions of the Creative Commons Attribution (CC BY) license (https://creativecommons.org/licenses/by/4.0/).

Abstract: Due to population aging, we are currently confronted with an increased number of chronic heart failure patients. The primary purpose of this study was to implement a noncontact system that can predict heart failure exacerbation through vocal analysis. We designed the system to evaluate the voice characteristics of every patient, and we used the identified variations as an input for a machine-learning-based approach. We collected data from a total of 16 patients, 9 men and 7 women, aged 65–91 years old, who agreed to take part in the study, with a detailed signed informed consent. We included hospitalized patients admitted with cardiogenic acute pulmonary edema in the study, regardless of the precipitation cause or other known cardiovascular comorbidities. There were no specific exclusion criteria, except age (which had to be over 18 years old) and patients with speech inabilities. We then recorded each patient's voice twice a day, using the same smartphone, Lenovo P780, from day one of hospitalization—when their general status was critical—until the day of discharge, when they were clinically stable. We used the New York Heart Association Functional Classification (NYHA) classification system for heart failure to include the patients in stages based on their clinical evolution. Each voice recording has been accordingly equated and subsequently introduced into the machine-learning algorithm. We used multiple machine-learning techniques for classification in order to detect which one turns out to be more appropriate for the given dataset and the one that can be the starting point for future developments. We used algorithms such as Artificial Neural Networks (ANN), Support Vector Machine (SVM) and K-Nearest Neighbors (KNN). After integrating the information from 15 patients, the algorithm correctly classified the 16th patient into the third NYHA stage at hospitalization and second NYHA stage at discharge, based only on his voice recording. The KNN algorithm proved to have the best classification accuracy, with a value of 0.945. Voice is a cheap and easy way to monitor a patient's health status. The algorithm we have used for analyzing the voice provides highly accurate preliminary results. We aim to obtain larger datasets and compute more complex voice analyzer algorithms to certify the outcomes presented.

Keywords: artificial intelligence; chronic heart failure; cardiogenic pulmonary edema; machine learning

1. Introduction

Age-related morphological and physiological changes lead to cardiogeriatric syndrome, predisposing the elder individual to develop Chronic Heart Failure (CHF) [1]. CHF is a significant public health issue, with a prevalence of over 37.7 million cases worldwide [2]. It is ranked by the substantial morbidity and mortality first and the significant annual healthcare and economic burden second [3,4].

CHF is the consequence of cardiac functional impairment secondary to many etiologies, commonly hypertension and coronary heart disease [5,6]. CHF symptoms, such as dyspnea, poor exercise tolerance, and fluid retention, strongly affect patients' quality of life [7]. The plurietiological substrate of heart failure has a critical variability depending on sex, ethnicity, age, comorbidities, and environment [8,9]. Globally, heart failure is one of the most important causes of hospitalization among adults over 65 years old, with medical costs ranging from USD 868 per patient in South Korea to USD 25,532 per patient in Germany, according to a study published in 2018 by Lesyuk W et al. [10]. The estimated lifetime cost of a chronic heart failure patient is 126,819 $ [11]. The situation in Romania is far from good; 4.7% of the population above 35 years old is diagnosed with CHF with an annual mortality rate of approximately 60% [3,12]. Once diagnosed with heart failure, a patient has an expected survival rate of 50% at five years and 10% at ten years [13,14].

However, the severity of the left ventricular dysfunction is associated with an even greater risk of sudden death [4]. Although the survival prognosis of heart failure is not good, the numbers have undergone a substantial improvement over time. [15]

1.1. Pathopyshiology of Acute Heart Failure

Heart failure is a clinical syndrome characterized by acute exacerbations resulting from gradual or rapid changes in the heart, with signs (elevated jugular venous pressure, pulmonary congestion) and symptoms (dyspnea, orthopnea, lower limb swelling) needing urgent therapy [16,17]. Acute heart failure's most frequent clinical tableaus are chronic heart failure decompensation, cardiogenic shock, and acute pulmonary edema [18].

The Cardiogenic Acute Pulmonary Edema (CAPE) develops secondary to a sharp increase in left ventricular pressure, impacting the left atrium retrogradely. Therefore, pressure in pulmonary capillaries results in fluid exudation in the intravascular compartment [19,20]. This mechanism leads to a low diffusion capacity in the lungs, causing dyspnea and fluid retention, which can progress into anasarca, depending on the severity of the cardiac dysfunction [21,22].

Anasarca represents a generalized form of edema, with subcutaneous tissue swelling throughout the body, including the swelling of the larynx, also known as the voice box [23].

The link between the phonation process and generalized edema was underlined in 2002, when Verdolini et al. stated that systemic dehydration mediates the augmentation of phonation threshold pressure [24]. In 2017, Murton et al. conducted a speech analysis on patients with heart failure and obtained significant speech accuracy improvement after pulmonary decongestion and clinical stabilization [25].

In terms of clinical decisions, management of acute heart failure aims to decrease the number of readmissions and long-term mortality [26]. Despite medical efforts, acute heart failure remains a pathology with a sober prognosis, and there is no therapy proven to have long-term mortality benefits [27]. To avoid rehospitalization, the need for better secondary prevention strategies is evident. [28]

1.2. Artificial Intelligence in Cardiology

Artificial intelligence is an engineering branch that uses novel concepts to resolve complex challenges [29]. As biology and medicine are rapidly becoming data-intensive, deep-learning algorithms have been used to assist physicians [30].

Twenty-first-century medicine is now spinning around the patient's individuality, and big data algorithms are efficient assistance tools in the medical environment [31]. Artificial intelligence should not be regarded as a futuristic phenomenon but rather as a tool that saves medical staff time and minimizes human error [30].

In a study conducted in 2017, Dawes et al. managed to predict outcome in pulmonary hypertension patients with an algorithm of three-dimensional patterns of systolic cardiac motion. The software copied the MRI data from 256 patients and learned which configurations were associated with early death or right heart failure. The algorithm used the short-axis cine images segmentation for the three-dimensional model. The prediction tool assessed survival using the median survival time and area under the curve with time-dependent receiver operating, for 1-year survival. Alongside conventional imaging and biological markers, this algorithm increased the accuracy of survival prediction [32].

The Artificial Intelligence-Clinical Decision Support System (AI-CDSS) is a hybrid (expert-driven and machine-learning-driven) tool designed to assist physicians in heart failure diagnosis. Dong-Ju Choi, Jin Joo Park et al. evaluated in their published study the diagnostic accuracy of AI-CDSS on a group of 97 patients with dyspnea. They assessed the concordance rate between the algorithm results and those of heart failure specialists. Out of the 97 patients, 44% had heart failure, with a concordance rate between AI-CDSS and heart failure specialists of 98%. On the other hand, the concordance rate between AI-CDSS and non-heart failure specialists was 76%. Finally, they underlined the usefulness of AI-CDSS in heart failure diagnosis, especially when a heart failure specialist is unavailable [33].

A recent review by Aixia Guo, Michael Pasque et al. summarized the recent findings and approaches of machine-learning techniques in heart failure diagnosis and outcome prediction. The review evaluated studies which used electronic health records, varying from demographic characteristics, medical treatment history, laboratory and imaging results to genetic profiles. They assert high-accuracy results of these prediction tools, taking into consideration at the same time the challenges that novel machine-learning models still need to overcome. Among the most common shortcomings in this area is the impossibility of full integration of the electronic health record (medical reports, a wide variety of imaging results, etc.). On the other hand, given that these algorithms are based on machine learning, patients with rare diseases and atypical profiles cannot benefit from this technology. Thus, it is necessary in the future to further enrich management techniques in order to provide interpretable and actionable models [34,35].

Our study offers a new perspective on the applicability of artificial intelligence in medicine. We pursue this software development in order to integrate it as a smartphone application in the near future. This application will run in the smartphone background, performing vocal analysis on heart failure patients. If it finds signs of heart failure decompensation, it will refer them to medical services. In this way, it will be possible to avoid severe presentations of acute heart failure, which require hospitalization and emergency treatment.

1.3. Main Contributions

The primary purpose of this study was to implement a noncontact system that can predict heart failure exacerbation through vocal analysis. The system was designed to evaluate every patient's voice characteristics, and the identified variations were used as an input for a machine-learning-based approach. This new concept proposes an implementation of a silent intelligent recorder in patients' home, capable of predicting heart failure decompensation.

Our preliminary results managed to highlight an important link between the phonation process and heart failure status. Voice is a cheap parameter that would prove extremely useful in the secondary prevention management of heart failure. In order to have effective secondary prevention campaigns in the future, we need an easy-to-use, fast-to-implement, cheap tool.

In our knowledge, there is currently no other open-source algorithm capable of predicting heart failure decompensation using artificial intelligence. The aim of our research study is to highlight the heart failure burden around the globe and the beneficial impact that a secondary prevention algorithm could have on frequent hospitalizations of heart failure patients.

2. Materials and Methods

2.1. Study Population

The selective criterion of inclusion was the cause of hospitalization. Patients presenting with cardiogenic acute pulmonary edema were selected regardless of the precipitation cause or other known cardiovascular comorbidities. Patients' enrollment in the study was voluntary, after a detailed presentation of the study design. The patients' data collection could not be completely anonymous, so the pseudoanonymization alternative was chosen. Thus, each participant was assigned an identifier, through which personal information is separated from the data collection of the study. All participants were informed about their right to privacy and about the private storage and use of their data. The study conducted did not present any potential psychological, social, physical or legal harm to patients. A total of 16 patients, 9 men and 7 women, aged 65–91 years old, agreed to participate in the study and signed a comprehensive informed consent. There were no specific exclusion criteria, except age (which had to be over 18 years old) and patients with speech inabilities.

2.2. Intervention

We recorded the voices of all patients twice a day, using a Lenovo P780 smartphone, from day one of hospitalization, until the day of discharge. We asked the patients to repeatedly pronounce two specific keywords (number thirty-three and vowel E) while recording. We attempted to minimize environmental noise as much as possible. The mean hospitalization period was seven days, with two recordings per day. We built a small database of 240 audio recordings. We classified them according to the New York Heart Association Functional Classification (Table 1) [36].

Table 1. New York Heart Association Functional Classification.

Class	Patient Symptoms
I	No limitation of physical activity. Ordinary physical activity does not cause undue fatigue, palpitation, dyspnea (shortness of breath)
II	Slight limitation of physical activity. Comfortable at rest. Ordinary physical activity results in fatigue, palpitation, dyspnea (shortness of breath).
III	Marked limitation of physical activity. Comfortable at rest. Less than ordinary activity causes fatigue, palpitations or dyspnea.
IV	Unable to carry on any physical activity without discomfort. Symptoms of heart failure at rest. If any physical activity is undertaken, discomfort increases.

2.3. Feature Extraction

Voice is a continuous-time signal; however, for computation, it is represented as a discrete-time signal. We measured the amplitude at equal distances in a set number of points per second, along with the continuous signal. We set the sampling rate at 48 kHz in this study. Sampling refers to the recording of the speech signals at a regular interval (Figure 1).

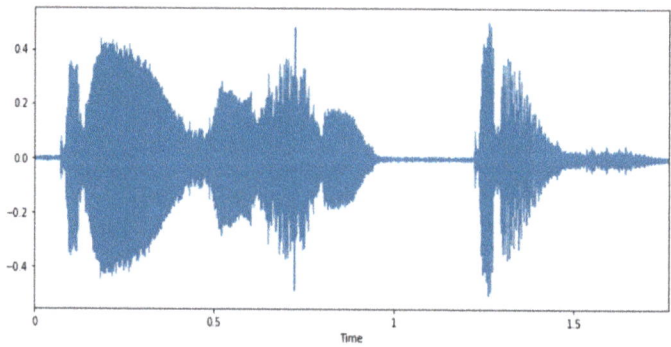

Figure 1. Original signal representing the samples amplitudes over time. In this audio, a female pronounced "33" once.

The raw data were processed to compute the input for the proposed machine-learning algorithms. Calculating the Mel-Frequency Cepstral Coefficients (MFCCs) is an essential step to extract the relevant voice features and reduce each file's dimension. Figure 2 presents the steps for MFCCs extraction, where Discrete Fourier Transform (DFT) is applied on the time signal generating the frequency spectrum. The logarithm function is used, and the Inverse DFT is computed. The final step is to add the Mel Cepstrum or Discrete Cosine Transform (DCT) [37] (Figure 2).

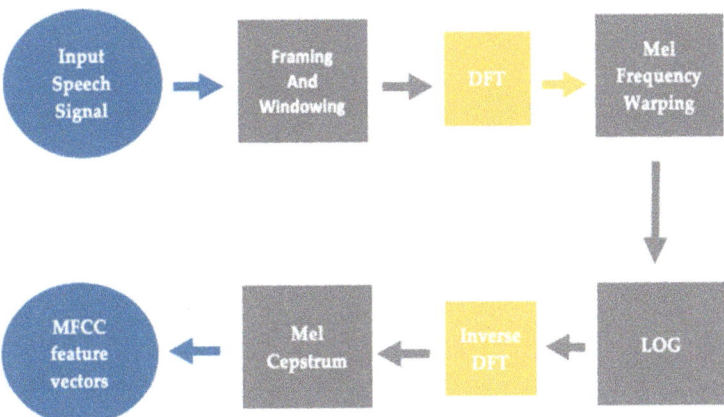

Figure 2. Steps involved in MFCC Features' extraction.

In the described method, the output is represented by up to 40 feature vectors; 20 feature vectors were used, graphically represented in Figure 3. As the dataset comprises different length audio files, the mean MFCC is computed for each feature. To minimize the noise impact, the values are normalized (Figure 3).

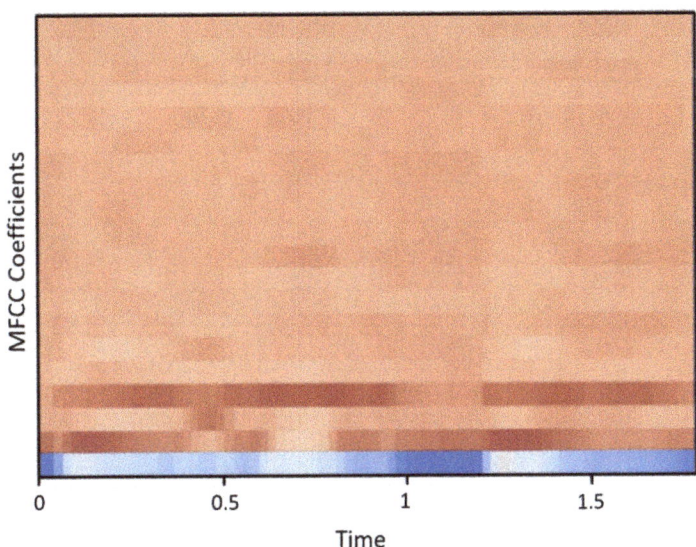

Figure 3. Visual representation of the 20 feature vectors—the Mel Frequency Cepstral Coefficients.

2.4. Machine-Learning Approaches

As a data analytic technique, machine-learning teaches computers to learn from experience, similar to human and animal nature. Machine-learning approaches use computational methods in order to absorb the data, without having to rely on predetermined equations as a model [38].

For classifying the audio files into the four heart-failure classes, we used multiple machine-learning techniques. Each method is generally explained below.

2.4.1. Support Vector Machine (SVM)

Support Vector Machine (SVM) is a machine-learning technique that analyzes data for classification and regression analysis using supervised learning models with associated learning algorithms. Being a nonprobabilistic binary linear classifier, SVM algorithm settles a given set of training examples into one of two categories. Consequently, SVM creates a gap between the two categories, in order to maximize the space between them. The new examples are then mapped into that space and predicted to a category, based on the gap side they fall in. SVM is a standard and suitable method for audio classification [39].

Figure 4 describes a schematic manner of the general SVM algorithm. There are multiple SVMs, using different mathematical functions (or kernels), as follows: linear, nonlinear, radial basis function (RBF), polynomial, and sigmoid. They were tested and evaluated to conclude which is the best kernel to use to determine heart-failure severity [40,41] (Figure 4).

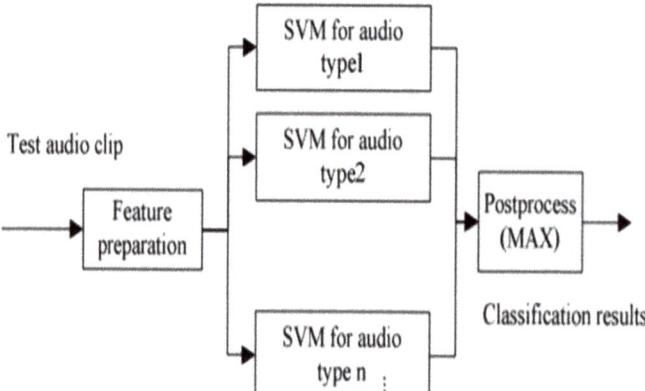

Figure 4. Classification procedure using SVM.

2.4.2. Artificial Neural Networks (ANN)

Artificial Neural Networks (ANN) represent computing systems inspired by the neural networks of animal brains. They are made up of nodes (artificial neurons) and connections that can transmit signals. These signals are represented by real numbers, and the output of each neuron is the sum of all its inputs. Usually, these artificial neurons are aggregated in layers. Each layer can produce different changes to its inputs. Correctly, the signal goes from the first to the last layer, often even repeatedly [42].

Figure 5a,b represent the used models, the chosen layers with the activation function specified for each of them: (Rectified Linear Activation Function, SoftMax, and Hyperbolic Tangent). A facile way to compute the model is by utilizing Keras, a high-level API that gives the user the necessary tools to build and evaluate the neural networks.

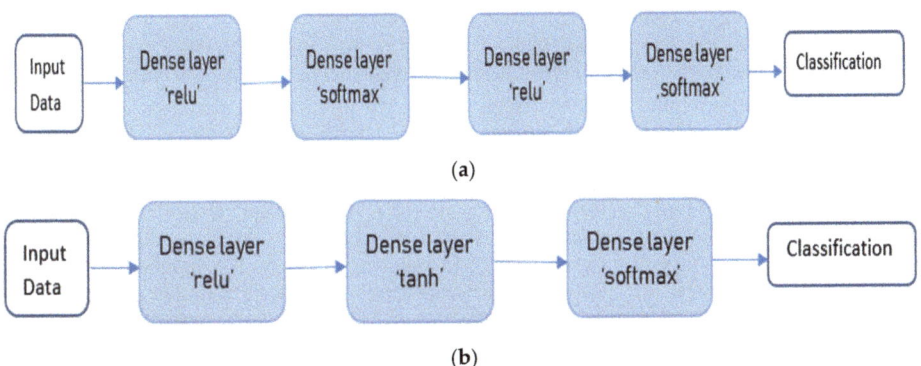

Figure 5. (**a**,**b**) The models used in the ANN method.

2.4.3. K-Nearest Neighbors (KNN)

K-Nearest Neighbors (KNN) represents a nonparametric classification method used in classification and regression. This algorithm performs classification based on distance, thus its function is only locally approximated and computation is postponed until function evaluation. If the analyzed units have different physical characteristics, it is recommended to normalize the data in order to improve its accuracy [43].

In our study, the classification is computed, and a new object is classified according to the votes of its neighbors. The 20 mean MFCCs extracted are used in this approach, and for this reason, it is employed as a 20-dimension classifier. This algorithm provides high accuracy for problems with unknown distributions [44].

The Principal Component Analysis (PCA) is computed to evaluate whether the noise is introduced and determine if it can be reduced. For model generation, a Grid Search is performed. For calculating a model with KNN, Scikit learn, an easy-to-use and efficient library from python, was selected.

The dataset was split into two parts for all three methods: the train set (80%) and the test set (20%).

3. Results

The study group has 16 patients, 9 men and 7 women. The small sample size of our study group is due to the COVID-19 pandemic. Our local hospital was dedicated to COVID-19 patients and it was not possible to continue enrolling new patients in the study. Consequently, we decided to move forward with the analysis of this group in order to see if the algorithm works.

Despite the small patient study group, we believe that the results obtained are relevant, considering the used algorithm. KNN is able to deliver high-accuracy results for small databases. The obtained results show a link between patients' vocal changes and heart failure status. Given these favorable preliminary results, we expect them to strengthen as the number of patients increases.

In terms of cardiovascular risk factors, the enrolled patients have a minimum age value of 65 years old, a maximum age value of 91 years old, with a mean value of 72.68 years old. An increased body mass index is found in 7 out of 16 patients, with a maximum value of 46.88 kg/m^2, corresponding to morbid obesity. High blood pressure and dyslipidemia are two very common risk factors in the study group: out of the 16 patients, 12 are known to have high blood pressure and/or dyslipidemia, with ambulatory treatment. Furthermore, 10 patients have type 2 diabetes, and 7 of these patients need insulin therapy (Table 2). The medical history of the 16 patients enrolled in the study revealed ischemic coronary heart disease in 16 out of 16 patients. Additionally, seven of them have history of percutaneous angioplasty, four have history of coronary artery bypass grafting and five were on ischemic visa drug therapy. All patients have heart failure, 10 of which have severe left ventricular systolic dysfunction (Table 3). The New York Heart Association functional classification (NYHA) of heart failure is a widely used tool in cardiologists' daily practice. It evaluates heart failure patients' symptom severity and the exertion threshold needed to provoke symptoms. Each patient was given a daily assessment on the NYHA scale, the result being associated with the voice recordings performed [36].

In order to be able to use the voice signals as input data for the proposed algorithm, the audio files were converted to vectors of numerical values. These values represent the audio signal's amplitude measured at equal intervals in the temporal space. Consequently, the audio files were converted to vectors of numbers. The different length files resulted in different sized vectors. Their processing led to the extraction of 22 representative values for 22 vocal characteristics (see Section 2.2 Feature Extraction). This process is mandatory in order for the final data collection to have files of the same size.

With the dataset available, the algorithms described in Sections 2.4.1–2.4.3 were tested, and the KNN algorithm was the most relevant as it generated the highest accuracy for classification. Additionally, the result was sustained by the confusion matrix available in (Table 4). This kind of matrix is used to validate the accuracy of the KNN classification method. The three columns from the matrix represent the three classes associated with the audio files. Each element from the diagonal represents the number of correctly classified data from each class and the other elements represent the erroneous ones.

Table 2. Cardiovascular risk factors of enrolled patients.

Patient No.	Age	Sex	Smoker Status	Body mass Index	Arterial Hypertension	Diabetes Mellitus Type 2	Dyslipidemia
1	75	F	No	24.21 kg/m²	Yes (grade 2)	Yes	Yes
2	71	F	Yes	34.66 kg/m²	Yes (grade 3)	No	Yes
3	73	M	No	38.06 kg/m²	Yes (grade 3)	Yes	Yes
4	76	M	No	24.8 kg/m²	Yes (grade 3)	No	No
5	70	M	Yes	27.65 kg/m²	Yes (grade 3)	No	Yes
6	65	M	No	27.7 kg/m²	Yes (grade 3)	Yes	Yes
7	91	M	No	24.68 kg/m²	Yes (grade 3)	Yes	Yes
8	70	M	No	31.04 kg/m²	No	No	Yes
9	66	F	Yes	44.17 kg/m²	Yes (grade 2)	Yes	No
10	79	F	No	23.43 kg/m²	Yes (grade 3)	Yes	No
11	75	M	Yes	26.23 kg/m²	No	No	No
12	78	M	Yes	26.89 kg/m²	Yes (grade 2)	No	Yes
13	67	M	Yes	30.86 kg/m²	Yes (grade 3)	Yes	Yes
14	74	F	No	44.92 kg/m²	No	Yes	Yes
15	67	F	Yes	33.58 kg/m²	Yes (grade 2)	Yes	Yes
16	66	F	Yes	46.88 kg/m²	No	Yes	Yes

The high accuracy obtained, having a value of 0.945, and the validation that was performed through the confusion matrix indicate that this method succeeded in classifying the data with high precision and is reliable for further development.

Alongside daily vocal analysis of the enrolled patients, their clinical and paraclinical monitoring was performed. Thus, weight at admission and discharge, daily diuresis, daily water intake and NTproBNP values were monitored. The clinical and paraclinical evolution of the patients enrolled in the study fits the results of the vocal analysis performed by the proposed algorithm (Table 5).

Table 3. Medical history of enrolled patients.

Patient NO.	Left Ventricular Ejection Fraction	IHD	IHD Type	Atrial Fibrillation	Aortic Valve Disease	Mitral Valve Disease	Tricuspid Valve Disease
1	15%	Yes	PCI	Yes	Metal prosthesis	Metal prosthesis	Tricuspid annuloplasty
2	50%	Yes	PCI	No	No	Easy mitral regurgitation	No
3	19%	Yes	CABG	No	No	Severe mitral regurgitation	Severe tricuspid regurgitation
4	35%	Yes	MTh.	No	Easy aortic regurgitation	Moderate mitral regurgitation	Moderate tricuspid regurgitation
5	30%	Yes	PCI	Yes	No	Moderate mitral regurgitation	Moderate tricuspid regurgitation
6	20%	Yes	PCI	No	No	Moderate mitral regurgitation	Moderate tricuspid regurgitation
7	40%	Yes	CABG	No	Moderate aortic stenosis	Severe mitral regurgitation	Easy tricuspid regurgitation
8	25%	Yes	MTh	No	No	Easy mitral regurgitation	No
9	40%	Yes	MTh	No	No	Moderate mitral regurgitation	Moderate tricuspid regurgitation
10	30%	Yes	MTh	Yes	No	Moderate mitral regurgitation	Easy tricuspid regurgitation
11	25%	Yes	CABG	Yes	Severe aortic stenosis	Metal prosthesis	Severe tricuspid regurgitation
12	50%	Yes	PCI	Yes	Moderate aortic regurgitation	Moderate mitral regurgitation	Moderate tricuspid regurgitation
13	45%	Yes	PCI	No	No	Easy mitral regurgitation	Easy tricuspid regurgitation
14	20%	Yes	MTh	Yes	No	Moderate mitral regurgitation	Moderate tricuspid regurgitation
15	40%	Yes	CABG	No	No	Moderate mitral regurgitation	Easy tricuspid regurgitation
16	10%	Yes	PCI	No	No	Moderate mitral regurgitation	Moderate tricuspid regurgitation

IHD = ischemic heart disease; IHD type = ischemic heart disease type; PCI = percutaneous coronary intervention; CABG = coronary artery bypass graft surgery; MTh = medical therapy.

Table 4. Approach score.

Method	Results
SVM	Accuracy obtained using radial basis function (rbf) kernel = 0.709 Accuracy obtained using linear kernel = 0.618 Accuracy obtained using polynomial kernel = 0.527
ANN	Model 1: Maximum value of the loss function obtained during testing: 1.1447 Maximum accuracy obtained during testing: 0.418 Model 2: Maximum value of the loss function obtained during testing: 1.3237 Maximum accuracy obtained during testing: 0.436
KNN	Model score obtained for KNN: 0.945 Confusion Matrix: [[20 0 2] [0 13 0] [1 0 19]]

Table 5. Evolution of water retention and NTproBNP during hospitalization.

Patient No.	Admission Weight	Discharge Weight	Mean Value of Daily Diuresis	Daily Water Supply	Ntprobnp Admission	Ntprobnp Discharge
1	62 kg	58 kg	2500 mL/24 h	2000 mL/day	3480 pg/mL	1200 pg/mL
2	78 kg	73 kg	3500 mL/24 h	1000 mL/day	4638 pg/mL	900 pg/mL
3	110 kg	102 kg	2600 mL/24 h	750mL/day	17,545 pg/mL	500 pg/mL
4	70 kg	65 kg	3000mL/24 h	2000 mL/day	3131 pg/mL	1000 pg/mL
5	78 kg	74 kg	3000 mL/24 h	1500 mL/day	>30.000 pg/mL	1200 pg/mL
6	96 kg	90 kg	3500 mL/24 h	1000 mL/day	1207 pg/mL	400 pg/mL
7	78 kg	71 kg	2700 mL/24 h	1000 mL/day	8987 pg/mL	700 pg/mL
8	95 kg	90 kg	3100 mL/24 h	1000 mL/day	4277 pg/mL	800 pg/mL
9	110 kg	103 kg	4000 mL/24 h	1500 mL/day	3664 pg/mL	650 pg/mL
10	60 kg	55g	3800 mL/24 h	1500 mL/day	5200 pg/mL	1105 pg/mL
11	85 kg	79 kg	3400 mL/24 h	1000 mL/day	15.300 pg/mL	940 pg/mL
12	85 kg	80 kg	3500 mL/24 h	1500 mL/day	4325 pg/mL	456 pg/mL
13	100 kg	94 kg	4000 mL/24 h	2000 mL/day	6800 pg/mL	670 pg/mL
14	115 kg	109 kg	4500 mL/24 h	1500 mL/day	2262 pg/mL	370 pg/mL
15	90 kg	82 kg	3800 mL/24 h	1000 mL/day	3797 pg/mL	800 pg/mL
16	120 kg	110 kg	4300 mL/24 h	1000 mL/day	10.939 pg/mL	589 pg/mL

4. Discussion

The purpose of this study was to prove that the phonation process suffers during acute heart failure. Therefore, the voice can be used as a prognostic marker and to monitor patients' health status.

The data of the patients admitted to the hospital for acute heart failure have been evaluated. The subject data have been analyzed from the critical status (first day of admission) to the stable status (day of discharge). Out of 16, severe left ventricular systolic dysfunction was noted in 10 patients, with a hypersodium diet as precipitating factor. In comparison, six patients have had moderate left ventricular systolic dysfunction associated with bronchopneumonia with or without moderate to severe valvulopathy (Table 4).

The machine-learning algorithm integrated the audio recordings from 15 patients. We used the last patient to test the algorithm, and he was classified accordingly and correctly after vocal analysis into the third NYHA stage at hospitalization and class II NYHA at discharge.

Numerous factors are known to contribute to the development of heart failure (HF). The potential causes include coronary artery disease, hypertension, cardiomyopathies, valvular and congenital heart disease, arrhythmias, alcohol and drugs, high output failure (anemia, thyrotoxicosis, Paget's disease, etc.), pericardial disease, and primary right heart failure [45]. The meta-analyses conducted by Jones et al. found an improvement in the survival rates secondary to CHF over the past 70 years. The estimated 1-year survival rate was 85.5%; however, the 5-year and 10-year survival rates were 56.7% and 34.9%, and most patients died directly from heart failure or cardiovascular diseases [46]. Although the risk of HF decompensation among older patients has declined over time, it remains one of the leading causes of hospitalization [47].

Cook et al. evaluated the annual global heart failure burden from all published sources and estimated it at $108 billion per annum in 2012. The direct costs accounted for $65 billion, and the indirect cost was $43 billion per annum. The mean immediate HF burden value for the high-income countries was 1.42% versus 0.11% for low- or middle-income countries [48,49]. The hospitalization expenses are the most significant cost component following the expenditures for the medication [50]. In hospitalization costs, room and board were the most important contributors, accounting for 43% of inpatient costs, followed by procedures, imaging, and laboratory testing [51]. Dialysis required the highest part of procedural costs, but it was needed only by a small number of patients [10].

Notable AI models with a successful history include echocardiogram images to identify patients with HF with preserved ejection fraction [7]. It is possible to predict the 1-year mortality from normal ECGs [8]. By reflecting the elevated potassium level in tall T-waves, AI models quantify the potassium regardless of the blood test [9]. The noninvasive cardio acoustic biomarkers were shown to offer reliable results in predicting the parameters of heart failure [10,11]. Misumi et al. used a machine-learning algorithm to examine the valuable predictors obtained from the left ventricular assistance device to provide a model for identifying aortic regurgitation [12].

Therefore, creating software for heart failure decompensation could be timesaving for clinicians and could play a vital role in improving patients' morbidity and mortality. In addition, it could prove to be a money-saving mechanism for healthcare systems and a pioneer in disease management technology [52].

5. Conclusions

We believe that our study serves as the first brick in the future construction of a software that will offer secondary prevention in chronic heart failure patients. Voice is an easy way to monitor a patient's health status as it is an easy-to-understand process, and it is not time- or money-consuming.

6. Limitations

The study sample is small, and consequently the obtained results are preliminary. Further research will be conducted in order to certify the outcomes presented. Additionally, patients enrolled in the study had to be capable of understanding and signing the comprehensive informed consent, a fact which had limited the enrollment of critical-state patients and low-educational background patients.

Author Contributions: Conceptualization, Ş.-S.B.; methodology, Ş.-S.B.; software, E.V., N.P., validation, Ş.-S.B. and M.-A.P.; formal analysis, M.-A.P.; writing, M.-A.P.; writing—review and editing, C.A.; visualization, L.-I.S.; supervision, C.-J.S.; project administration, C.-J.S. All authors have read and agreed to the published version of the manuscript.

Funding: This research received no external funding.

Institutional Review Board Statement: The study was conducted according to the guidelines of the Declaration of Helsinki, and approved by the Ethics Committee of "Carol Davila" University of Medicine and Pharmacy, Bucharest, Romania (protocol code PO-35-F-03, date 12 July 2021).

Informed Consent Statement: Informed consent was obtained from all subjects involved in the study.

Data Availability Statement: Data available on request due to ethical restrictions. The data presented in this study are available on request from the corresponding author. The data are not publicly available due to ethical restrictions.

Conflicts of Interest: The authors declare no conflict of interest.

References

1. Naylor, M.D.; Brooten, D.A.; Campbell, R.L.; Maislin, G.; McCauley, K.M.; Schwartz, J.S. Transitional care of older adults hospitalized with heart failure: A randomized controlled trial. *J. Am. Geriatr. Soc.* **2004**, *52*, 675–684. [CrossRef]
2. Ziaeian, B.; Fonarow, G.C. Epidemiology and aetiology of heart failure. *Nat. Rev. Cardiol.* **2016**, *13*, 368–378. [CrossRef] [PubMed]
3. Andrei, C.A.; Oancea, B.; Nedelcu, M.; Sinescu, R.D. Predicting Cardiovascular Diseases Prevalence Using Neural Networks. *Econ. Comput. Econ. Cybern. Stud. Res.* **2015**, *49*, 73–84.
4. Lee, H.; Oh, S.H.; Cho, H.; Cho, H.J.; Kang, H.Y. Prevalence and socio-economic burden of heart failure in an aging society of South Kirea. *BMC Cardiovasc. Disord.* **2016**, *16*, 215. [CrossRef] [PubMed]
5. Bui, A.L.; Horwich, T.B.; Fonarow, G.C. Epidemiology and risk profile of heart failure. *Nat. Rev. Cardiol.* **2011**, *1*, 30–41. [CrossRef] [PubMed]
6. Roger, V.L. Epidemiology of heart failure. *Circ. Res.* **2013**, *113*, 646–659. [CrossRef]
7. Brennan, E.J. Chronic heart failure nursing: Integrated multidisciplinary care. *Br. J. Nurs.* **2018**, *27*, 681–688. [CrossRef] [PubMed]
8. Porcel, J.M. Pleural effusions from congestive heart failure. *Semin. Respir. Crit. Care Med.* **2010**, *31*, 689–697. [CrossRef]
9. Natanzon, A.; Kronzon, I. Pericardial and pleural effusions in congestive heart failure- anatomical, pathophysiologic and clinical considerations. *Am. J. Med. Sci.* **2009**, *338*, 211–216. [CrossRef]
10. Lesyuk, W.; Kriza, C.; Kolominsky-Rabas, P. Cost-of-illness studies in heart failure: A systematic review 2004–2016. *BMC Cardiovasc. Disord.* **2018**, *18*, 74. [CrossRef]
11. Heidenreich, P.A.; Albert, N.M.; Allen, L.A.; Bluemke, D.A.; Butler, J.; Fonarow, G.C.; Ikonomidis, J.S.; Khavjou, O.; Konstam, M.A.; Maddox, T.M.; et al. Forecasting the impact of heart failure in the United States: A policy statement from the American Heart Association. *Circ. Heart Fail.* **2013**, *6*, 606–609. [CrossRef]
12. Chioncel, O.; Tatu-Chitoiu, G.; Christodorescu, R.; Coman, I.M.; Deleanu, D.; Vinereanu, D.; Macarie, C.; Crespo, M.; Laroche, C.; Fereirra, T.; et al. Characteristic of patients with heart failure from Romania enrolled in—ESC-HF Long-term (ESC-HF-LT) Registry. *Rom. J. Cardiol.* **2015**, *25*, 1–8.
13. Van Nuys, K.E.; Xie, Z.; Tysinger, B.; Hlatky, M.A.; Goldman, D.P. Innovation in Heart Failure Treatment: Life expectancy, Disability and Healt Disparities. *JACC Heart Fail.* **2018**, *6*, 401–409. [CrossRef] [PubMed]
14. Bytyci, I.; Bajraktari, G. Mortality in heart failure patients. *Anatol. J. Cardiol.* **2015**, *15*, 63–68. [CrossRef] [PubMed]
15. Ni, H.; Xu, J. Recent trends in heart failure-related Mortality: United States 2000–2014. In *NCHS Data Brief*; National Center for Health Statistics: Hyattsville, MD, USA, 2015; Volume 231, pp. 1–8.
16. King, M.; Kingery, J.; Casey, B. Diagnosis and evaluation of heart failure. *Am. Fam. Physician* **2012**, *85*, 1161–1168.
17. Kurmani, S.; Squire, I. Acute Heart Failure: Definition, Classification and Epidemiology. *Curr. Heart Fail. Rep.* **2017**, *14*, 385–392. [CrossRef]
18. Gheorghiade, M.; Zannad, F.; Sopko, G.; Klein, L.; Piña, I.L.; Konstam, M.A.; Massie, B.M.; Roland, E.; Targum, S.; Collins, S.P.; et al. Acute heart failure syndromes: Current state and framework for future research. *Circulation* **2005**, *112*, 3958–3968. [CrossRef]
19. Dobbe, L.; Rahman, R.; Elmassry, M.; Paz, P.; Nugent, K. Cardiogenic Pulmonary Edema. *Am. J. Med. Sci.* **2019**, *358*, 389–397. [CrossRef]
20. Tsuchiya, N.; Griffin, L.; Yabuuchi, H.; Kawanami, S.; Shinzato, J.; Murayama, S. Imaging findings of pulmonary edema: Part 1. Cardiogenic pulmonary edema and acute respiratory distress syndrome. *Acta Radiol.* **2020**, *61*, 184–194. [CrossRef]
21. Vergani, G.; Cressoni, M.; Crimella, F.; L'Acqua, C.; Sisillo, E.; Gurgitano, M.; Liguori, A.; Annoni, A.; Carrafiello, G.; Chiumello, D. A Morphological and Quantitative Analysis of Lung CT Scan in Patients with Acute Respiratory Distress Syndrome and in Cardiogenic Pulmonary Edema. *J. Intensive Care Med.* **2020**, *35*, 284–292. [CrossRef] [PubMed]
22. Sacchetti, A.D.; Harris, R.H. Acute cardiogenic pulmonary edema. What's the latest in emergency treatment? *Postgrad Med.* **1998**, *103*, 145–166. [CrossRef]
23. Trayes, K.P.; Studdiford, J.S.; Pickle, S.; Tully, A.S. Edema: Diagnosis and management. *Am. Fam. Physician* **2013**, *88*, 102–110. [PubMed]
24. Verdolini, K.; Min, Y.; Titze, I.R.; Lemke, J.; Brown, K.; van Mersbergen, M.; Jiang, J.J.; Fisher, K. Biological Mechanisms Underlying Voice Changes Due to Dehydration. *J. Speech Lang. Heart Res.* **2002**, *45*, 268–281. [CrossRef]
25. Murton, O.M.; Hillman, R.E.; Mehta, D.D. Acoustic speech analysis of patients with decompensated heart failure: A pilot study. *J. Acoust. Soc. Am.* **2017**, *142*, EL401–EL407. [CrossRef]
26. Toback, M.; Clark, N. Strategies to improve self-management in heart failure patients. *Contemp. Nurse* **2017**, *53*, 105–120. [CrossRef] [PubMed]
27. Andrews, A.M.; Russell, C.L.; Cheng, A.L. Medication Adherence Interventions for Older Adults with Heart Failure: A systematic Review. *J. Gerontol. Nurs.* **2017**, *43*, 37–45. [CrossRef]
28. Savarese, G.; Lund, L.H. Global Public Health Burden of Heart Failure. *Card. Fail. Rev.* **2017**, *3*, 7–11. [CrossRef]
29. Johnson, K.; Soto, J.T.; Glicksberg, B.; Shameer, K.; Miotto, R.; Ali, M.; Ashley, E.; Dudley, J.T. Artificial Intelligence in Cardiology. *J. Am. Coll. Cardiol.* **2018**, *71*, 2668–2679. [CrossRef]
30. Bonderman, D. Artificial intelligence in cardiology. *Wien. Klin. Wochenschr.* **2017**, *129*, 866–868. [CrossRef] [PubMed]

31. Ramesh, A.N.; Kambhampati, C.; Monson, R.T., Jr.; Drew, P.J. Artificial intelligence in medicine. *Ann. R. Coll. Surg. Engl.* **2004**, *86*, 334–338. [CrossRef]
32. Dawes, T.J.W.; de Marvao, A.; Shi, W.; Fletcher, T.; Watson, G.M.J.; Wharton, J.; Rhodes, C.J.; Howard, L.S.G.E.; Gibbs, J.S.R.; Rueckert, D.; et al. Machine Learning of Three-dimensional Right Ventricular Motion Enables Outcome Prediction in Pulmonary Hypertension: A Cardiac MR Imaging Study. *Radiology* **2017**, *283*, 381–390. [CrossRef]
33. Choi, D.-J.; Park, J.J.; Ali, T.; Lee, S. Artificial intelligence for the diagnosis of heart failure. *npj Digit. Med.* **2020**, *3*, 1–6. [CrossRef] [PubMed]
34. Guo, A.; Pasque, M.; Loh, F.; Mann, D.L.; Payne, P.R.O. Heart Failure Diagnosis, Readmission, and Mortality Prediction Using Machine Learning and Artificial Intelligence Models. *Curr. Epidemiol. Rep.* **2020**, *7*, 212–219. [CrossRef]
35. Khader, S.; Johnson, K.W.; Yahi, A.; Miotto, R.; Li, L.; Ricks, D.; Jebakaran, J.; Kovatch, P.; Sengupta, P.P.; Gelijns, S.; et al. Predictive modeling of hospital readmission rates using electronic medical record-wide machine learning: A case-study using Mount Sinai Heart Failure Cohort. *Pac. Symp. Biocomput.* **2017**, *22*, 276–287.
36. Dolgin, M.; New York Heart Association; Criteria Committee. *Nomenclature and Criteria for Diagnosis of Diseases of the Heart and Great Vessels*, 9th ed.; Little Brown & Co.: Boston, MA, USA, 1994; pp. 253–256.
37. Magre, S.B.; Janse, P.V.; Desmukh, R.R. A review on Feature Extraction and Noise Reduction Technique. *Int. J. Adv. Res. Comput. Sci. Softw. Eng.* **2014**, *4*, 352–356.
38. Sidey-Gibbons, J.A.M.; Sidey-Gibbons, C.J. Machine learning in medicine: A practical introduction. *BMC Med. Res. Methodol.* **2019**, *19*, 1–18. [CrossRef]
39. Cortes, C.; Vapnik, V.N. Support-vector networks. *Mach. Learn.* **1995**, *20*, 273–297. [CrossRef]
40. Zhang, R.; Li, B.; Peng, T. Audio classification based on SVM-UBM. In Proceedings of the 9th International Conference on Signal Processing Beijing, Beijing, China, 26–29 October 2008; pp. 1586–1589.
41. Hofmann, T.; Schölkopf, B.; Smola, A.J. Kernel methods in machine learning. *Ann. Stat.* **2008**, *36*, 1171–1220. [CrossRef]
42. Schmidhuber, J. Deep Learning in Neural Networks: An Overview. *Neural Netw.* **2015**, *61*, 85–117. [CrossRef] [PubMed]
43. Hastie, T.; Tibshirani, R.; Friedman, J. *The Elements of Statistical Learning: Data Mining, Inference, and Prediction: With 200 Full-Color Illustrations*; Springer: New York, NY, USA, 2001.
44. Lin, Y.; Wang, J. Research on the Text Classification Based on SVM-KNN. In Proceedings of the 2014 IEEE 5th International Conference on Software Engineering and Service Science, Beijing, China, 27–29 June 2014.
45. Groenewegen, A.; Rutten, F.H.; Mosterd, A.; Hoes, A.W. Epidemiologyand of heart failure. *Eur. J. Heart Fail.* **2020**, *22*, 1342–1356. [CrossRef] [PubMed]
46. Jones, N.R.; Roalfe, A.K.; Adoki, I.; Hobbs, F.D.R.; Taylor, C.J. Survival of patients with chronic heart failure in the community: A systematic review and meta-analysis. *Eur. J. Heart Fail.* **2019**, *21*, 1306–1325. [CrossRef]
47. Dharmarajan, K.; Rich, M.W. Epidemiology, Pathophysiology and Prognosis of Heart Failure in Older Adults. *Heart Fail. Clin.* **2017**, *13*, 417–426. [CrossRef]
48. Cook, C.; Cole, G.; Asaria, P.; Jabbour, R.; Francis, D.P. The annual global economic burden of heart failure. *Int. J. Cardiol.* **2014**, *171*, 368–376. [CrossRef]
49. Zugck, C.; Muller, A.; Helms, T.M.; Wildau, H.J.; Becks, T.; Hacker, J.; Haag, S.; Goldhagen, K.; Schwab, J.O. Health economic impact of heart failure: An analysis of the nationwide German database. *Dtsch. Med. Wochenschr.* **2010**, *135*, 633–638. [CrossRef]
50. Delgado, J.F.; Oliva, J.; Llano, M.; Pascual-Figal, D.; Grillo, J.J.; Comín-Colet, J.; Díaz, B.; de la Concha, L.M.; Martí, B.; Peña, L.M. Health care and non-health care costs in the treatment of patients with symptomatic chronic heart failure in Spain. *Rev. Esp. Cardiol.* **2014**, *67*, 643–650. [CrossRef]
51. Dunlay, S.M.; Shah, N.D.; Shi, Q.; Morlan, B.; VanHouten, H.; Long, K.H.; Roger, V.L. Lifetime costs of medical care after heart failure diagnosis. *Circ. Cardiovasc. Qual. Outcomes* **2011**, *4*, 68–75. [CrossRef]
52. Jadczyk, T.; Wojakowski, W.; Tendera, M.; Henry, T.D.; Egnaczyk, G.; Shreenivas, S. Artificial Intelligence Can Improve Patient Management at the Time of a Pandemic: The Role of Voice Technology. *J. Med. Internet Res.* **2021**, *23*, e22959. [CrossRef] [PubMed]

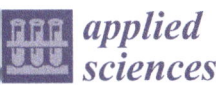

Article

Nonlinear Random Forest Classification, a Copula-Based Approach

Radko Mesiar [1,2] and Ayyub Sheikhi [3,*]

[1] Department of Mathematics and Descriptive Geometry, Faculty of Civil Engineering, Slovak University of Technology in Bratislava, Radlinskeho 11, 810 05 Bratislava, Slovakia; radko.mesiar@stuba.sk
[2] Institute for Research and Applications of Fuzzy Modeling, University of Ostrava, 30. Dubna 22, 701 03 Ostrava, Czech Republic
[3] Department of Statistics, Faculty of Mathematics and Computer, Shahid Bahonar University of Kerman, Kerman 7616913439, Iran
* Correspondence: sheikhy.a@uk.ac.ir

Abstract: In this work, we use a copula-based approach to select the most important features for a random forest classification. Based on associated copulas between these features, we carry out this feature selection. We then embed the selected features to a random forest algorithm to classify a label-valued outcome. Our algorithm enables us to select the most relevant features when the features are not necessarily connected by a linear function; also, we can stop the classification when we reach the desired level of accuracy. We apply this method on a simulation study as well as a real dataset of COVID-19 and for a diabetes dataset.

Keywords: random forest; copula; mutual information; classification; COVID-19

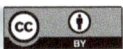

1. Introduction

Dimension reduction is a major area of interest within the field of data mining and knowledge discovery, especially in high-dimensional analysis. Recently, the issue of machine learning has received considerable attention; hence, a number of researchers have sought to perform more accurate dimension reductions in this issue [1,2]. While dimension reduction tries to reduce the dimension of data by selecting some functions of the original dataset, feature selection is one of its special cases, which selects the most important features among all of them. There are many areas of statistics and machine learning that benefit from feature selection techniques. From the statistics point of view, Han and Liu et al. (2013) [3] and Basabi (2008) [4] have applied feature selection for multivariate time series. Debashis et al. (2008) [5] have investigated feature selection and regression in high-dimensional problems.

It is known that selecting the most important and relevant features is the main aim in decision tree/random forest algorithms. Although there are many classification approaches proposed in the literature, they rarely deal with the possible existence of nonlinear relations between attributes. On the other hand, note that mutual information-based filter methods have gained popularity due to their ability to capture the non-linear association between dependent and independent variables in a machine learning setting. Mutual information based on a copula function will be a good choice to carry out a feature selection in which the results are stable against noises and outliers [6,7]. So, one of the major aims of this work is using feature selection in a classification context based on a copula function, especially in random forest classification.

Random forests are commonly used machine learning algorithm, which are a combination of various independent decision trees that are trained independently on a random subset of data and use averaging to improve the predictive accuracy and control over-/under-fitting [8–11]. In this work, in order to extract the most important features in random forest, we use associated copula of features. In this regard, the connection copula between the exploratory variables as well as the associated copula of exploratory attributes and the class labeled attribute are considered. The rest of the paper is organized as follows: we review preliminaries and introduce our method in the next section; we illustrate our algorithm considering simulated data as well as two real datasets in Section 3; finally, Section 4 is devoted to some concluding remarks.

2. Preliminaries and Related Works

The application of feature selection in machine learning and data mining techniques has been extensively considered in the literature. Kabir et al. (2020) [12] used a neural network to carry out a feature selection, while Zheng et al. (2020) [11] used a feature selection approach in a deep neural network. Li et al. (2017) [13] reviewed the feature selection techniques in data mining; see also the book of Lin and Motoda (2012) [14]. For more information, we refer to Hastie et al. (2009) [3], Chao et al. (2019) [15] and Sheikhpour et al. (2017) [16].

Peng et al. (2019) [17] and Yao et al. (2020) [18] have discussed random forest-based feature selection. It is known that the dependence structure between features plays an important role in dimension reduction. Huag et al. (2009) [19] carried out a dimension reduction based on extreme dependence between attributes. Paul et al. (2017) [5] used feature selection for outcome prediction in medical sciences. Zhang and Zhou (2010) [20] investigated multi-label dimensionality reduction features by maximizing the dependence between the original feature description and the associated class labels; see also Zhong et al. (2018) [21]. Shin and Park (2011) [22] analyzed a correlation-based dimension reduction.

In this work, we use dependence structures between variables to find the best feature selection and construct an agglomerative information gain of random forest. We apply our algorithm to classify influenza and COVID-19 patients. Iwendi et al. (2020) [23] carried out a COVID-19 patient health prediction using a random forest algorithm. Li et al. (2020) [13] applied machine learning methods to generate a computational classification model for discriminating between COVID-19 patients and influenza patients only based on clinical variables. See also Wu et al. (2020) [24], Ceylan (2020) [25] and Li et al. (2020) [13] and references therein for more information. Azar et al. (2014) [26] applied a random forest classifier for lymph diseases. See also Subasi et al. (2017) [27] for chronic kidney disease diagnosis using random forest; Açıcı et al. (2017) [28] for a random forest method to detect Parkinson disease; Jabbar et al. (2016) [29] for a prediction of heart disease using random forest. Additionally, a review work of Remeseiro et al. (2019) [30] may be helpful regarding this subject.

Sun et al. (2020) [31] have implemented a mutual information-based feature selection.

Assume that $F_{X_1,X_2,...,X_d}$ is the joint multivariate distribution function of the random vector $X = (X_1, X_2, \ldots, X_d)$ and F_{X_i}, $i = 1, 2, \ldots, d$, are the related marginal distribution functions. A grounded d-increasing uniformly marginal function $C : [0,1]^d \to [0,1]$ is called a copula of X whenever it couples the multivariate distribution function $F_{X_1,X_2,...,X_d}$ to its marginals F_{X_i}, $i = 1, 2, \ldots, d$, i.e.,

$$F_{X_1,X_2,...,X_d}(x_1, x_2, \ldots, x_d) = C_X(F_{X_1}(x_1), F_{X_2}(x_2), \ldots, F_{X_d}(x_d)). \tag{1}$$

Note that if X is a continuous random vector, then the copula C_X is unique. For more details concerning copulas, their families and association measures, we recommend Nelsen (2006) [32] and Durante and Sempi (2016) [33]. Merits of copulas and dependence measures in dimension reduction have been discussed in the literature. See, for instance, Snehalika et al. (2020) [34] and Chang et al. (2016) [35] for copula-based feature selection; Ozdemir et al. (2017) [36] and Salinas-Gutiérrez et al. (2010) [37] for classification algorithms using copulas; Marta et al. (2017) [38] and Lascio et al. (2018) [39] for copula-based clustering approaches; Houari et al. (2106) [40] and Kluppelberg and Kuhn (2009) [41] for copula functions used in dimension reduction.

A well-known measure of uncertainty in a probability distribution is its average Hartley information measure called (Shannon) entropy. For a discrete random variable X with values $x_1, x_2, \ldots, x_n$ and mass density function $p(.)$, its entropy is defined as:

$$H(X) = -\sum_{i=1}^{n} p(x_i) \log p(x_i), \tag{2}$$

and for a continuous random variable X, its (differential) entropy is given by:

$$H(X) = -\int_{\mathcal{X}} p(x) \log p(x) dx, \tag{3}$$

where $\mathcal{X}$ is the support of X. Similarly, for a (continuous) multivariate random vector X of dimension k with the multivariate density $p(X)$, the entropy is defined as:

$$H(X) = -\oint_{\mathcal{X}} p(X) \log p(X) dX, \tag{4}$$

where $\oint$ is an k-integral on $\mathcal{X}$. For two random variables X and Y with joint distribution $p(x, y)$, the conventional information gain (IG) or mutual information (MI) is defined as:

$$I(X, Y) = \int_{\mathcal{X}} \int_{\mathcal{Y}} p(x, y) \log \frac{p(x, y)}{p(x)p(y)} dx dy, \tag{5}$$

which is used to measure the amount of information shared by X and Y together, with convention $\frac{0}{0} = 1$. Moreover, one may generalize this concept to a continuous random vector $X = (X_1, X_1, \ldots, X_k)$ as:

$$I(X) = \oint_{\mathcal{X}} p(X) \log \frac{p(X)}{\prod_{i=1}^{k} p(x_i)} dX, \tag{6}$$

Ma and Sun (2011) [42] defined the concept of "copula entropy". Based on their definition, for a multivariate random vector X, which is associated with copula density $c(u)$, its copula entropy is:

$$h_c(X) = -\oint_u c(u) \log c(X) du.$$

Additionally, they have pointed out that the mutual information is a copula entropy. Indeed we have the following lemmas

Lemma 1. Ref. [32] *For a multivariate random vector X with the multivariate density $p(X)$ and copula density $c_X(u)$,*

$$I(X) = -h_c(X).$$

Finally, the conditional mutual information is useful to express the mutual information of two random vectors conditioned by a third random vector. If we have a k-dimensional random vector X, m-dimensional random vector Y and n-dimensional random vector Z, such that $X \sim p_X(x)$, $Y \sim p_Y(y)$, $Z \sim p_Z(z)$, $(X, Z) \sim p_{X,Z}(x, z)$, $(Y, Z) \sim p_{Y,Z}(y, z)$ and $(X, Y, Z) \sim p_{X,Y,Z}(x, y, z)$, then mutual information of X,Y given Z which is referred to as "conditional information gain" or "conditional mutual information" of variables X and Y given Z is obtained as:

$$I(X, Y|Z) = \oint_z \oint_y \oint_x p_{X,Y,Z}(x, y, z) \log \frac{p_Z(z) p_{X,Y,Z}(x, y, z)}{p_{X,Z}(x, z) p_{Y,Z}(, y, z)} dx dy dz. \tag{7}$$

3. Copula-Based Random Forest

The connection between mutual information and copula function has been investigated in the literature. We can also represent the conditional mutual information via the copula function through the following proposition:

Proposition 1. *If the random vector (X, Y, Z) is associated with copula $C_{X,Y,Z}(u, v, w)$, then Equation (7) is*

$$I(X, Y|Z) = h_c(X, Z) + h_c(Y, Z) - h_c(X, Y, Z) - h_c(Z) \tag{8}$$

Proof of Proposition 1. By an appropriate equivalent modification of the argument of the log function in the integrand of (7), we readily obtain:

$$I(X, Y|Z) = \oint_Z \oint_Y \oint_X p_{X,Y,Z}(x, y, z) \log \frac{p_Z(z) p_{X,Y,Z}(x, y, z)}{p_{X,Z}(x, z) p_{Y,Z}(, y, z)} dx dy dz$$

$$= -h(X, Z) - h(Y, Z) + h(X, Y, Z) + h(Z)$$

$$= h_c(X, Z) + h_c(Y, Z) - h_c(X, Y, Z) - h_c(Z).$$

The last equality comes from one of the results of Ma and Sun (2011), which proves that for $X = (X_1, X_2, \ldots, X_n)$,

$$h(X) = \sum_{i=1}^{n} h(X_i) + h_c(X).$$

In order to use the mutual information in the decision trees, assume we have a dataset $D = \{(x_1, y_1), (x_2, y_2), \ldots, (x_n, y_n)\}$, where $x_i \in \mathcal{X}$ is the i-th input or observation and $y_i \in \mathcal{Y}$ is the corresponding outcome variable. In a machine learning approach, the major goal is constructing (or finding) a classification map $f : \mathcal{X} \to \mathcal{Y}$ which takes the features $x \in \mathcal{X}$ of a data point as its input and outputs a predicted label. The special case of the outcome variable is a class label $y_i \in \{-1, 1\}$; i.e., it has two possible values, such as: negative/positive, pathogenic/benign, patient/normal, etc. The general objective function that must be maximized is:

$$J_{CMI}(X_k) = I(X_k, Y) - \beta \sum_{i=1}^{n} I(X_i, X_k) - \gamma \sum_{i=1}^{n} I(X_i, X_j|Y) \tag{9}$$

where $I(X_k, Y)$ measures the relation between term X_k and target variable Y, $I(X_i, X_k)$ quantifies the redundancy between X_i and X_k; while $I(X_i, X_j|Y)$ measures the complementarity between terms X_i and X. $\square$

Similar to Proposition 1, one may state the Equation (9) based on copula as:

$$J_{CMI}(X_k) = h_c(X_k, Y) + \beta \sum_{i=1}^{n} h_c(X_i, X_k)$$

$$- \gamma \sum_{i=1}^{n} [h_c(X_i, Y) + h_c(X_k, Y) - h_c(X_i, X_k, Y) - h_c(Y)]$$

$$= (1 - \gamma(n+1)) h_c(X_k, Y) + n\gamma h(Y)$$

$$+ \beta \sum_{i=1}^{n} h_c(X_i, X_k) - \gamma \sum_{k \neq i=1}^{n} h_c(X_i, Y) + \gamma \sum_{i=1}^{n} h_c(X_i, X_k, Y),$$

where the first term of the last part of equality refers to the relevancy of the new feature X_k. Peng et al. (2019) [17] introduced the "Minimum Redundancy Maximum Relevance (mRMR)" criterion to set the value of β to be the reverse of the number of selected features and $\gamma = 0$. We generalize their results by simplifying $J_{CMI}(X_k)$. In particular, we have the following criterion, which we have to maximize:

$$J_{MRMR}(X_k) = I(X_k, Y) - \frac{1}{|S|}\sum_{i=1}^{n} I(X_i, X_k) = -h_c(X_k, Y) + \frac{1}{|S|}\sum_{i=1}^{n} h_c(X_i, X_k) \qquad (10)$$

From this formula, it can be seen that mRMR tries to select features that have high correlation to the target variable while they are mutually far away from each other, and in this case, the couple of functions plays an important role in the connection between the input and class level variables.

Since decision trees are prone to overfitting and do not globally find an optimal solution, their generalization, random forests, are suggested to overcome these disadvantages. Our algorithm considers the dependence between attributes to provide the best feature selection set and embeds these selected features to a random forest procedure. In this approach, we first use the dependence between attributes to choose the max-dependent as well as the max-relevant features to the class label and eliminate the max-redundant features. From the point of view of these three criteria, our approach is equivalent to the method presented by Peng et al. (2019) [17].

The confusion matrix is a metric that is often used to measure the performance of a classification algorithm. It is also called a contingency table and in a binary classification it is a 2 × 2 table, as shown in Figure 1.

$$Sensitivity = \frac{TP}{TP + FN}. \qquad (11)$$

$$Specificity = \frac{TN}{TN + FP}. \qquad (12)$$

$$Accuracy = \frac{TP + TN}{TP + TN + FP + FN}. \qquad (13)$$

		Predicted Class	
		Positive	Negative
Actual Class	Positive	True Positives (TP)	False Negatives (FN)
	Negative	False Positives (FP)	True Negatives (TN)

Figure 1. Confusion matrix.

We use our copula-based random forest to find the most relevant features and carry out a classification task. For this, using the copula function which connects input variables with each other as well as with the class variable, we find the most important variables by maximizing of these three criterions and then, based on their priorities, we embed them to a random forest approach to classify the class label feature. We continue our selection to find the most important feature until we reach the desired level of criteria. Traditional criteria can define some values of accuracy/sensitivity/specificity. Inspired by Snehalika et al. (2020) [34], Algorithm 1 presents a pseudo code of this method. Without loss of generality, we consider that the criterion is the accuracy. The algorithm for the sensitivity and specificity is the same.

Algorithm 1. Algorithm of copula-based random forest classification.

Result Data: data set $\mathcal{D} = (X, Y)$, threshold value δ.
Result: Selected feature set $\mathcal{S}$, Classification results.
1 Initialization: $\mathcal{S} = 0$, $accuracy = 0$, F = all features,
2 while $accuracy \leq \delta$ do
3 $x_R = \underset{X_k \in F \setminus S}{argmax} \left[-h_c(X_k, Y) + \frac{1}{|S|} \sum_{i=1}^{n} h_c(X_i, X_k) \right]$;
4 $\mathcal{S} = \mathcal{S} \cup x_R$;
5 $F = F \setminus \mathcal{S}$;
6 Perform a random Forrest classification;
7 the accuracy of random forest classification using 13;
8 $accuracy = Acc_{new} + accuracy$;
9 end

4. Numerical Results

A simulated dataset as well as real data analysis is presented to illustrate our method.

4.1. Simulation Study

In order to carry out a simulation study, we generated data from normal distribution with copula dependence. Our considered copulas were Gaussian, t and Gumbel copulas; see, e.g., Nelsen (2006) [32]. Using the copula library, we first generated $n = 10,000$ random samples $x_1, \ldots, x_{10}$ from a 10-variate Gaussian copula where all off-diagonal elements of their correlation matrix equal to $\rho = 0.85$ and their marginals follow the standard normal distribution. In a similar fashion, again, we generated another 10 variates $x_{11}, \ldots, x_{20}$ independent from the first 10 variables. Then, for simulating from t-copula, we generated 10-variates $x_{21}, \ldots, x_{30}$ from t-copula with all correlation values equal to $\rho = 0.85$, $df = 19$ [43] and their marginals follow the standard normal distribution. Finally, a bivariate Gumbel copula with $\theta = 5$ [44] and normal marginals were generated and inserted into x_{31}, x_{32}. A schematic heatmap plot of these 32 features is shown in Figure 2. Using a linear combination, we added values of these feathers and made the outcome variable. In order to obtain a class-valued variable, we recoded the negative values of the outcome variable to "0" and other values to "1".

Using Algorithm 1, we started with $n = 2$ features. The most important features to classify y were x_{26} and x_{32} with sensitivity = 0.869, specificity = 0.867 and accuracy = 0.875. Continuing the selection of the most relevant features has led us to x_{26}, x_{32} and x_{31} as the first three relevant features. In order to obtain unbiased results, we performed a 10-fold cross validation, and in each fold, we left out 1000 cases as a test group and the remainder for the train set. Averages of sensitivity, specificity and accuracy were calculated to assess the algorithm. Table 1 shows the most relevant and least redundant features with their evaluation scales sensitivity, specificity and accuracy. This table helps us to assess our algorithm by monitoring its running time as well as its comparison with other algorithms. Since, after selecting the features, we use the traditional random forest approach, it is reasonable that we compare our results with the results of the traditional random forest approach. Comparing the last two rows of Table 1, we deduce that the results of our algorithm and the traditional random forest algorithm are the same.

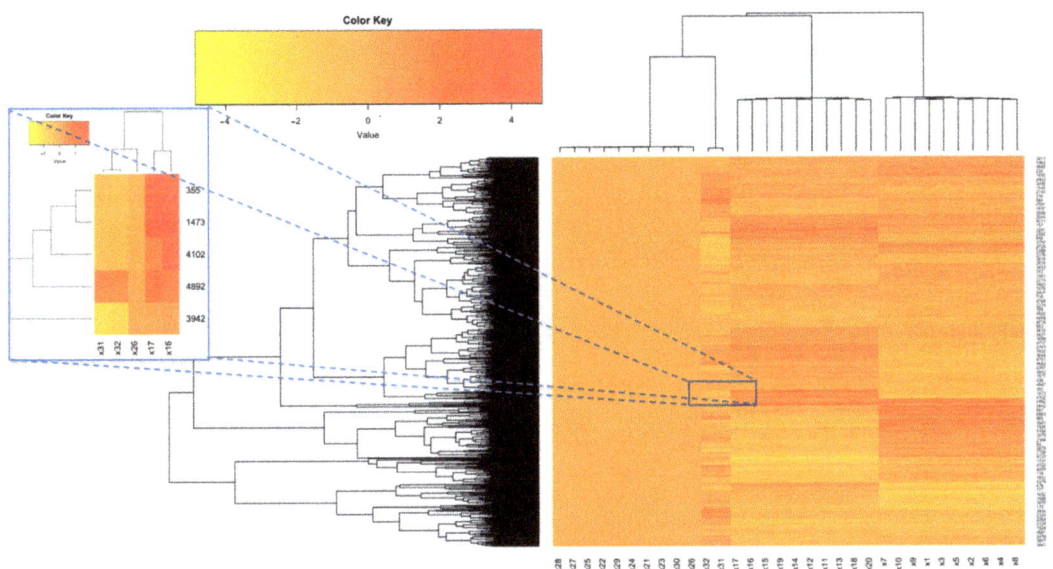

Figure 2. Heatmap plots of simulated data.

Table 1. Selected feature with their measures of assessment in simulate data.

n	Relevant Attributes	Sensitivity	Specificity	Accuracy	Running Time
2	x26, x32	0.869	0.867	0.875	4.51
3	x26, x32, x31	0.879	0.869	0.879	4.91
4	x26 x32 x31 x16	0.880	0.873	0.880	5.12
5	x26, x32, x31, x16, x13	0.881	0.878	0.881	5.55
6	x26, x32, x31, x16, x13, x12	0.888	0.880	0.886	5.83
7	x26, x32, x31, x16, x13, x12, x20	0.891	0.888	0.891	6.33
8	x26, x32, x31, x16, x13, x12, x20, x18	0.893	0.892	0.892	6.55
10	x26, x32, x31, x16, x13, x20, x12, x18, x17, x14	0.898	0.895	0.893	6.92
15	x26, x32, x31, x16, x13, x12, x20, x18, x14, x17 x15, x11, x19, x3, x7	0.908	0.896	0.901	8.34
20	x26, x32, x31, x16, x13, x12, x20, x18, x14, x17 x11, x15, x19, x3, x7, x9, x8, x5, x6, x1	0.918	0.909	0.917	11.30
25	x26, x32, x31, x16, x13, x12, x20, x18, x17, x14, x11, x15, x19, x3, x7, x8, x9, x6, x5, x1 x4, x2, x10, x27, x29	0.929	0.939	0.934	13.61
32	All attributes: x1, x2, … ,x32	0.982	0.979	0.981	16.75
32	Traditional random forest	0.982	0.979	0.981	16.75

Additionally, from the running time point of view, as seen from the last column of the table, for a small number of attributes, the running time (based on seconds) is negligible, and by increasing the number of attributes, the running time increases significantly. From the pros and cons point of view of the proposed approach, as understood from this table, there is a design-of-experiment approach that physicians may encounter. They can regulate the number of desired attributes to carry out a reasonable random forest classification based on the percentage of accuracy, specificity and sensitivity. Evidently, as seen from the last column of Table 1, after selecting attributes using copula, such a classification algorithm will run fast for a small number of attributes; one may think this is an operation research problem. Specifically, the sample size, the number of attributes and the complexity of relationship between attributes play important roles in such a classification procedure. So, from the point of view of the practical implications, these results enable researchers to specify the number of attributes based on the desired levels of sensitivity, specificity and accuracy, and if the relationship between attributes is not complicated, one can choose a greater number of attributes and achieve more accuracy, and vice versa.

4.2. COVID-19 Dataset

Li et al. (2020) [13], in a meta-analysis, merged 151 datasets of COVID-19 including patient symptoms and routine test results. Nineteen clinical variables were included as explanatory inputs. The variables included age, sex, serum levels of neutrophil (continuous and ordinal), serum levels of leukocytes (continuous and ordinal), serum levels of lymphocytes (continuous and ordinal), results of CT scans, results of chest X-rays, reported symptoms (diarrhea, fever, coughing, sore throat, nausea and fatigue), body temperature, and underlying risk factors (renal diseases and diabetes) [13]. By applying machine learning methods, they reanalyzed these data and investigated correlation between explanatory variables and generated a computational classification model for discriminating between COVID-19 patients and influenza patients based on clinical variables alone.

In a COVID-19 patient case, an agglomerative approach test may help diagnosis of illness. We used our copula-based feature selection to identify the most effective attributes to make a discrimination between COVID-19 patients and influenza patients. We started with two attributes. The most relevant attributes were "age" and "fatigue". We then applied these two attributes to separate the COVID-19 and influenza patients and obtained evaluation values sensitivity, specificity and accuracy, respectively as 0.755, 0.864 and 0.836. Seeking the three most important classification attributes lead us to "age", "fatigue" and "nausea/vomiting" with sensitivity equaling 0.840, specificity equaling 0.886 and accuracy equaling 0.873. Table 2 summarizes the 10 most important features with their classification evaluation's scores. As understood from this table, there is a design-of-experiment approach that a physician may encounter. In fact, the required percentage of information determines the number and types of tests of patients. For example, if there is a required 85% accuracy of classification only, then it is enough to know "age", "fatigue" and "nausea/vomiting" of patients, while for 91.4% accuracy, we need to test the 15 most important attributes.

Table 2. Selected features with their measures of assessment in COVID-19 dataset.

n	Names of Attributes	Sensitivity	Specificity	Accuracy
2	Age, Fatigue	0.755	0.864	0.836
3	Age, Fatigue, Nausea/Vomiting	0.840	0.886	0.873
4	Age, Fatigue, Nausea/Vomiting, Diarrhea	0.826	0.875	0.860
5	Age, Fatigue, Nausea/Vomiting, Diarrhea, Sore Throat	0.783	0.891	0.860
10	Age, Fatigue, Nausea/Vomiting, Diarrhea, Sore Throat, X-ray Results, Shortness of Breath, Neutrophil, Serum Levels of White Blood Cell, Risk Factors	0.735	0.922	0.865
15	Age, Fatigue, Nausea/Vomiting, Diarrhea, Sore Throat, X-ray Results, Shortness of Breath, Neutrophil, Serum Levels of White Blood Cell, Risk Factors, Temperature, Coughing, Lymphocytes, Neutrophil Categorical, Sex	0.873	0.929	0.914

4.3. Diabetes 130-US Hospitals Dataset

In this subsection, we assess our approach in a big data analysis. We apply our algorithm to classify the Diabetes 130-US hospitals dataset [45]. This dataset represents 10 years (1999–2008) of clinical care at 130 US hospitals and integrated delivery networks. It is comprised of 101,721 observations of 50 features representing patient and hospital outcomes. The data contains such attributes as "race", "gender", "age", "admission type", "time in hospital" and another 45 attributes. Detailed descriptions of all the attributes are provided in Strack et al. (2014).

We used the "diabetesMed" variable (0 and 1) as our response/target class variable and applied the other attributes to classify patients into two groups: no medical prescription needed and medical prescription needed. Similar to the previous subsection, the results are summarized in Table 3.

Table 3. Selected features with their measures of assessment in Diabetes 130-Us hospital dataset.

n	Names of Attributes	Sensitivity	Specificity	Accuracy
2	num_medications, num_procedures	0.742	0.756	0.708
3	num_medications, num_procedures, A1Cresult	0.766	0.771	0.780
5	num_medications, num_procedures, A1Cresult, epaglinide, max_glu_serum	0.837	0.806	0.801
10	num_medications, number_diagnoses, age, A1Cresult, repaglinide, max_glu_serum, weight, glimepiride, rosiglitazone, pioglitazone	0.921	0.948	0.871
20	num_medications, number_diagnoses, age, A1Cresult, repaglinide, max_glu_serum, weight, glimepiride, rosiglitazone, pioglitazone, glyburide, number_emergency, glipizide, number_outpatient, race, metformin, diag_2, readmitted, repaglinide, diag_3	0.981	0.977	0.972
50	All attributes	0.986	0.981	0.978

5. Conclusions

A copula-based algorithm has been employed in a random forest classification. In this regard, the most important features were extracted based on their associated copulas. The simulation study as well as real data analysis have shown that the proposed couple-based algorithm may be helpful when the explanatory variables are connected nonlinearly and when we are going to extract the most important features instead of all features.

The idea of this paper may be extended in some manners. One may use this idea in a multi-class random forest classification. Additionally, a random forest regression considering the connecting copula of features will be useful. Moreover, the associated copula of features in order classification tasks such as the support vector machine, discriminant analysis and naive Bayes classification will be of interest. Many extensions of random forest have been investigated by several authors, for example, boosted random forest, deep dynamic random forest, ensemble learning methods random forest, etc. Each extension of the random forest classification may be combined with our approach to obtain better results. We are going to extend these results in a longitudinal dataset in which the outcome variables are connected using some copulas.

Author Contributions: Conceptualization, R.M. and A.S. All authors have read and agreed to the published version of the manuscript.

Funding: APVV-18-0052 and VEGA 1/0006/19.

Institutional Review Board Statement: Not applicable.

Informed Consent Statement: Not applicable.

Data Availability Statement: https://archive.ics.uci.edu/ml/datasets/diabetes+130-us+hospitals+for+years+1999-2008 (accessed on 2 June 2021).

Acknowledgments: The work of the first author was supported by the project APVV-18-0052 and VEGA 1/0006/19. Additionally, the authors wish to thank the anonymous reviewers for the comments and suggestions that have led to a significant improvement of the original manuscript.

Conflicts of Interest: The authors declare no conflict of interest.

References

1. Han, M.; Liu, X. Feature selection techniques with class separability for multivariate time series. *Neurocomputing* **2013**, *110*, 29–34. [CrossRef]
2. Breiman, L. Random forests. *Mach. Learn.* **2001**, *45*, 5–32. [CrossRef]
3. Hastie, T.; Tibshirani, R.; Friedman, J. *The Elements of Statistical Learning: Data Mining, Inference, and Prediction*; Springer Science & Business Media: Berlin, Germany, 2009.
4. Chakraborty, B. Feature selection for multivariate time series. In Proceedings of the IASC 2008 4th World Conference of IASC on Computational Statistics and Data Analysis, Yokohama, Japan, 5–8 December 2008; pp. 227–233.
5. Paul, D.; Su, R.; Romain, M.; Sébastien, V.; Pierre, V.; Isabelle, G. Feature selection for outcome prediction in oesophageal cancer using genetic algorithm and random forest classifier. *Comput. Med. Imaging Graph.* **2017**, *60*, 42–49. [CrossRef]
6. Battiti, R. Using mutual information for selecting features in supervised neural net learning. *IEEE Trans. Neural Netw.* **1994**, *5*, 537–550. [CrossRef]
7. Li, J.; Cheng, K.; Wang, S.; Morstatter, F.; Trevino, R.P.; Tang, J.; Liu, H. Feature selection: A data perspective. *ACM Comput. Surv.* **2017**, *50*, 1–45. [CrossRef]
8. Biau, G.; Scornet, E. A random forest guided tour. *Test* **2016**, *25*, 197–227. [CrossRef]
9. Cutler, A.; Cutler, D.R.; Stevens, J.R. Random forests. In *Ensemble Machine Learning*; Springer: Berlin, Germany, 2012; pp. 157–175.
10. Lall, S.; Sinha, D.; Ghosh, A.; Sengupta, D.; Bandyopadhyay, S. Stable feature selection using copula-based mutual information. *Pattern Recognit.* **2021**, *112*, 107697. [CrossRef]
11. Chen, Z.; Pang, M.; Zhao, Z.; Li, S.; Miao, R.; Zhang, Y.; Feng, X.; Feng, X.; Zhang, Y.; Duan, M.; et al. Feature selection may improve deep neural networks for the bioinformatics problems. *Bioinformatics* **2020**, *36*, 1542–1552. [CrossRef]
12. Kabir, M.M.; Islam, M.M.; Murase, K. A new wrapper feature selection approach using neural network. *Neurocomputing* **2010**, *73*, 3273–3283. [CrossRef]
13. Li, W.T.; Ma, J.; Shende, N.; Castaneda, G.; Chakladar, J.; Tsai, J.C.; Apostol, L.; Honda, C.O.; Xu, J.; Wong, L.M.; et al. Using machine learning of clinical data to diagnose COVID-19. *medRxiv* **2020**, *20*, 247.
14. Liu, H.; Motoda, H. *Feature Selection for Knowledge Discovery and Data Mining*; Springer Science & Business Media: Berlin, Germany, 2012; Volume 454.
15. Chao, G.; Luo, Y.; Ding, W. Recent advances in supervised dimension reduction: A survey. *Mach. Learn. Knowl. Extr.* **2019**, *1*, 341–358. [CrossRef]
16. Sheikhpour, R.; Sarram, M.A.; Gharaghani, S.; Chahooki, M.A.Z. A survey on semi-supervised feature selection methods. *Pattern Recognit.* **2017**, *64*, 141–158. [CrossRef]
17. Peng, X.; Li, J.; Wang, G.; Wu, Y.; Li, L.; Li, Z.; Bhatti, A.A.; Zhou, C.; Hepburn, D.M.; Reid, A.J.; et al. Random forest based optimal feature selection for partial discharge pattern recognition in hv cables. *IEEE Trans. Power Deliv.* **2019**, *34*, 1715–1724. [CrossRef]
18. Yao, R.; Li, J.; Hui, M.; Bai, L.; Wu, Q. Feature selection based on random forest for partial discharges characteristic set. *IEEE Access* **2020**, *8*, 159151–159161. [CrossRef]
19. Haug, S.; Klüppelberg, C.; Kuhn, G. Copula structure analysis based on extreme dependence. *Stat. Interface* **2015**, *8*, 93–107.
20. Zhang, Y.; Zhou, Z.H. Multilabel dimensionality reduction via dependence maximization. *ACM Trans. Knowl. Discov. Data* **2010**, *4*, 1–21. [CrossRef]
21. Zhong, Y.; Xu, C.; Du, B.; Zhang, L. Independent feature and label components for multi-label classification. In *2018 IEEE International Conference on Data Mining (ICDM)*; IEEE: Piscataway, NJ, USA, 2018; pp. 827–836.
22. Shin, Y.J.; Park, C.H. Analysis of correlation based dimension reduction methods. *Int. J. Appl. Math. Comput. Sci.* **2011**, *21*, 549–558. [CrossRef]
23. Iwendi, C.; Bashir, A.K.; Peshkar, A.; Sujatha, R.; Chatterjee, J.M.; Pasupuleti, S. COVID-19 patient health prediction using boosted random forest algorithm. *Front. Public Health.* **2020**, *8*, 357. [CrossRef] [PubMed]
24. Wu, J.; Zhang, P.; Zhang, L.; Meng, W.; Li, J.; Tong, C.; Li, Y.; Cai, J.; Yang, Z.; Zhu, J.; et al. Rapid and accurate identification of covid-19 infection through machine learning based on clinical available blood test results. *medRxiv* **2020**. [CrossRef]
25. Ceylan, Z. Estimation of COVI-19 prevalence in Italy, Spain, and France. *Sci. Total Environ.* **2020**, *729*, 138817. [CrossRef]
26. Azar, A.T.; Elshazly, H.I.; Hassanien, A.E.; Elkorany, A.M. A random forest classifier for lymph diseases. *Comput. Methods Programs Biomed.* **2014**, *113*, 465–473. [CrossRef]
27. Subasi, A.; Alickovic, E.; Kevric, J. Diagnosis of chronic kidney disease by using random forest. In *CMBEBIH 2017*; Springer: Berlin, Germany, 2017; pp. 589–594.
28. Açıcı, K.; Erdaş, Ç.B.; Aşuroğlu, T.; Toprak, M.K.; Erdem, H.; Oğul, H. A random forest method to detect parkinsons disease via gait analysis. In *International Conference on Engineering Applications of Neural Networks*; Springer: Berlin, Germany, 2017; pp. 609–619.

29. Jabbar, M.A.; Deekshatulu, B.L.; Chandra, P. Prediction of heart disease using random forest and feature subset selection. In *Innovations in Bio-Inspired Computing and Applications*; Springer: Berlin, Germany, 2016; pp. 187–196.
30. Remeseiro, B.; Bolon-Canedo, V. A review of feature selection methods in medical applications. *Comput. Biol. Med.* **2019**, *112*, 103375. [CrossRef]
31. Sun, L.; Yin, T.; Ding, W.; Qian, Y.; Xu, J. Multilabel feature selection using ml-relieff and neighborhood mutual information for multilabel neighborhood decision systems. *Inf. Sci.* **2020**, *537*, 401–424. [CrossRef]
32. Nelsen, R.B. *An Introduction to Copulas*; Springer Science & Business Media: Berlin, Germany, 2006.
33. Durante, F.; Sempi, C. *Principles of Copula Theory*; CRC Press: Boca Raton, FL, USA, 2015.
34. Snehalika, L.; Debajyoti, S.; Abhik, G.H.; Debarka, S.; Sanghamitra, B. Feature selection using copula-based mutual information. *Pattern Recognit.* **2021**, *112*, 107697.
35. Chang, Y.; Li, Y.; Ding, A.; Dy, J. A robust-equitable copula dependence measure for feature selection. In Proceedings of the Artificial Intelligence and Statistics, Cadiz, Spain, 9–11 May 2016; pp. 84–92.
36. Ozdemir, O.; Allen, T.G.; Choi, S.; Wimalajeewa, T.; Varshney, P.K. Copula-based classifier fusion under statistical dependence. *IEEE Trans. Pattern Anal. Mach. Intell.* **2017**, *40*, 2740–2748. [CrossRef]
37. Salinas-Gutiérrez, R.; Hernández-Aguirre, A.; Rivera-Meraz, M.J.; Villa-Diharce, E.R. Using gaussian copulas in supervised probabilistic classification. In *Soft Computing for Intelligent Control and Mobile Robotics*; Springer: Berlin, Germany, 2010; pp. 355–372.
38. Martal, D.F.L.; Durante, F.; Pappada, R. Copula—Based clustering methods. In *Copulas and Dependence Models with Applications*; Springer: Cham, Switzerland, 2017; pp. 49–67.
39. Di Lascio, F.M.L. Coclust: An R package for copula-based cluster analysis. *Recent Appl. Data Clust.* **2018**, *93*, 74865.
40. Houari, R.; Bounceur, A.; Kechadi, M.T.; Tari, A.K.; Euler, R. Dimensionality reduction in data mining: A copula approach. *Expert Syst. Appl.* **2016**, *64*, 247–260. [CrossRef]
41. Klüppelberg, C.; Kuhn, G. Copula structure analysis. *J. R. Stat. Soc. Ser. B* **2009**, *71*, 737–753. [CrossRef]
42. Ma, J.; Sun, Z. Mutual information is copula entropy. *Tsinghua Sci. Technol.* **2011**, *16*, 51–54. [CrossRef]
43. Demarta, S.; McNeil, A.J. The t copula and related copulas. *Int. Stat. Rev.* **2005**, *73*, 111–129. [CrossRef]
44. Wang, L.; Guo, X.; Zeng, J.; Hong, Y. Using gumbel copula and empirical marginal distribution in estimation of distribution algorithm. In *Third International Workshop on Advanced Computational Intelligence*; IEEE: Piscataway, NJ, USA, 2010; pp. 583–587.
45. Strack, B.; DeShazo, J.P.; Gennings, C.; Olmo, J.L.; Ventura, S.; Cios, K.J.; Clore, J.N. Impact of HbA1c Measurement on Hospital Readmission Rates: Analysis of 70,000 Clinical Database Patient Records. *BioMed Res. Int.* **2014**, *2014*, 781670. [CrossRef]

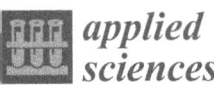

Article

A Novel Unsupervised Computational Method for Ventricular and Supraventricular Origin Beats Classification

Manuel M. Casas [1], Roberto L. Avitia [1,*], Jose Antonio Cardenas-Haro [2], Jugal Kalita [3], Francisco J. Torres-Reyes [4], Marco A. Reyna [1] and Miguel E. Bravo-Zanoguera [1]

1. Bioengineering Department, Engineering Faculty, Autonomous University of Baja California, Mexicali 21280, Mexico; manuel.martinez.casas@uabc.edu.mx (M.M.C.); mreyna@uabc.edu.mx (M.A.R.); mbravo@uabc.edu.mx (M.E.B.-Z.)
2. Department of Computer Science, Western Illinois University, Macomb, IL 61455, USA; a-cardenas-haro@wiu.edu
3. Department of Computer Science, University of Colorado, Colorado Springs, CO 80918, USA; jkalita@uccs.edu
4. Department of Computer Science, Autonomous University of San Luis Potosi, San Luis Potosí 78300, Mexico; francisco.torres@uaslp.mx
* Correspondence: ravitia@uabc.edu.mx

Abstract: Arrhythmias are the most common events tracked by a physician. The need for continuous monitoring of such events in the ECG has opened the opportunity for automatic detection. Intra- and inter-patient paradigms are the two approaches currently followed by the scientific community. The intra-patient approach seems to resolve the problem with a high classification percentage but requires a physician to label key samples. The inter-patient makes use of historic data of different patients to build a general classifier, but the inherent variability in the ECG's signal among patients leads to lower classification percentages compared to the intra-patient approach. In this work, we propose a new unsupervised algorithm that adapts to every patient using the heart rate and morphological features of the ECG beats to classify beats between supraventricular origin and ventricular origin. The results of our work in terms of F-score are 0.88, 0.89, and 0.93 for the ventricular origin beats for three popular ECG databases, and around 0.99 for the supraventricular origin for the same databases, comparable to supervised approaches presented in other works. This paper presents a new path to make use of ECG data to classify heartbeats without the assistance of a physician despite the needed improvements.

Keywords: beats classification; ECG; algorithms; ML

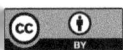

1. Introduction

The electrocardiogram (ECG), the electrical activity of the heart, has been studied extensively because of its high relevance in clinical practice. In most cases, it can provide insights into the heart condition. Common but important events physicians track are the arrhythmias, which are any disturbance in rate, regularity, site of origin, or conduction of the heart signal activity. An arrhythmia can be a single aberrant beat or a sustained rhythmic disturbance that can be present through a time period. The ECG is the best tool to diagnose these irregularities from the heart signals [1].

ECG signal is represented in a waveform graph shape, and it is considered the heart's primary source of information, as well as the primary source for detection of cardiac irregularities [2]. An arrhythmia may lead to severe heart disease such as atrial premature contraction (APC), premature ventricular contraction (PVC), right bundle branch block (RBBB), etc. [3,4]. At present, a topic that is becoming highly relevant in the application of deep learning (AI) in health are the so-called computer-aided detection (CADe) and diagnosis (CADx) in which, through a system based on recognition of patterns in images, meaning lesions in complex structures can be identified and classified through the different shapes and intensity levels in the pixels; some examples of this are the CADe/CADx systems developed for detection of lung and breast cancer, colonoscopy, etc. [5–8], but there are still no applications thus far for the classification and diagnosis of cardiac arrhythmias.

As an example of arrhythmia, we have the ventricular extrasystoles, which are a reflection of the activation of the ventricles from a site below the AV node. Its outcome is linked to an underlying disease, and there could be three causes for it: reentry, increased automatism, and triggered activity.

The increased automatism suggests an ectopic group of cells in the ventricle. This process is the underlying mechanism of arrhythmias secondary to hyperkalemia. Reentry occurs in patients with underlying scarring ischemic heart disease or myocardial ischemia. This mechanism can produce isolated ectopic beats or trigger ventricular tachycardia and eventually sudden cardiac death [9,10]. Moreover, nowadays, a new trend is emerging in the deep learning (DL))-based ECG heartbeat classification, and several scientists present their efforts in this field. Although extensive experimental work is carried out on this topic, it is not suitable yet for real-time scenarios. Their approaches are not optimally efficient to cover the inter-patient variability issue in ECG signals [11,12].

Although ECG signals have been used for diagnosis for over a century, manually tracking these arrhythmias over even a thousand heartbeats is an infeasible task, even for expert physicians, because of the amount of time required to perform such endeavors. These kinds of tasks require automated mechanisms to detect and classify all these events. This is why AI is now an extremely relevant and important part of the algorithms for automated learning in electrocardiographic signals [13–15].

On an ECG, rhythm refers to the part of the heart that is controlling the initiation of electrical activity. Under normal circumstances, the sinoatrial node (SAN) initiates electrical activity because it undergoes spontaneous depolarization first at a rate of 60–100 bpm. When a rhythm originates from above the ventricles in the atria, it is termed a supraventricular (SVB) rhythm (narrow QRS or <120 ms), and when a rhythm originates from within the ventricles, it is termed a ventricular (VB) rhythm (broad QRS or >120 ms); these characteristics are represented in Figure 1.

The Association for the Advancement of Medical Instrumentation (AAMI) provides guidelines to classify heartbeats in an ECG signal into normal beats (N), supraventricular beats (SVB), ventricular beats (VB), fusion beats (FB), and unclassified beats (QB) [16,17]. However, because of their rarity in patients, the last two types of heartbeats are not usually included, and both QB and FB are relabeled simply as VB, leaving the task to classify only between NB, SVB, and VB.

An issue is the way research approaches the use of data sets. There are two accepted approaches to the problem, namely, inter- and intra-patient methodologies [18].

Works related to the inter-patient paradigm have lower performance against intra-patient works because of the use of different patients' heartbeats in training, validation, and testing sets. However such works reflect the reality accurately since the inevitable variabilities among patients are incorporated in their results.

In this research, we present a review of previous work wherein it is shown that until nowm it has not been possible to overcome the variabilities among patients and train a generalized model from the databases available. The guidance of a physician is still needed to develop a patient adaptive model. This means that in the future, physicians would need to label new data because the signal for every individual patient changes in shape and heart rate, and the old parameters of the algorithm may need to be updated.

In this article, a novel unsupervised method is introduced that classifies between beats of supraventricular origin (SVBo), formed by the NB and SVB classes, and beats of ventricular origin (VBo), formed by the VB and FB. This approach does not require the assistance of a physician since it tries to capture the inherent patterns in the signal, and it uses heartbeat features from previous works across patients. Based on our experiments, it was concluded that this methodology works best when they are at least 40 VBo. The present approach may be used as a first step to distinguish between the remaining NB and SVB in future experiments.

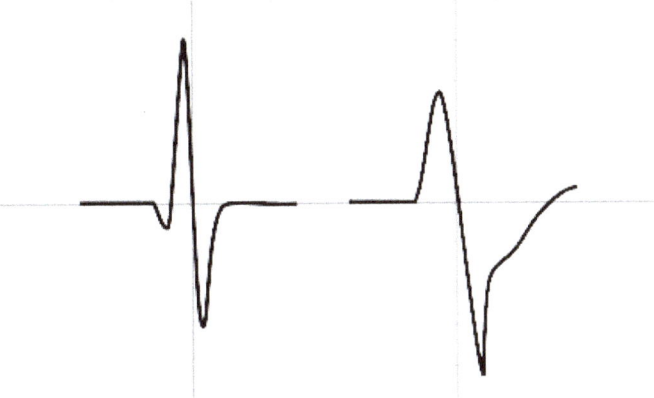

Figure 1. A supraventricular origin beat shows a narrow QRS (**left**) and a ventricular origin beat appears to be similar to a broad QRS (**right**).

The silhouette coefficient was implemented in MATLAB and used at the beginning to evaluate the quality of the clustering based on some parameters. For the experiments, an algorithm for clustering was implemented in MATLAB, and since this is an adaptive model for self-organizing maps, meaning that we could not use the silhouette score in general, and we would have to use it for every particular case or patient, which would yield just a distribution with no information worth for our purposes, as explained in Section 3.7, we chose between some parameters from the outcome that we derived from the comparison against the labels. In a future study with a modified algorithm, we aim to use the silhouette coefficient for the fine-tuning of the algorithm and better parameters.

2. Previous Research

Chazal et al. [19] extracted features in the time domain including heart rate and waveform descriptors of the ECG signal on both leads available in the MITBIH Arrhythmia Database. They used a linear discriminant classifier that outperforms their past work at that time. Llamedo et al. [20] presented a global classifier using the same training set as in Chazal et al. [19] but included two more databases to further test their method. He used the heart rate and features extracted from discrete wavelet transforms. He tested various sets of features and two different Bayesian linear classifiers ending with the linear discriminant classifier. Llamedo et al. [21] modified their past work to include more than two leads, using the same features and classifier. He used the INCART database in which every record has 12 leads. Using all the leads available, he outperformed their past work using this database. This is the only database available with 12 leads. Ye et al. [22] classified all types of heartbeats in the MITBIH database using the AAMI classification scheme. The morphological features used are coefficients of DWT and the result of applying independent components analysis, reducing the dimensionality with principal components analysis. The heart rate was also used as a feature. The classifier used is a support vector machine that combines the two leads of the MITBIH database. Once the features are extracted, the patients' heartbeats are used for training and testing resulting in overoptimistic results of nearly 100%. However, the same model trained and tested as Chazal et al. [19] and Llamedo et al. [20,21] produced lower performance because of the variabilities among patients. Their results are comparable to Chazal et al. [19] and Llamedo et al. [20,21]. Mar et al. [23] principally worked on feature selection to classify ECG signals. They used a number of features in the temporal domain, morphological waveform features, statistical features, and features from the temporal–frequency domain using the DWT. The sequential forward floating search algorithm was used to determine relevant features, along with a linear discriminant classifier.

Once the optimal features are extracted, they are used to classify through a multilayer perceptron. The results are comparable to Chazal et al. [19], Llamedo et al. [20,21], and Ye et al. [22].

It is mentioned in [24] that general classification models are highly unreliable with ECG signals and are not widely used in practice. In order to overcome this problem faced by the intra-patient methodology, an adaptive patient model may be more effective because the patterns within a single patient are much easier to capture than in the inter-patient methodology. Such work involves the use of a certain number of beats previously labeled by a physician to train a learning algorithm. Works presented in [24,25] obtain results above 95% in almost all the cases, and some very close to 100%, in both precision and recall for the AAMI types of heartbeats.

Only Llamedo et al. [26] and Al Rahhal et al. [27] showed results without initial expert labeling. Wiens et al. [24] tested their algorithm developed using active learning with the same patients' beats against the software from HAMILTON and with the advantage that it does not require data from the patient, but it only recognizes premature ventricular beats. Wiens et al. [24] outperformed HAMILTON. Llamedo et al. [26] modified their previous work in [21], which uses a general classifier by including a clustering algorithm, the K-means method. This modification slightly improves the performance, compared to their previous work, and also allows an expert to contribute to the output of the algorithm. The final results are around 95% with the help of the expert for each patient record. Al Rahhal et al. [27] used active classification through the deep learning approach. They suppressed the low frequency parts of the heartbeat and processed those employing an autoencoder algorithm to represent the signal in a lower dimension. A final softmax function is recorded similar to that in Chazal et al. [19], Llamedo et al. [20,21,27], Ye et al. [22], and Mar et al. [23]. Their results with beats labeled by an expert is close to 100% for every database they tested, while the automatic results when they used only the trained algorithm are much lower, representing the variability among patients. The only drawback is that a physician is needed to locate these labels on the ECG signal and as the heart's beats rhythm and signals may change over time, future relabeling may be required to tune the trained model. Other interesting and related approaches are proposed in [15,28–30]; these deal with abnormalities in ECG segments based on supervised learning.

3. Materials and Methods

3.1. ECG Databases

All experiments were performed using selected records from public databases available in Physionet [31]. Each database has different files that correspond to the digitized signals, the information about the patients' annotations, and the labels for heartbeats in the records. The following databases were used:

(a) MIT-BIH Arrhythmia database (MITBIH), consisting of 48 half-hour signals recorded with two channels each one sampling at 360 samples per second with 11-bit resolution over 10 mV. The annotations for each heartbeat were made by cardiologists.

(b) MIT-BIH Supraventricular Arrhythmia database (SUPRA), made up of 78 records, each 30 min long. Each record has two-lead signals, sampled at 120 Hz, with annotation files produced automatically first and then corrected by a medical student.

(c) St. Petersburg Institute of Cardiological Technics (INCART) 12-lead Arrhythmia database, built up of 75 annotated records, each consisting of 12-lead signals sampled at 257 Hz for 30 min.

Following the labels suggested by the AAMI and the subsequent classification proposed in Llamedo and other works [20,21,26], the heartbeats were relabeled to NB, SB, and VB. For the purpose of this first unsupervised work, the later labels were changed to their anatomic origin in the heart as SVBo and VBo.

3.2. Summary Approach

The algorithm requires a series of preprocessing and processing steps in order to cluster and distinguish the beats of supraventricular and ventricular origin. Figure 2 provides a high-level illustration of the processing pipeline divided into stages. In the first stage, Data extraction and cleaning, the patient signal is preprocessed and every beat of each record is sliced to form a matrix to work on. In stage 2, Clustering and descriptors, the clustering is performed and a set of different descriptors are computed to characterize each cluster (the expanded version of this stage is shown in Figure 3). The labeling processing is in stage 3, Classification, where the descriptors are used to compute a series of proportions for each cluster, and if these proportions reach a certain threshold, the cluster is classified as SVBo; otherwise, it is classified as VBo.

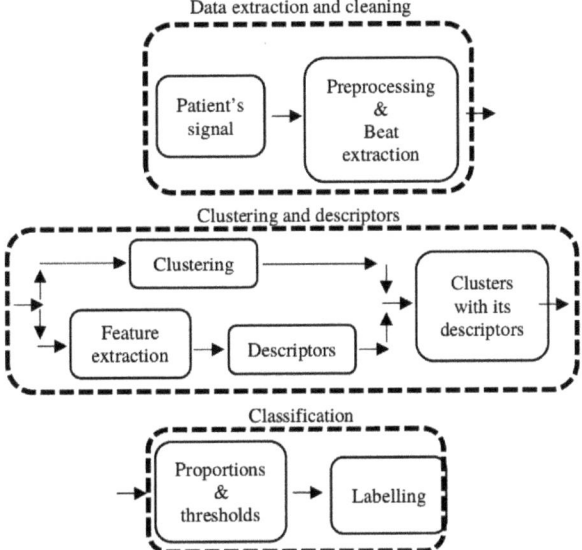

Figure 2. A high-level illustration of the processing pipeline.

Three important assumptions for the algorithm are as follows:
(a) With a significant number of VBo, the clustering algorithm is able to separate the signals;
(b) If a trend is computed on the R–R interval signal, almost all the beats above this trend are going to be SVBo and most of the VBo occur below the trend, along with the rest of SVBo;
(c) In the feature space, the SVBo signals are grouped together because they share similar waveform shapes, and the VBo signals are spread all over the feature space.

These assumptions were used to compute the descriptors and subsequently the proportions for the labeling of the clusters.

3.3. Data Extraction and Cleaning

The preprocessing of the signals is an important task to allow the extraction of useful information from them and for further analysis. The following four preprocessing procedures were performed:
(a) Baseline wander removal;
(b) Beat extraction;
(c) Normalization;
(d) Resample of signals.

The baseline wander is generated by a low-frequency signal. Removing this noise benefits the extraction of time-domain features. For this task, the Discrete wavelet transform (DWT) is employed. Via the DWT coefficients, the ECG signal can be described in both time and frequency. The values of the coefficients are the results of passing the ECG signal through a series of high pass filters (HPFs) and low pass filters (LPFs). Depending on the wavelet applied, the LPF has specific coefficient values. The HPF is derived from the LPF as follows:

$$HPF[L-1-k] = [-1]^k LPF[k] \qquad (1)$$

where L is the length of the filter in the number of samples, and k are the coefficients of the filter. Each pair of filters can be represented as follows:

$$A[n] = \sum_{k=0}^{K} LPF[k]x[n-k] \qquad (2)$$

$$D[n] = \sum_{k=0}^{K} HPF[k]x[n-k] \qquad (3)$$

The filter has a half downsample after it to make the DWT efficient, represented as follows:

$$A_o[n] = A[2n] \qquad (4)$$

$$D_o[n] = D[2n] \qquad (5)$$

where n is the length of the signal produced. The DWT sends the signal through a cascade of HPF and LPF, resulting in an average signal detailed and differentiated for classification.

Following the recommendations in [32], the signal was decomposed into the ninth level using Daubechies wavelet family and the wavelet Daubechies 6 (db6), where the frequency in this level was about 0–0.351 Hz [32] levels of resolution. The signal proceeds through all the necessary levels to isolate the energy of the noise. To eliminate the baseline wander from the ECG, the signal was constructed from the eighth coefficient to the first, replacing the coefficients of the ninth with zeros. Figure 4 shows the denoising process of the ECG signal.

The heartbeats were extracted from the denoised signal. Every record had a file indicating the heartbeat location in the sample and its type. After analyzing the research and results of Martis et al. [32], which uses a window of approximately 552 ms and the research and results of Marinucci et al. [33] that uses a window of 700 ms, in our case, we considered a slightly wider window, i.e., 730 ms–330 ms before the R peak and 400 ms after it—which were enough to cover the heartbeats of our test signals, making sure the whole beat and its characteristic waveform are totally covered. Every beat has a length of 0.73 s but because the sampling frequency varies among the databases, the length in samples varies depending on the database employed:

(a) MITBIH ECG signals consisted of 263 samples;
(b) INCART consisted of 188 samples;
(c) SUPRA had 93 samples.

Finally, the signal values were normalized between 0 and 1 and resampled at 360 Hz, the sampling frequency of the MITBIH database signals. This was carried out following the recommendations of Llamedo et al. [26].

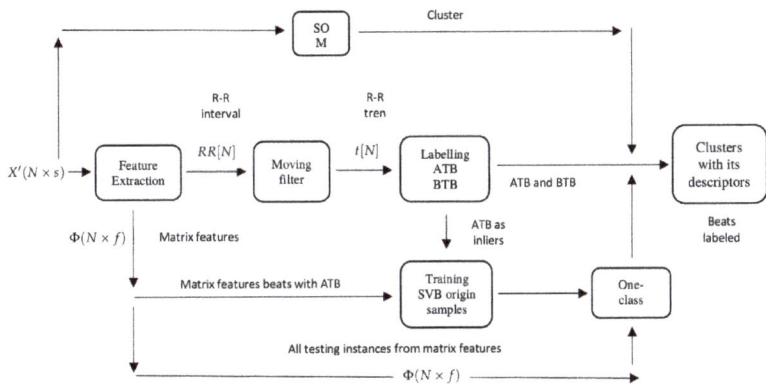

Figure 3. Expanded version of the stage "clustering and descriptors" of Figure 2.

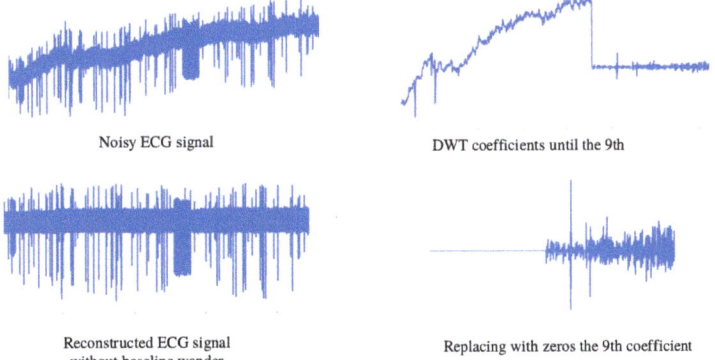

Figure 4. Illustration of denoising an ECG signal.

3.4. Clustering and Descriptors

In the clustering and descriptors step, three major procedures were performed according to the assumptions previously stated.

Firstly, the signals were clustered in groups. This work proposes that the clustering algorithm, self-organizing maps (SOM), is able to distinguish between SVBo and VBo, then the problem is reduced to classifying the clusters in SVBo or VBo using a set of descriptors. The SOM is an arrangement of neurons connected in a single-layer network, with most of the cases presented in a two-dimensional network. It is characterized by soft competition between neurons in the output layer, where a winner neuron and its neighbors are updated at every iteration in the training. The SOM learns the distribution and topology of the input vectors, generally mapping data R^n onto a regular bidimensional grid. A parametric reference vector $m_i \in R^n$ is associated with every node i in the map. Every input x is compared with every node, and the closest match is selected, and then the input is mapped onto that location $c = argmin_i \|x - m_i\|$. Nodes topographically close to others in the array will learn from the same input with the following formula:

$$m_i(t+1) = m_i(t) + \infty * h_{c,i}(t)[x(t) - m_i(t)] \tag{6}$$

The heartbeats extracted are sliced from the 60th to 170th sample and clustered, using the self-organizing map (SOM) algorithm. The time frame extracted from the heartbeats ensures that the hearbeat QRS complex is used for clustering, which is an important differentiator between the SVBo and VBo.

Secondly, this work stated that if we computed the trend of the heart rate in a window time, most of the heartbeats above the trend are SVBo, and most of the VBo will be located below the trend. The heart rate is computed taking the distance in samples from the heartbeats that the R peak selected and the previous one. All databases identify a heartbeat with its R peak location; thus, every R peak is already identified in the data. The trend $t[N]$ is computed using a moving average filter as follows:

$$y[n] = \sum_{k=0}^{K} w[k]x[n-k] \qquad (7)$$

where k represents the index terms of the signal, $w[k]$ represents the window signal, $x[n-k]$ is the signal value that is being filtered shifting k terms, and $y[n]$ is the filtered output signal. RR features such as mean, kurtosis, and SD were not part of the inputs for final clustering. RR intervals as features were used as an initial reference to preclassify the clusters as "normal" if they were above the red trend line, as can be seen in Figure 5 and explained in Section 3.4.

The beats above the trend level are labeled as above-the-trend beats (ATBs), and they are used in the third step as SVBo, and all those below are labeled as below-the-trend beats (BTBs). These labels become descriptors for each cluster. In Figure 5, a patient's R–R interval, its trend, and the labeling of ATB and BTB in the heart rate are shown.

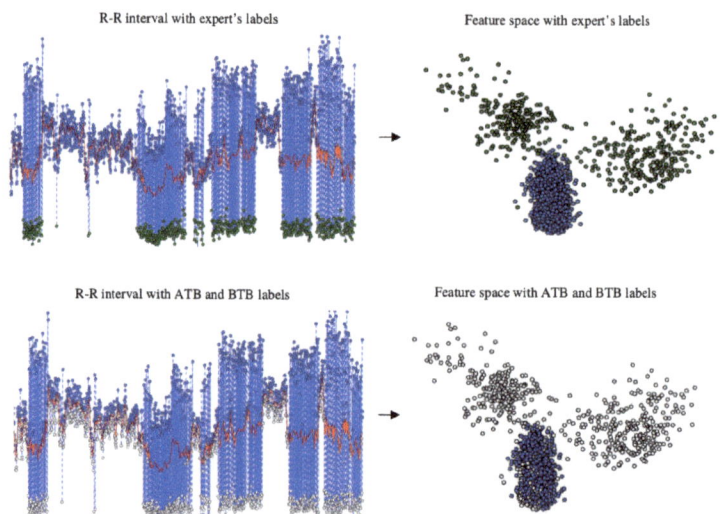

Figure 5. Comparison of real label and label above and below the trend. The blue marks indicate SVBo and ATB, green marks indicate VBo, and white are BTB.

The third assumption is that, in the feature space, most of SVBo are grouped and VBo are scattered. With the help of the second assumption, most heartbeats identified above the trend are labeled as SVBo and with this one class, the one-class SVM (OC-SVM) classifier algorithm is trained to create a nonlinear discriminant function to include more SVBo, and the rest of the heartbeats are classified as VBo. The OC-SVM separates the data using a subset of the class identified as reference for outliers by some prior value specified $v \in (0,1)$. The solution is to estimate a function f, which is a discriminant between the points marked as outliers and the insiders. The function f can be seen as

$$f(x) = \begin{cases} SVM_o & \text{if } x \in S \\ VB_o & \text{if } x \in \tilde{S} \end{cases} \qquad (8)$$

where the SVM_o are identified as the subset inside the function and VBo outside. For this, it is necessary to resolve the quadratic programming function

$$min\left(\frac{1}{2}\|w\|^2 + \frac{1}{vN}\sum_{i=1}^{N}\xi_i - \rho\right) \qquad (9)$$

subject to

$$w \cdot \phi(x_i) \geq \rho - \xi_i$$
$$i = 1, 2, \ldots, N$$
$$x_i \geq 0$$

where $\phi : X \rightarrow H$ represents a kernel map, which transforms the training examples to another space, N is the maximum number of training samples, w and ρ are the weight and offset parameterizing the hyperplane in the feature space, and ξ_i is the classic slack variable from the standard support vector machines to prevent over-fitting.

Resolving the quadratic problem, the decision boundary is as follows:

$$f(x) = sign(w \cdot \phi(x_i) - \rho) \qquad (10)$$

The matrix $X'(s) \in R^{N \times S}$ containing the heartbeats is converted into feature space $\Phi(N \times f)$, where f is the feature dimension used. In this work, different sets of features were used in experimentation and will be explained in the next sections. In order to help to distinguish which clusters are SVBo or VBo, a partial number of SVBo are identified utilizing One-Class SVM. The ATBs are used as SVBo class, the only class in this step, and the OC-SVM creates a discriminant function to englobe similar heartbeats. Furthermore, Figure 5 shows the beats above the trend located in a feature space. Figure 6 shows different decision boundaries in a feature space created with different hyperparameters in the OC-SVM. The beats identified as SVBo from the one-class SVM serve as well as descriptors to characterize each cluster.

In Table 1, an example of data separated in clusters with its descriptors is displayed; this is from the same signal used for Figures 5 and 6.

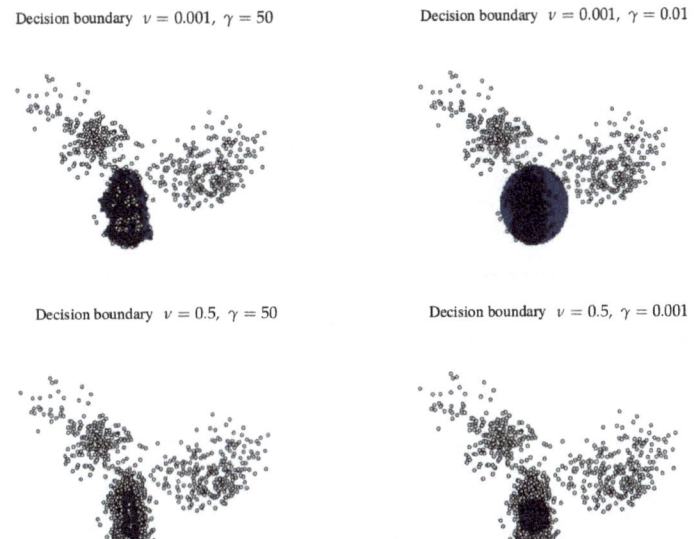

Figure 6. Illustration of different decision boundaries using different hyperparameter values in one-class SVM.

Table 1. Example of ECG signal separated in clusters and its descriptors.

Cluster (cl_j)	# Beats in Cluster (cl_j)	# ATB in Cluster (cl_j)	# BTB in Cluster (cl_j)	# SVBo Identified
1	227	0	227	0
2	292	195	97	273
3	346	216	130	221
4	478	316	162	385
5	451	299	152	394
6	229	0	229	0

3.5. Classification

To determine if a cluster cl^j is SVBo or VBo, three proportions $P_i^{cl^j}$, where $i = 1, 2, 3$ and cl^j is a cluster, are computed using the descriptors previously defined. Each proportion $P_i^{cl^j}$ is compared with its corresponding d_i threshold and the results from the comparisons are used to label that cl^j as SVBo or VBo. The first proportion, $P_1^{cl^j}$ is computed as follows in Equation (11):

$$P_1^{cl^j} = \frac{\#SVBo}{\#beats \text{ in } cl^j} \tag{11}$$

This proportion is the percentage of SVBo identified in the cluster by the one-class SVM algorithm. If the proportion surpasses the threshold d_1, then the cl^j is labeled as being SVBo.

The second proportion, $P_2^{cl^j}$ is shown in the next Equation (12).

$$P_2^{cl^j} = \frac{\#SVBo}{\#beats \text{ in } cl^j} \tag{12}$$

This proportion represents the error of the one-class SVM in labeling the SVBo or the error of SOM clustering SVBo with VBo. It is expected that clusters that are VBo only have mostly BTB and much less ATB. However, some of SVBo may be mixed in a cluster of VBo, and the one-class SVM may identify them as VBos. In such cases, comparing the rate between the number of SVBo in this cluster and the total number of BTB with its threshold d_2 tells us what type of cluster it is. A majority of BTB will not let the proportion reach the threshold. If the cluster does not contain any BTB, this proportion is not computed. $P_3^{cl^j}$ is shown in (13).

$$P_3^{cl^j} = \frac{\#ATB}{\#beats \text{ in } cl^j} \tag{13}$$

Lastly, as mentioned before, because it is hypothesized that most of the ATBs are SVBo because a great number of beats are NB in many signals, this rate represents the relation between the ATB and the number of beats in this cluster. The values of the thresholds are determined experimentally, as will be explained. If any of these thresholds are reached, the cluster is labeled as SVBo; otherwise, it is represented as VB.

3.6. Hyperparameters and Features

The approach has a great number of hyperparameters, changing their values may change the output of the approach. The SOMs parameters include the following:

1. Type of grid for cluster nodes;
2. Number of neurons;
3. Number of neighbors;
4. Number of iterations;
5. Learning rate.

As the SOM is a clustering algorithm, in this case, a reproducibility experiment was performed to ensure that the results can be reproduced multiple times to guarantee its use outside this study.

The one-class SVM has the hyperparameter ν, which determines the proportion of beats outside of the decision function. The kernel employs the radial basis function

(RBF) that uses the γ hyperparameter, which plays an important role in determining the decision boundary.

Additionally, the threshold d_i to determine if a cluster is SVBo or VBo needs to be specified as well.

The default hyperparameters used for SOM training have a neighbor size of 3 and a hexagonal grid topology with 200 iterations.

Furthermore, the hyperparameters whose values are determined experimentally are as follows:

1. The dimension of the grid of SOM;
2. The ν in the One-Class SVM algorithm;
3. γ for the RBF kernel;
4. The thresholds d_i.

Different subsets of features were extracted and merged together to form the final features set to be experimented with to reach the highest classification performance. The first feature subset is the DWT db3 coefficients of the QRS complex; the second feature subset is DWT db6 coefficients of the whole beat; the third feature subset feature is statistical computations of the sections before, after, and within the QRS complex; the fourth feature subset is the statistical computations of the QRS complex. The statistical computations are the mean, the standard deviation, the maximum, the minimum, the skewness, and the kurtosis. The final feature sets to experiment with were as follows: feature set 1 is the PCA transformation of the first features subset; feature set 2 is the PCA transformation of the second feature subset; feature set 3 is the merged of the first and fourth feature subsets; feature set 4 is the fourth feature subset; feature set 5 is the PCA transformation of the third feature subset; feature set 6 is the merged of the first and third feature subsets; features set 7 is the merge of the second and fourth feature subsets.

Table 2 summarizes the basic features and the set of features created with all these.

Table 2. Subset and Set of Features Formed.

Features	Description
subset feature 1	QRS complex + DWT db3
subset feature 2	Whole beat + DWT db6
subset feature 3	Sections + SO + HOS
subset feature 4	QRS complex + SO + HOS
feature set 1	feature 1 + PCA
feature set 2	feature 2 + PCA
feature set 3	feature 1 + feature 4
feature set 4	feature 4
feature set 5	feature 3 + PCA
feature set 6	feature 1 + feature 3
feature set 7	feature 2 + feature 4

3.7. Experimentation Setup

Figure 7 shows the experimental setup. First, five types of topologies were used in SOM to determine which one is more appropriate for the given data: 2×2, 3×2, 3×3, 4×3, and 4×4. Each type of SOM was run five times using the set of the default hyperparameters ($\nu = 0.1$, $\gamma = 1.5$, $d_1 = 0.5$, $d_2 = 0.7$, and $d_3 = 0.3$) and with the default set of features (DWT + PCA of the QRS complex of the signals) to determine the reproducibility of the results. These parameter values and features were selected because they produce good results in the first trials. Experimenting with these variables as defaults gave us an insight into the proper topology to use for this task.

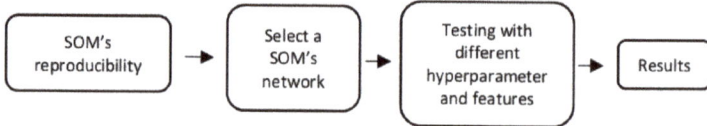

Figure 7. Experiment setup.

Once a topology was selected, the set of features and parameters were determined first using three different values for each hyperparameter for each set of features for each database, and the best three sets of features were selected. Then, we experimented with five different values of hyperparameters and the best one was selected to obtain the final results to compare it with prior works.

3.8. Evaluation

Because of the high imbalance among the classes, the results are in terms of sensitivity (S) also known as recall and positive predictive value (P^+) also known precision, as presented in [26]. In addition, the F-score is presented here, which is the harmonic mean of these two parameters. F-score is computed as given in Equation (14).

$$F = 2 * \frac{S \times P^+}{S + P^+} \qquad (14)$$

The F-score (F) can be seen as a measure of combined performance involving both S and P^+. With values between 0 and 1, highest performance with 1, each S and P^+ needs to be high to have a high F-score. In other words, it involves a balance between these two performance measures.

The searches for the best SOM topology and the best set of features and parameters values possible result in a great number of results in terms of S, P^+, and F. As for specific values of parameters and specific selection of features, the performance varies for each database, and changing these can cause increased or decreased performances.

The purpose of these experiments is to set the hyperparameters' values that can maintain the best balance possible among the performance for the three databases. To achieve this, a modification of the F-score formula is made to compare the performance of each F-score for each database. We call it F-general (Fg), and the equation is shown in (15).

$$Fg = 3 * \frac{F_{SUPRA} \times F_{MITBIH} \times F_{INCART}}{F_{SUPRA} + F_{MITBIH} + F_{INCART}} \qquad (15)$$

This equation is motivated by the way F-score is computed, from a precision value and recall. It is also a harmonic mean of the three F-scores for the three databases. The reason we used this equation is that we looked for hyperparameters and features not biased towards any of the databases. The purpose is to have a generalized set of hyperparameters and features that could balance the performance among the databases. This equation was applied to select the SOM network, the hyperparameters, and set of features.

4. Results

Table 3 shows the results of inserting every patients' signal through the algorithm for each network topology proposed with the default hyperparameters and set of features.

In order to ensure the reproducibility of the results, in terms of S and P^+, the mean and the standard deviation were taken from the five runs of every database for every network topology.

Table 3. SOM Reproducibility Experiments Results.

	SOM Topology	VBo	SVBo		VBo	
		S	P+	S	P+	F Score
SUPRA	2×2	0.85905	0.78189	0.98632	0.99191	0.81866
		0.0002	0.00052	0.00004	0.00001	0.0003
	3×2	0.89814	0.79383	0.98654	0.99115	0.84277
		0.00216	0.00071	0.00019	0.00407	0.00109
	3×3	0.89386	0.77637	0.9853	0.99389	0.83095
		0.0046	0.00717	0.00067	0.00026	0.00299
	4×3	0.87991	0.79268	0.98368	0.99083	0.7909
		0.03701	0.09298	0.00667	0.00414	0.00551
	4×4	0.90934	0.68555	0.97617	0.99473	0.78168
		0.00798	0.014	0.00152	0.00046	0.01005
MITBIH	2×2	0.8075	0.94047	0.99576	0.98423	0.86893
		0.00027	0.00013	0.00001	0.00002	0.00021
	3×2	0.83549	0.91752	0.99377	0.986	0.87458
		0.00108	0.0031	0.00026	0.001	0.00116
	3×3	0.84905	0.88435	0.99078	0.98753	0.86631
		0.00207	0.00994	0.00092	0.00016	0.00378
	4×3	0.8544	0.84955	0.98738	0.98792	0.85177
		0.00229	0.02786	0.00273	0.00018	0.01351
	4×4	0.86079	0.85686	0.98807	0.98845	0.85879
		0.0023	0.01002	0.001	0.00018	0.00436
INCART	2×2	0.89461	0.94787	0.9936	0.9864	0.92047
		0.00119	0.0005	0.00006	0.00015	0.00071
	3×2	0.92128	0.91843	0.98936	0.98976	0.91985
		0.00178	0.00336	0.00048	0.00023	0.00188
	3×3	0.92325	0.88574	0.98452	0.98997	0.9041
		0.00231	0.00296	0.00043	0.0003	0.00231
	4×3	0.92732	0.86486	0.98116	0.99046	0.89498
		0.00226	0.00752	0.00122	0.00029	0.00381
	4×4	0.92359	0.87453	0.98277	0.99	0.89839
		0.00042	0.00249	0.00039	0.00005	0.00129

It can be seen that the standard deviation from the runs of every topology of every database has a value near zero, which means minimum or insignificant changes between the results within the topology but not between topologies.

In order to select one, Table 4 presents the F of the VB origin because the results in the SVB origin are nearly 1 in every database. For the SUPRA database, the two F highest values are obtained with the topologies 3×2, and 3×3 with 0.8427 and 0.8309, respectively. With the MITBIH database, the highest valued topologies are 2×2, 3×2 and 3×3, with F-scores of 0.8689, 0.8745, and 0.8663, respectively. The INCART database produces the highest values with the 2×2 and 3×2 topologies, with 0.9204 and 0.9198 F-scores values, respectively. The 3×2 topology has the highest performances for SUPRA and MITBIH databases compared to other topologies, while for INCART, the 2×2 topology is just slightly above 3×2. However, the Fg of each database shows that the 3×2 topology has the highest performance for the three databases, and because of that, this SOM network was used to run the next experiments involving the selection of the parameters and set of features.

As the default parameters gave good results in the first tests, other similar and close values were tested as upper and lower bound values, with sets of features as presented before, in order to find better combination of hyperparameters and features to improve our results. The test values for each parameter are as follows: $\nu = 0.001, 0.1, 0.5$; $\gamma = 0.001, 1.5, 3$; $d_1 = 0.4, 0.5, 0.6$; $d_2 = 0.5, 0.6, 0.7$; $d_3 = 0.2, 0.3, 0.4$. Each parameter has three different values, giving rise to 243 experiments for each set of features for each record in every database. In each experiment, the S, P^+, and F for each set of features (for each database) were computed, and only the highest performance in terms of F are shown in Table 5.

Table 4. Selecting the Best of SOM Topology.

	SUPRA	MITBIH	INCART	F-General
2 × 2	0.81866	0.86893	0.92047	0.75318503
3 × 2	0.84277	0.87458	0.91985	0.77126533
3 × 3	0.83095	0.86631	0.9041	0.75056012
4 × 3	0.7909	0.85177	0.89498	0.71276568
4 × 4	0.78168	0.85879	0.89839	0.71262883

Results with the highest values are in Table 5, and these are presented for each set of features. For example, parameters for feature set $1 = \nu = 0.1$, $\gamma = 1.5$, $d_1 = 0.4$, $d_2 = 0.5$, $d_3 = 0.3$. The Fg is computed from with each VBos F of every database for every set of features. The best three were set of features 1, 3, and 4. It is important to mention that these features involve only the QRS complex, which, in fact, is very accurate medically in distinguishing the heartbeat between SVBo and VBo.

Table 5. Selecting the Best Three Features.

	SUPRA	MITBIH	INCART	F-General
feature set 1	0.8892	0.8755	0.9214	0.801129807
feature set 2	0.8602	0.8755	0.928	0.787117392
feature set 3	0.8892	0.8755	0.9214	0.801129807
feature set 4	0.8957	0.8723	0.9468	0.817466775
feature set 5	0.8946	0.8721	0.8687	0.771506723
feature set 6	0.8184	0.7725	0.9029	0.686694226
feature set 7	0.8608	0.8721	0.8919	0.765261291

As the hyperparameters values for the three different sets of features were nearly the same, just varying $d_2 = 0.6$ in feature set 4 and $d_2 = 0.5$ in feature set 1 and 3, the final hyperpameter values to experiment with were as follows: $\nu = 0.05, 0.1, 0.15, 0.25, 0.3$; $\gamma = 1, 1.25, 1.5, 2, 2.5$; $d_1 = 0.3, 0.35, 0.4, 0.45, 0.5$; $d_2 = 0.55, 0.575, 0.6, 0.625, 0.65$; $d_3 = 0.25, 0.275, 0.3, 0.325, 0.35$. In this case, 3125 experiments were performed for each set of features for each database.

In order to select the best set of features with parameters, Table 6 presents the Fg values computed with the highest F for each database for each set of features. The hyperparameters of each feature set presented the best F were as follows: feature set $1 = \nu = 0.05$, $\gamma = 2.25$, $d_1 = 0.45$, $d_2 = 0.55$, $d_3 = 0.35$; feature set $3 = \nu = 0.1$, $\gamma = 1.25$, $d_1 = 0.3$, $d_2 = 0.55$, $d_3 = 0.3$; feature set $4 = \nu = 0.15$, $\gamma = 1$, $d_1 = 0.35$, $d_2 = 0.55$, $d_3 = 0.3$. It has to be noticed that even though these set of features were selected with almost the same parameters values, they ended up with completely different and Fg values. The best set of features with its parameters was feature set 4, with 0.8220%. With this, the experimentation concludes with a SOM network of 3 × 2 neurons, with feature set 4 and the parameters $v = 0.15, \gamma = 1, d_1 = 0.35, d_2 = 0.55, d_3 = 0.3$.

Table 6. Example of ECG signal separated in clusters and its descriptors.

	SUPRA	MITBIH	INCART	F-General
feature set 1	0.9005	0.8655	0.9276	0.80519243
feature set 3	0.8892	0.8862	0.9187	0.80614369
feature set 4	0.89569357	0.8862	0.9394	0.8220299

The results of all the databases are compared with similar works in Table 7. The approach was tested also with two databases derived from the MITBIH database, as in [21,27]. Even though some other authors such as Kiranyaz et al. [34] claim that the average detection accuracies of both VB and SPV ectopic beats were over 97% using the MIT-BIH arrhythmia database, for both training and testing of the algorithm, this shows that the supervised algorithms so far continue being of higher precision or accuracy.

In Figure 8, the performance of the algorithm for 109 records that have at least 40 VBos is shown. The histogram shows that 89 out of 109 records have at least a 0.85 F-score, and 60 out of 109 are over 0.95 F-score. These records are 30 min long; in other words, there are approximately 1500 and up to 2500 heartbeats depending on the heart rate. These records represent most of the VBos in the three databases.

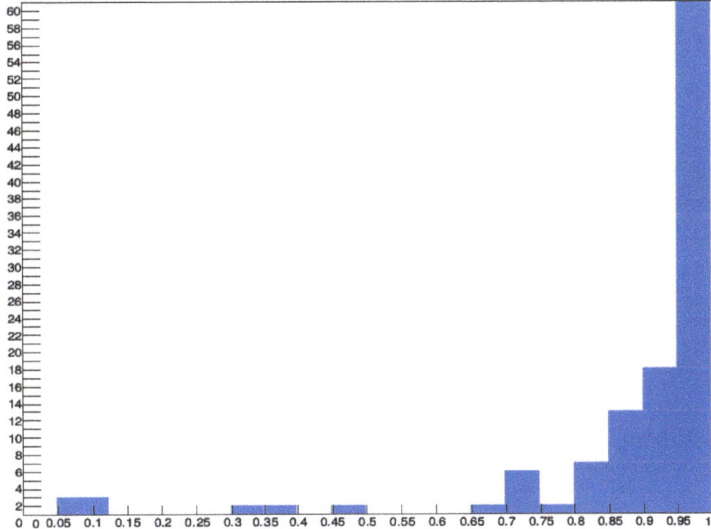

Figure 8. F-score performance with at least 40 VoB.

Table 7. Comparing results with similar works.

Type of Model	Data	Work	NB S	NB P+	SVB S	SVB P+	SVBo (N B and SVB) S	SVBo (N B and SVB) P+	VBo (VB and FB) S	VBo (VB and FB) P+	F-Score for VBo
Generalized Models	MITBIH-AR DS2	Mar [9]	0.90	0.99	0.83	0.34			0.87	0.61	0.7171
		Chazal [5]	87	99	0.759	0.385			0.777	0.819	0.7974
		Llamedo [7]			0.77	0.39			0.81	0.87	0.8389
		Ye [8]			0.608	0.523			0.815	0.631	0.7112
		This work					0.9996	0.9848	0.8039	0.9945	0.8891
	MITBIH-AR DS2	Llamedo [11]	0.93 ± 0	0.99 ± 0	0.77 ± 0	0.39 ± 0			0.82 ± 0	0.70 ± 0	0.7552
		This work					0.9996	0.9848	0.8039	0.9945	0.8891
	MITBIH-AR common tests records	Al Rahhal [12]			0.115	0.132			0.847	0.871	0.8588
		This work					0.9928	0.9797	0.8309	0.9335	0.8792
Patient adaptive (no training data from the same patient)	MITBIH	Llamedo [11]	0.96 ± 0	0.98 ± 0	0.76 ± 2	0.43 ± 2			0.80 ± 2	0.82 ± 3	0.8098
		Al Rahhal [12]			0.41	0.429			0.91	0.795	0.8486
		HAMILTON [10]							0.928	0.795	0.8563
		This work					0.9957	0.9865	0.8360	0.9428	0.8862
	SUPRA	Llamedo [11]	0.94 ± 0	0.97 ± 0	0.47 ± 3	0.50 ± 1			0.82 ± 0	0.54 ± 1	0.6511
		Al Rahhal [12]			0.880	0.1431			0.6519	0.931	0.1639
		This work					0.9938	0.9941	0.8981	0.8930	0.8956
	INCART	Llamedo [11]	0.89 ± 0	0.99 ± 0	0.74 ± 4	0.8 ± 0			0.88 ± 0	0.96 ± 1	0.9182
		Al Rahhal [12]			0.1558	0.0254			0.7511	0.3763	0.5013
		This work					0.9946	0.9899	0.9220	0.9575	0.9394

5. Discussion

One of the main differences among all works is the percentage of P^+ in VBo, where our approach produces percentages above 90%, with the exception of the SUPRA database with 0.8930%. This means that a great number of beats classified as VBo are indeed VBo.

The F-score of this work outperforms the general classifier models. Martis et al. [23] and Ye et al. [22] present the lowest F-score because of their P^+ around 0.60, plunging the F-score value, while Chazal et al. [19] and Llamedo et al. [20] maintain similar values for both S and P^+, with F-score of 0.79 and 0.83 respectively. The inevitable variability between patients lowers the performance of these general classifiers. The results for this work are higher, with 0.88, because it presents a P^+ near 100%.

An additional comparison is made with works where they present models that can be adapted to a patient. The results to be compared are the models before physician's help is provided for the adaptive algorithms, otherwise, their results are nearly 95%. Only Llamedo et al. [26] and Al Rahhal et al. [27] presented this type of results, and Wiens et al. [24] presented the performance of the HAMILTON software on the MIT-BIH database for comparative results. As in the general models, the performance on the F-score for VBo in the algorithm proposed was superior over these methods. No patterns in their results exist showing misclassification measurements, which vary depending on the database. For example, Llamedo presents balanced results in the MIIBIH database, while a very low 0.54 in P^+ is presented in the SUPRA database, and in the INCART database, the P^+ is 0.96 against a 0.88 for S. Meanwhile, Al Ranhal et al. [27] have very similar results with the HAMILTON software, with a low performance of 0.79% for the MITBIH database in P^+, 0.93 for the SUPRA database for the same measurement, and very lower, 0.37, in the INCART database. Our approach has higher performance because it maintains an S always above 0.9 for P^+ in every database; in this way, the derived F-score presents a superior performance. Overall, our approach has produced better results in F-score for VBo, compared to these studies.

The physicians' need for constant monitoring of the arrhythmias presented the opportunity for the creation of algorithms or methodologies that perform automatic measurements of arrythmia. Different approaches have been used by the scientific community, such as the intra- and inter-patient paradigms. Such approaches have historically employed manual data tagging by an expert. The works of Llamedo et al. [20] and Al Rahhal et al. [27] were the first to show results from prelabeled data.

Those studies showed progress, compared to previous studies, but they maintained the limitation of not being able to overcome the variations between patients or to train a general model that uses the available databases, as explained in Section 3.1. Our work introduces a new unsupervised method that classifies beats of SVBo origin, formed by classes NB and SVB, and beats of ventricular origin VBo, formed by VB and FB. This method does not require the assistance of an expert physician, as it captures the inherent patterns found in the captured signal and makes use of the heartbeat characteristics captured from previous patient studies.

Previous works need labels in order to create a heartbeat classifier. A general classifier, created by heartbeat samples from other patients, may not be the best solution as the inevitable variability lowers the performance of the classifier. Even though the adaptive patient classifiers are a promising solution in classifying arrhythmias, it needs a physician to identify a certain number of heartbeats to feed the algorithm for every patient.

In this work, a new unsupervised algorithm was proposed to classify between supraventricular and ventricular heartbeats in a single patient, in a window time, without previous labels provided by a physician.

Three assumptions were proposed to implement this algorithm. A never used one was that most of the heartbeats above a computed trend in the heart rate are of supraventricular nature. This can be used as a new feature in future works.

6. Conclusions

In this work, a new unsupervised algorithm was proposed to classify between supraventricular and ventricular heartbeats without the need for any labeling by a physician. A new feature is using as a reference the trend in the heart rate to classify the heartbeats above that trend as of "supraventricular" nature.

The results of this algorithm show better performance against other generalized models and/or adaptive patient models without the need for a physician's assistance.

These results show a promising path for unsupervised models to classify these types of heartbeats, and it can be seen as a milestone to develop further stages for classification between supraventricular heartbeats and normal heartbeats.

This comes from the fact that this model adapts itself to the patient's heartbeats waveform. Our algorithm works better without the need for a large number of VBo heartbeats. These results show a promising path for unsupervised models to be used as classifying indicators for SVBo and VBo types of heartbeats.

No other similar work has been developed thus far, though some improvements in the algorithm are needed to reach higher performance in precision and recall metrics. Although the purpose of this research is to develop an adaptive system granting better results, compared to those from other authors, we also concluded that the silhouette criterion can be applied in a new research study or proposal in the classification of ECG signals, which, to the best of our knowledge, nobody has performed thus far.

Author Contributions: Conceptualization and formal analysis, M.M.C. and R.L.A.; Methodology, J.K.; Data Curation, J.A.C.-H.; Investigation, M.A.R. and F.J.T.-R.; Funding acquisition and resources, M.E.B.-Z.; Software, J.A.C.-H. All authors have read and agreed to the published version of the manuscript.

Funding: The APC was funded by the Autonomous University of Baja California.

Institutional Review Board Statement: Not applicable.

Informed Consent Statement: Not applicable.

Acknowledgments: We want to express our gratitude to the National Council of Science and Technology (Conacyt) for the provided funding, scholarships, and materials in support of this research.

Conflicts of Interest: The authors declare that there is no conflict of interest regarding the publication of this paper.

Ethics Approval: This research as well as the human data used in it was approved by the Committee of Ethics in Research of the General Hospital of Mexicali, B.C.; Mexico.

References

1. Thaler, M.S. *The Only EKG Book You'll Ever Need*, 8th ed.; Wolters Kluwer: Philadelphia, PA, USA, 2015.
2. Mitra, M.; Samanta, R. Cardiac Arrhythmia Classification Using Neural Networks with Selected Features. *Procedia Technol.* **2013**, *10*, 76–84. [CrossRef]
3. Haldar, N.A.H.; Khan, F.A.; Ali, A.; Abbas, H. Arrhythmia classification using Mahalanobis distance based improved Fuzzy C-Means clustering for mobile health monitoring systems. *Neurocomputing* **2017**, *220*, 221–235. [CrossRef]
4. Martínez-Casas, M.; Avitia, R.L.; Gonzalez-Navarro, F.F.; Cárdenas-Haro, J.A.; Reyna, M.A. Bayesian Classification Models for Premature Ventricular Contraction Detection on ECG Traces. *J. Healthc. Eng.* **2018**, *2018*, 2694768. [CrossRef]
5. Firmino, M.; Angelo, G.; Morais, H.; Dantas, M.R.; Valentim, R. Computer-aided detection (CADe) and diagnosis (CADx) system for lung cancer with likelihood of malignancy. *Biomed. Eng. Online* **2016**, *15*, 2. [CrossRef]
6. Hann, A.; Troya, J.; Fitting, D. Current status and limitations of artificial intelligence in colonoscopy. *UEG J.* **2021**. [CrossRef]
7. Aswiga, R.; Aishwarya, R.; Shanthi, A. Augmenting Transfer Learning with Feature Extraction Techniques for Limited Breast Imaging Datasets. *J. Digit. Imaging* **2021**. [CrossRef]
8. Ruikar, D.D.; Santosh, K.; Hegadi, R.S.; Rupnar, L.; Choudhary, V.A. 5K+ CT Images on Fractured Limbs: A Dataset for Medical Imaging Research. *J. Med. Syst.* **2021**, *45*, 51. [CrossRef] [PubMed]
9. Noheria, A.; Deshmukh, A.; Asirvatham, S. Ablating Premature Ventricular Complexes: Justification, Techniques, and Outcomes. *Methodist DeBakey Cardiovasc. J.* **2015**, *11*, 109–120. [CrossRef]

10. Priori, S.G.; Blomström-Lundqvist, C.; Mazzanti, A.; Blom, N.; Borggrefe, M.; Camm, J.; Elliott, P.M.; Fitzsimons, D.; Hatala, R.; Hindricks, G.; et al. 2015 ESC Guidelines for the management of patients with ventricular arrhythmias and the prevention of sudden cardiac death: The Task Force for the Management of Patients with Ventricular Arrhythmias and the Prevention of Sudden Cardiac Death of the European Society of Cardiology (ESC)Endorsed by: Association for European Paediatric and Congenital Cardiology (AEPC). *Eur. Heart J.* **2015**, *36*, 2793–2867. [CrossRef]
11. Oh, S.L.; Ng, E.Y.; Tan, R.S.; Acharya, U.R. Automated diagnosis of arrhythmia using combination of CNN and LSTM techniques with variable length heart beats. *Comput. Biol. Med.* **2018**, *102*, 278–287. [CrossRef]
12. Pandey, S.K.; Janghel, R.R. ECG Arrhythmia Classification Using Artificial Neural Networks. In *Proceedings of 2nd International Conference on Communication, Computing and Networking*; Krishna, C.R., Dutta, M., Kumar, R., Eds.; Springer: Singapore, 2019; pp. 645–652.
13. Mincholé, A.; Camps, J.; Lyon, A.; Rodríguez, B. Machine learning in the electrocardiogram. *J. Electrocardiol.* **2019**, *57*, S61–S64. [CrossRef]
14. Mincholé, A.; Rodriguez, B. Artificial intelligence for the electrocardiogram. *Nat. Med.* **2019**, *25*, 22–23. [CrossRef]
15. Tong, Y.; Sun, Y.; Zhou, P.; Shen, Y.; Jiang, H.; Sha, X.; Chang, S. Locating abnormal heartbeats in ECG segments based on deep weakly supervised learning. *Biomed. Signal Process. Control* **2021**, *68*, 102674. [CrossRef]
16. AAMI ECAR. *Recommended Practice for Testing and Reporting Performance Results of Ventricular Arrhythmia Detection Algorithms*; Association for the Advancement of Medical Instrumentation: Arlington, VA, USA, 1987; Volume 69
17. Association for the Advancement of Medical Instrumentation (AAMI). *Testing and Reporting Performance Results of Cardiac Rhythm and ST Segment Measurement Algorithms*; ANSI/AAMI EC38; Association for the Advancement of Medical Instrumentation: Arlington, VA, USA, 1998; Volume 1998
18. Luz, E.J.D.S.; Schwartz, W.R.; Cámara-Chávez, G.; Menotti, D. ECG-based heartbeat classification for arrhythmia detection: A survey. *Comput. Methods Prog. Biomed.* **2016**, *127*, 144–164. [CrossRef]
19. De Chazal, P.; O'Dwyer, M.; Reilly, R.B. Automatic classification of heartbeats using ECG morphology and heartbeat interval features. *IEEE Trans. Biomed. Eng.* **2004**, *51*, 1196–1206. [CrossRef]
20. Llamedo, M.; Martínez, J.P. Heartbeat Classification Using Feature Selection Driven by Database Generalization Criteria. *IEEE Trans. Biomed. Eng.* **2011**, *58*, 616–625. [CrossRef] [PubMed]
21. Llamedo, M.; Khawaja, A.; Martinez, J.P. Cross-database evaluation of a multilead heartbeat classifier. *IEEE Trans. Inf. Technol. Biomed.* **2012**, *16*, 658–664. [CrossRef] [PubMed]
22. Ye, C.; Kumar, B.V.; Coimbra, M.T. Heartbeat classification using morphological and dynamic features of ECG signals. *IEEE Trans. Biomed. Eng.* **2012**, *59*, 2930–2941. [PubMed]
23. Mar, T.; Zaunseder, S.; Martínez, J.P.; Llamedo, M.; Poll, R. Optimization of ECG classification by means of feature selection. *IEEE Trans. Biomed. Eng.* **2011**, *58*, 2168–2177. [CrossRef] [PubMed]
24. Wiens, J.; Guttag, J. Active Learning Applied to Patient-Adaptive Heartbeat Classification. In *Advances in Neural Information Processing Systems*; Lafferty, J., Williams, C., Shawe-Taylor, J., Zemel, R., Culotta, A., Eds.; Curran Associates, Inc.: Red Hook, NY, USA, 2010; Volume 23.
25. Alvarado, A.S.; Lakshminarayan, C.; Principe, J.C. Time-based compression and classification of heartbeats. *IEEE Trans. Biomed. Eng.* **2012**, *59*, 1641–1648. [CrossRef] [PubMed]
26. Llamedo, M.; Martínez, J.P. An Automatic Patient-Adapted ECG Heartbeat Classifier Allowing Expert Assistance. *IEEE Trans. Biomed. Eng.* **2012**, *59*, 2312–2320. [CrossRef]
27. Al Rahhal, M.M.; Bazi, Y.; AlHichri, H.; Alajlan, N.; Melgani, F.; Yager, R.R. Deep learning approach for active classification of electrocardiogram signals. *Inf. Sci.* **2016**, *345*, 340–354. [CrossRef]
28. Chen, S.; Hua, W.; Li, Z.; Li, J.; Gao, X. Heartbeat classification using projected and dynamic features of ECG signal. *Biomed. Signal Process. Control* **2017**, *31*, 165–173. [CrossRef]
29. Nasim, A.; Sbrollini, A.; Morettini, M.; Burattini, L. Extended Segmented Beat Modulation Method for Cardiac Beat Classification and Electrocardiogram Denoising. *Electronics* **2020**, *9*, 1178. [CrossRef]
30. Neves, I.; Folgado, D.; Santos, S.; Barandas, M.; Campagner, A.; Ronzio, L.; Cabitza, F.; Gamboa, H. Interpretable heartbeat classification using local model-agnostic explanations on ECGs. *Comput. Biol. Med.* **2021**, *133*, 104393. [CrossRef] [PubMed]
31. Goldberger, A.L.; Amaral, L.A.N.; Glass, L.; Hausdorff, J.M.; Ivanov, P.C.; Mark, R.G.; Mietus, J.E.; Moody, G.B.; Peng, C.K.; Stanley, H.E. PhysioBank, PhysioToolkit, and PhysioNet: Components of a New Research Resource for Complex Physiologic Signals. *Circulation* **2000**, *101*, e215–e220, doi: 10.1161/01.CIR.101.23.e215. [CrossRef]
32. Martis, R.J.; Acharya, U.R.; Min, L.C. ECG beat classification using PCA, LDA, ICA and Discrete Wavelet Transform. *Biomed. Signal Process. Control* **2013**, *8*, 437–448. [CrossRef]
33. Marinucci, D.; Sbrollini, A.; Marcantoni, I.; Morettini, M.; Swenne, C.A.; Burattini, L. Artificial Neural Network for Atrial Fibrillation Identification in Portable Devices. *Sensors* **2020**, *20*, 3570. [CrossRef]
34. Kiranyaz, S.; Ince, T.; Gabbouj, M. Real-time patient-specific ECG classification by 1-D convolutional neural networks. *IEEE Trans. Biomed. Eng.* **2015**, *63*, 664–675. [CrossRef]

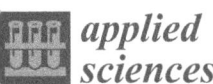

Article

On Combining Feature Selection and Over-Sampling Techniques for Breast Cancer Prediction

Min-Wei Huang [1,2,†], Chien-Hung Chiu [3,†], Chih-Fong Tsai [4] and Wei-Chao Lin [3,5,*]

1. Department of Physical Therapy and Graduate Institute of Rehabilitation Science, China Medical University, Taichung 406040, Taiwan; hminwei@gmail.com
2. Department of Psychiatry, Chiayi Branch, Taichung Veterans General Hospital, Chiayi 60090, Taiwan
3. Department of Thoracic Surgery, Chang Gung Memorial Hospital, Linkou 333423, Taiwan; b9102067@cgmh.org.tw
4. Department of Information Management, National Central University, Taoyuan 320317, Taiwan; cftsai@mgt.ncu.edu.tw
5. Department of Information Management, Chang Gung University, Taoyuan 33302, Taiwan
* Correspondence: viclin@gap.cgu.edu.tw
† These authors contributed equally.

Citation: Huang, M.-W.; Chiu, C.-H.; Tsai, C.-F.; Lin, W.-C. On Combining Feature Selection and Over-Sampling Techniques for Breast Cancer Prediction. *Appl. Sci.* **2021**, *11*, 6574. https://doi.org/10.3390/app11146574

Academic Editors: Stefano Silvestri and Francesco Gargiulo

Received: 16 June 2021
Accepted: 15 July 2021
Published: 17 July 2021

Publisher's Note: MDPI stays neutral with regard to jurisdictional claims in published maps and institutional affiliations.

Copyright: © 2021 by the authors. Licensee MDPI, Basel, Switzerland. This article is an open access article distributed under the terms and conditions of the Creative Commons Attribution (CC BY) license (https://creativecommons.org/licenses/by/4.0/).

Abstract: Breast cancer prediction datasets are usually class imbalanced, where the number of data samples in the malignant and benign patient classes are significantly different. Over-sampling techniques can be used to re-balance the datasets to construct more effective prediction models. Moreover, some related studies have considered feature selection to remove irrelevant features from the datasets for further performance improvement. However, since the order of combining feature selection and over-sampling can result in different training sets to construct the prediction model, it is unknown which order performs better. In this paper, the information gain (IG) and genetic algorithm (GA) feature selection methods and the synthetic minority over-sampling technique (SMOTE) are used for different combinations. The experimental results based on two breast cancer datasets show that the combination of feature selection and over-sampling outperform the single usage of either feature selection and over-sampling for the highly class imbalanced datasets. In particular, performing IG first and SMOTE second is the better choice. For other datasets with a small class imbalance ratio and a smaller number of features, performing SMOTE is enough to construct an effective prediction model.

Keywords: breast cancer; data mining; machine learning; feature selection; over-sampling; class imbalance

1. Introduction

Breast cancer, which is cancer that develops from breast tissue, is one of the important problems in the medical domain. It is the second most severe cancer among all of the cancers that have already been discovered. Some factors have been found to cause breast cancer, such as obesity, a lack of physical exercise, alcoholism, hormone replacement therapy during menopause, ionizing radiation, a family history of breast cancer, etc. [1]. In practice, many medial institutes have paid much attention to the early detection of breast cancer.

In related literatures, many data mining and machine learning techniques have been used to develop various kinds of breast cancer prediction models. Among them, some focus on the improvement of learning models and some focus on data pre-processing steps. For example, convolutional neural networks (CNN), as one representative of a deep learning technique, were modified to improve their prediction performance [2,3]. On the other hand, some studies focus on feature selection for filtering out irrelevant features from a given dataset for the construction of more effective classifiers [4,5] and data sampling for re-balancing class imbalanced datasets in order to decrease the effect of skewed class distribution in the learning process [6,7].

For related works of feature selection, Sasikala et al. [8] propose a novel feature selection method based on the genetic algorithm to select a gene subset from high dimensional gene data, which causes different classifiers perform better than the ones without feature selection. In [9], a genetic algorithm is used for feature selection, where the selected subset is used to construct different classifiers for performance comparisons. On the other hand, Jiang and Jin [10] use a gradient boosting decision tree with Bayesian optimization to remove the irrelevant and redundant features from gene expression data. Raj et al. [11] compare several feature selection methods to determine the best one to combine with the random forest classifier.

For related works on class imbalance learning, Zhang et al. [12] propose a clustering-based under-sampling method to select informative samples from the clusters identified in the majority and minority classes, and the decision tree based on this boosting technique is employed for the prediction model. In [13], eighteen different under- and over-sampling methods are used to balance related class imbalanced cancer datasets, in which the over-sampling methods perform better than the under-sampling ones. Cai et al. [14] apply the synthetic minority over-sampling technique (SMOTE) to balance the training dataset and employ the stacking ensemble method to combine multiple classifiers, which achieved better performance than conventional methods. Rani et al. [15] investigated the effect of performing SMOTE on five different classifiers to determine the best one for breast cancer prediction.

According to Fernandez et al. [16], SMOTE over-sampling can benefit from the use of feature selection, where feature selection is performed over the class imbalanced dataset to select a subset feature of it, and then the reduced dataset is over-sampled to make it contain the same size of the data samples as in the majority and minority classes. Recently, Solanki et al. [17] propose the contrary procedure that SMOTE be performed first to re-balance the breast cancer dataset, and then wrapper-based feature selection methods can be applied to reduce the feature dimensions.

However, to the best of our knowledge there is not any study examining the performances of both procedures to combine feature selection and over-sampling for breast cancer prediction. Therefore, the research objective of this paper is to compare these two combination orders with two baselines by employing feature selection and over-sampling individually. Particularly, filter and wrapper-based feature selection methods are combined with SMOTE for performance comparison. In addition, one small- and one large-scale breast cancer datasets are used in order to understand the performance of different approaches.

The contribution of this paper is two-fold. First, the procedures of combining the feature selection and over-sampling steps are compared in terms of breast cancer prediction, which has never been done before. Second, the best combination procedure and combined algorithms that will be identified in this paper can be used as one the representative baseline methods for future research.

The rest of this paper is organized as follows. Section 2 overviews related literature on feature selection and over-sampling. Section 3 describes the two different combination procedures and the experimental setup. Section 4 presents the experimental results, and Section 5 concludes the paper.

2. Literature Review

2.1. Feature Selection

Feature selection is an important data pre-processing step in data mining and knowledge discovery from databases. It focuses on selecting representative features from a given training set, which have higher discriminative power to make classifiers better able to distinguish between different classes. Moreover, another advantage of feature selection is to reduce feature dimensionality, which lowers the computational complexity during the classifier training stage [5,18].

In general, feature selection algorithms are composed of four basic steps, which are a generation procedure to generate the candidate feature subset, an evaluation function to evaluate the effectiveness of the feature subset, a stopping criterion to determine when to stop the previous steps, and a validation procedure to examine whether the feature subset is valid [19].

Existing feature selection algorithms can be divided into filter, wrapper, and embedded methods depending on how they combine the feature selection search with the construction of the classifiers. In filter methods, the relevance of features such as distance, consistency, dependency, information, and correlation are assessed,. That is, the feature relevance score is calculated, in which low-scoring features are removed. Some representative methods include relief, the Fisher score, and information gain.

In wrapper methods, a specific classification algorithm is used to determine the quality of different subsets of features. Since the space of feature subsets can grow exponentially with the number of features, heuristic search methods are used to guide the search for an optimal subset. Therefore, wrapper methods are very computationally intensive, especially when the construction of the chosen classifier requires a high computational cost. One representative wrapper method is the genetic algorithm.

In embedded methods, feature selection is incorporated as part of the classifier training process. That is, the feature selection method is embedded in the modeling algorithm, where the classifier is used to evaluate the quality of the selected subset of features. Embedded methods have the advantage of including interaction with the classification model, while at the same time being far less computationally intensive than wrapper methods. One representative wrapper method is the decision tree classifier.

2.2. Over-Sampling

In practice, the class imbalanced dataset problem usually occurs since the number of data samples in one class are significantly different from those of the other one; say the imbalance ratio is 1:100. For the example of breast cancer datasets, they do not usually contain both the malignant and benign patient classes, denoted as the minority and majority classes, respectively. Without dealing with the class imbalance problem, most machine learning models aim at maximizing the accuracy of its classification rule by ignoring the minority class examples, with the classification of all testing examples being organized into the majority class [6].

In general, there are three types of solutions to the class imbalance problem, which are algorithm level, data level, and cost-sensitivity methods. Among them, the data level methods based on data sampling techniques are usually considered first since they are used independently of the classifier [6]. Data sampling techniques focus on re-balancing the given training set. Particularly, under- and over-sampling techniques have been used, in which the former is for reducing the size of the majority class, whereas the latter is used for enlarging the size of the minority class. Among them, the synthetic minority over-sampling technique (SMOTE) is one representative method, which has been used as the baseline in many related studies [16].

The aim of SMOTE is to produce new synthetic examples for the minority class. For example, a minority class instance i is selected as the basis to create new synthetic data. According to a specific distance metric, usually the Euclidean distance, the number of the neighbors nearest to i are chosen from the training set, e.g., i_1, i_2, and i_3. Next, a randomized interpolation is conducted to obtain new synthetic data, i.e., s_1, s_2, and s_3.

3. Research Methodology
3.1. Two Combination Orders for Feature Selection and Over-Sampling

In this paper, two orders of combining the feature selection and over-sampling steps are compared by being given a training set, denoted as TR, which is composed of M and N

majority and minority class data samples, respectively, and each data sample is represented by k dimensional features. For the first order, i.e., performing feature selection first and over-sampling second, a chosen feature selection algorithm is employed to select some representative features from the TR. As a result, a reduced feature subset of TR is produced, denoted as $TR_{reduced}$, where each data sample is represented by o dimensional features ($k > o$). Next, the over-sampling algorithm is used to generate M–N synthetic data samples for the minority class, leading to a balanced training set, denoted as $TR_{reduced\_balanced}$, which is composed of $2M$ data samples. That is, the number of data samples in the majority and minority classes are the same.

On the other hand, for the second combination order, the over-sampling algorithm is used first to re-balance the training set, i.e., TR, which results in a balanced training set, denoted as $TR_{balanced}$. $TR_{balanced}$ is composed of $2M$ data samples, and each data sample is represented by k dimensional features. Next, the chosen feature selection algorithm is performed over $TR_{balanced}$, leading to a reduced feature subset of $TR_{balanced}$, denoted as $TR_{balanced\_reduced}$. In $TR_{balanced\_reduced}$, each data sample is represented by p dimensional features ($k > p$). Note that the number of features in $TR_{reduced\_balanced}$ by the first combination order and $TR_{balanced\_reduced}$ by the second combination order are not necessarily the same, i.e., $o \neq p$.

Therefore, the performances of the classifiers trained by $TR_{reduced\_balanced}$ and $TR_{balanced\_reduced}$ can be compared individually based on the same testing set. Moreover, other classifiers trained by $TR_{reduced}$ through performing feature selection alone and $TR_{balanced}$ through performing over-sampling alone are regarded as the baseline approaches for further performance comparison.

3.2. Experimental Setup

3.2.1. Datasets

In order to examine the performances of both orders of combining feature selection and over-sampling, two related breast cancer datasets are considered. The first one is based on the KDD Cup 2008 breast cancer dataset (https://www.kdd.org/kdd-cup/view/kdd-cup-2008 (accessed on 15 February 2021)), which contains 102294 data samples, and each data sample is represented by 117 different image features, which are extracted from 4 X-ray images per patient. Particularly, the class imbalance ratio is 163.2.

The second dataset is based on the Breast Cancer Wisconsin Dataset downloaded from the UCI Machine Learning Repository (https://archive.ics.uci.edu/ml/datasets/breast+cancer+wisconsin+%28original%29 (accessed on 15 February 2021)). It is composed of 699 data samples, in which each data sample is represented by 10 features including clump thickness, uniformity of cell size, uniformity of cell shape, marginal adhesion, single epithelial cell size, bare nuclei, bland chromatin, normal nucleoli, and mitoses. In addition, the class imbalance ratio is 1.86.

To train and test the classifier, the 5-fold cross validation method is used to divide each dataset into 80% and 20% training and testing sets. This means that every subset will be trained and tested five times, and the average prediction accuracy can obtained consequently be. In other words, each patient data will be used as the training and testing data example. In addition, the class imbalance ratio of the training set in each fold is controlled to be the same as the original dataset.

3.2.2. The Feature Selection and Over-Sampling Methods

In this paper, the information gain (IG) as the filter method and the genetic algorithm (GA) as the wrapper method are used for feature selection. Particularly, these two methods have been used in many research problems, including text classification [20], gene expression microarray analysis [21], intrusion detection [22], financial distress prediction [23], software defect prediction [24], etc.

IG evaluates the gain of each variable in the context of the target variable, which is based on calculating the reduction in entropy. That is, the feature ranking stage focuses on ranking the subsets of features by high information gain entropy in decreasing order. In GA, an initial set of candidate solutions (i.e., individuals) are created and their corresponding fitness values are calculated for the later cross-over and mutation steps. Specifically, the individuals are subsets of predictors, and the fitness values are measures of the model performance.

Analyses were performed using the WEKA data mining software package. Most related parameters are based on its default values, except for the genetic algorithm, where the population size, crossover rate, and mutation rate were set as 50, 0.8, and 0.01, respectively [25].

On the other hand, the over-sampling method is based on SMOTE. It has been widely used as a baseline over-sampling method for breast cancer datasets [14–17]. The percentage of synthetic instances was set to make the two datasets become balanced datasets where the malignant and benign classes contain the same numbers of data samples. Other related parameters were based on the default values of WEKA.

3.2.3. The Classifier Design

After the original training set TR was pre-processed by different approaches, i.e., $TR_{reduced\_balanced}$, $TR_{balanced\_reduced}$, $TR_{balanced}$, and $TR_{reduced}$, they were used to train the support vector machine (SVM) classifier for performance comparisons. In related literature, SVM has been widely used as the baseline classifier for breast cancer prediction [26–29].

The implementation of SVM was based on the RBF kernel function, and its related parameters were based on the default values of WEKA.

4. Experimental Results

4.1. The KDD Cup 2008 Breast Cancer Dataset

Figure 1 shows the AUC (area under the ROC curve) rates of different approaches. In addition, Figure 2 shows the type I errors of the different approaches, which represent the error of miss-classifying the malignant cases into the benign class. Note that IG+SMOTE and GA+SMOTE mean the combination order of performing feature selection first and over-sampling second, whereas SMOTE+IG and SMOTE+GA represent the opposite combination order. In addition, the baseline represents using the original training set without performing any feature selection or over-sampling steps to train the SVM classifier.

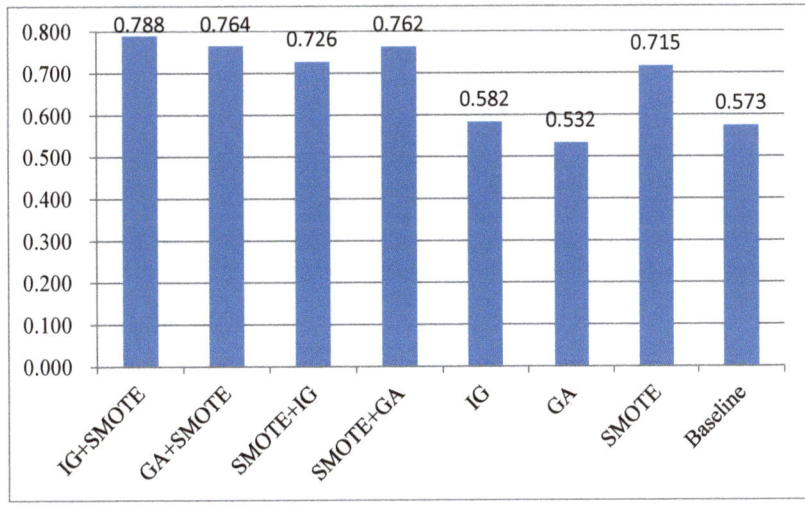

Figure 1. AUC rates of different approaches over the KDD Cup 2008 breast cancer dataset.

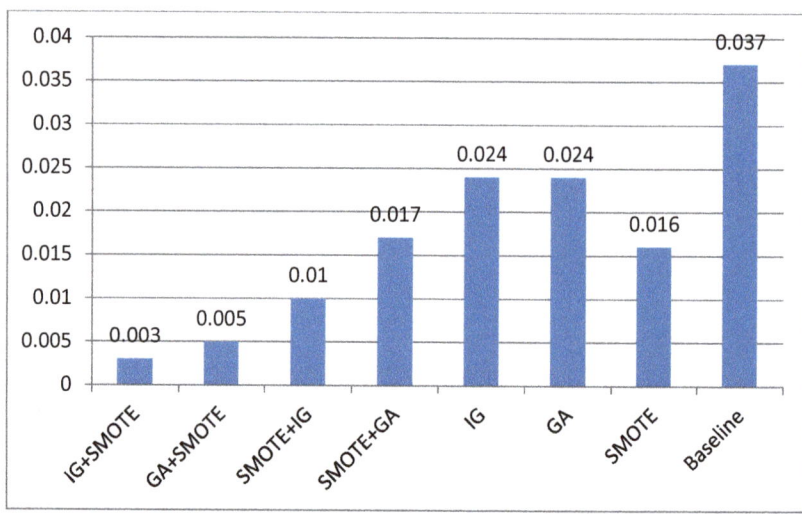

Figure 2. The type I errors of different approaches over the KDD Cup 2008 breast cancer dataset.

As we can see, the combinations of feature selection and over-sampling can allow the SVM to provide higher AUC rates and related lower type I errors than the ones with feature selection and over-sampling alone at the baseline. More specifically, the combination order of performing feature selection first and over-sampling second outperforms the opposite combination order. In particular, IG+SMOTE is the best combined approach, which causes the SVM to provide an AUC rate of 0.788 and a type I error rate of 0.003, which significantly outperforms the others ($p < 0.05$). On the other hand, for the feature reduction result, using IG and GA produce the selection of 94 and 14, respectively.

4.2. The Breast Cancer Wisconsin Dataset

Figures 3 and 4 show the AUC rates and the type I errors of different approaches, respectively. Different from the previous results, the approach that performed the best for the AUC was SMOTE (i.e., 0.962), whereas the second one was the baseline (i.e., 0.960). On the other hand, the approach that performed the best for the type I error is SMOTE+IG (i.e., 0.032), whereas the second-best ones are the baseline and SMOTE (i.e., 0.037). The other approaches producing similar AUC results were IG (i.e., 0.959), IG+SMOTE (i.e., 0.957) and SMOTE+IG (i.e., 0.955), whereas IG+SMOTE and IG produced similar type I errors, which were 0.038 and 0.044. These approaches do not have a significant level of performance difference. In particular, for the feature reduction result, using IG and GA produce 8 and 1 selected features, respectively.

The experimental results based on two different breast cancer datasets indicate that when the collected dataset is highly class imbalanced and contains a certain number of features, it is better to consider the combination of feature selection and over-sampling. Particularly, performing feature selection first and over-sampling second is likely to cause the classifier to provide higher accuracy than performing over-sampling first and feature selection second.

On the other hand, if the imbalance ratio of the collected dataset is not very high and it does not contain a large number of features, there is no need to consider the combination of feature selection and over-sampling. On the contrary, performing over-sampling to rebalance the dataset is enough to allow the classifier to provide relatively good performance.

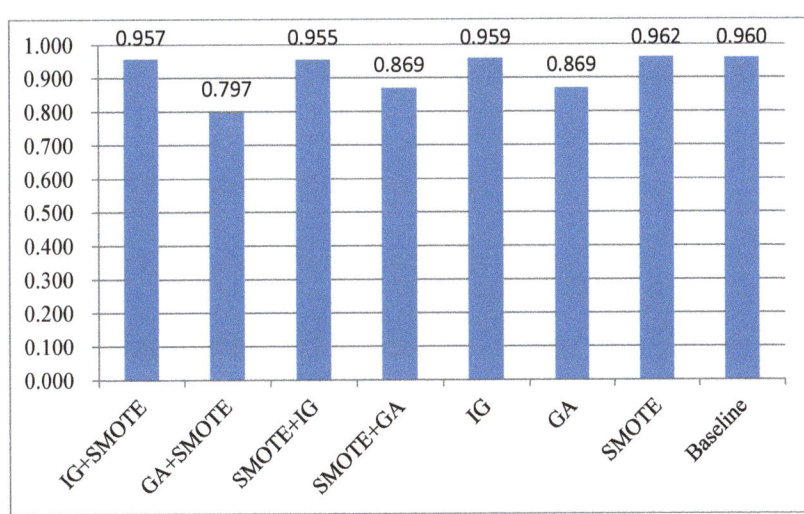

Figure 3. AUC rates of different approaches over the Breast Cancer Wisconsin Dataset.

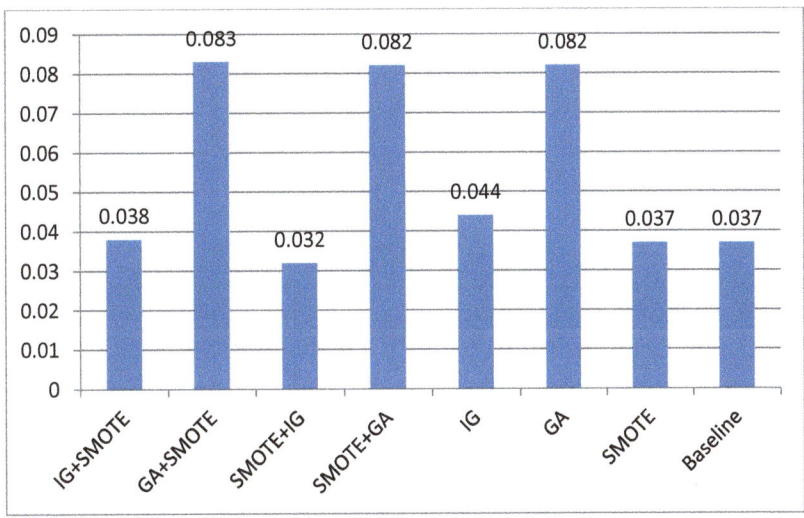

Figure 4. The type I errors of different approaches over the Breast Cancer Wisconsin Dataset.

5. Conclusions

Feature selection aims at selecting representative features from a given training set, whereas over-sampling is for re-balancing the class imbalanced training set. In this paper, the order of combining feature selection and over-sampling for breast cancer prediction are compared in terms of classification accuracy. In order to assess the performances of different combination approaches, the information gain (IG) and the genetic algorithm (GA) as the filter and wrapper-based feature selection methods and the synthetic minority over-sampling technique (SMOTE) were employed for creation of the combinations. Moreover, two breast cancer datasets with significantly different class imbalance ratios and number of features were used for the experiments.

Regarding the experimental results, for the highly imbalanced dataset containing a large number of features, performing both feature selection and over-sampling can cause the SVM classifier provide higher AUC rates than performing feature selection and over-sampling alone as well as at the baseline. In particular, it is recommended to execute feature selection first and over-sampling second. On the contrary, for the dataset with the low imbalance ratio and small number of features, performing over-sampling alone is the better choice.

Author Contributions: Conceptualization, C.-H.C. and M.-W.H.; methodology, C.-H.C. and C.-F.T.; software, W.-C.L.; validation, C.-F.T., W.-C.L., and M.-W.H.; formal analysis, C.-H.C., C.-F.T., and M.-W.H.; resources, C.-H.C.; data curation, C.-F.T.; writing—original draft preparation, C.-H.C., C.-F.T., and M.-W.H.; writing—review and editing, M.-W.H. and C.-H.C.; supervision, C.-H.C.; project administration, M.-W.H.; funding acquisition, W.-C.L. All authors have read and agreed to the published version of the manuscript.

Funding: This research was funded by the Ministry of Science and Technology of Taiwan, grant MOST 109-2410-H-182-012 and Chang Gung Memorial Hospital, Linkou, grant BMRPH13.

Institutional Review Board Statement: Not applicable.

Informed Consent Statement: Not applicable.

Data Availability Statement: The data that support the findings of this study are openly available in https://www.kdd.org/kdd-cup/view/kdd-cup-2008 (accessed on 15 February 2021) and https://archive.ics.uci.edu/ml/datasets/breast+cancer+wisconsin+%28original%29 (accessed on 15 February 2021).

Acknowledgments: The work was supported in part by the Ministry of Science and Technology of Taiwan under Grant MOST 109-2410-H-182-012 and in part by Chang Gung Memorial Hospital, Linkou under Grant BMRPH13.

Conflicts of Interest: The authors declare no conflict of interest.

References

1. Aydiner, A.; Igci, A.; Soran, A. *Breast Cancer: A Guide to Clinical Practice*; Springer: Berlin, Germany, 2019.
2. Zhang, Y.-D.; Satapathy, S.C.; Guttery, D.S.; Gorriz, J.M.; Wang, S.-H. Improved breast cancer classification through combining graph convolutional network and convolutional neural network. *Inf. Process. Manag.* **2021**, *58*, 102439. [CrossRef]
3. Zhang, Y.-D.; Pan, C.; Chen, X.; Wang, F. Abnormal breast identification by nine-layer convolutional neural network with parametric rectified linear unit and rank-based stochastic pooling. *J. Comput. Sci.* **2018**, *27*, 57–68. [CrossRef]
4. Chandrashekar, G.; Sahin, F. A survey on feature selection methods. *Comput. Electr. Eng.* **2014**, *40*, 16–28. [CrossRef]
5. Saeys, Y.; Inza, I.; Larrañaga, P. A review of feature selection techniques in bioinformatics. *Bioinformatics* **2007**, *23*, 2507–2517. [CrossRef] [PubMed]
6. Galar, M.; Fernandez, A.; Barrenechea, E.; Bustince, H.; Herrera, F. A Review on Ensembles for the Class Imbalance Problem: Bagging-, Boosting-, and Hybrid-Based Approaches. *IEEE Trans. Syst. Man, Cybern. Part C Appl. Rev.* **2012**, *42*, 463–484. [CrossRef]
7. López, V.; Fernández, A.; García, S.; Palade, V.; Herrera, F. An insight into classification with imbalanced data: Empirical results and current trends on using data intrinsic characteristics. *Inf. Sci.* **2013**, *250*, 113–141. [CrossRef]
8. Sasikala, S.; Balamurugan, S.A.A.; Geetha, S. A Novel Feature Selection Technique for Improved Survivability Diagnosis of Breast Cancer. *Procedia Comput. Sci.* **2015**, *50*, 16–23. [CrossRef]
9. Alickovic, E.; Subasi, A. Breast cancer diagnosis using GA feature selection and Rotation Forest. *Neural Comput. Appl.* **2017**, *28*, 753–763. [CrossRef]
10. Jiang, Q.; Jin, M. Feature Selection for Breast Cancer Classification by Integrating Somatic Mutation and Gene Expression. *Front. Genet.* **2021**, *12*, 629946. [CrossRef] [PubMed]
11. Raj, S.; Singh, S.; Kumar, A.; Sarkar, S.; Pradhan, C. Feature selection and random forest classification for breast cancer disease. In *Data Analytics in Bioinformatics*; Wiley: Hoboken, NJ, USA, 2021; pp. 191–210.
12. Zhang, J.; Chen, L.; Tian, J.-X.; Abid, F.; Yang, W.; Tang, X.-F. Breast Cancer Diagnosis Using Cluster-based Undersampling and Boosted C5.0 Algorithm. *Int. J. Control. Autom. Syst.* **2021**, *19*, 1998–2008. [CrossRef]
13. Fotouhi, S.; Asadi, S.; Kattan, M.W. A comprehensive data level analysis for cancer diagnosis on imbalanced data. *J. Biomed. Inform.* **2019**, *90*, 103089. [CrossRef] [PubMed]
14. Cai, T.; He, H.; Zhang, W. Breast Cancer Diagnosis Using Imbalanced Learning and Ensemble Method. *Appl. Comput. Math.* **2018**, *7*, 146. [CrossRef]
15. Rani, K.U.; Ramadevi, G.N.; Lavanya, D. Performance of synthetic minority oversampling technique on imbalanced breast cancer data. In Proceedings of the 3rd International Conference on Computing for Sustainable Global Development, New Delhi, India, 16–18 March 2016; pp. 1623–1627.

16. Fernandez, A.; Garcia, S.; Herrera, F.; Chawla, N.V. SMOTE for Learning from Imbalanced Data: Progress and Challenges, Marking the 15-year Anniversary. *J. Artif. Intell. Res.* **2018**, *61*, 863–905. [CrossRef]
17. Solanki, Y.; Chakrabarti, P.; Jasinski, M.; Leonowicz, Z.; Bolshev, V.; Vinogradov, A.; Jasinska, E.; Gono, R.; Nami, M. A Hybrid Supervised Machine Learning Classifier System for Breast Cancer Prognosis Using Feature Selection and Data Imbalance Handling Approaches. *Electronics* **2021**, *10*, 699. [CrossRef]
18. Guyon, I.; Elisseeff, A. An introduction to variable and feature selection. *J. Mach. Learn. Res.* **2003**, *3*, 1157–1182.
19. Dash, M.; Liu, H. Feature selection for classification. *Intell. Data Anal.* **1997**, *1*, 131–156. [CrossRef]
20. Pintas, J.T.; Fernandes, L.A.F.; Garcia, A.C.B. Feature selection methods for text classification: A systematic literature review. *Artif. Intell. Rev.* **2021**, 1–52. [CrossRef]
21. Lazar, C.; Taminau, J.; Meganck, S.; Steenhoff, D.; Coletta, A.; Molter, C.; De Schaetzen, V.; Duque, R.; Bersini, H.; Nowe, A. A Survey on Filter Techniques for Feature Selection in Gene Expression Microarray Analysis. *IEEE Trans. Comput. Biol. Bioinform.* **2012**, *9*, 1106–1119. [CrossRef]
22. Davis, J.J.; Clark, A.J. Data preprocessing for anomaly based network intrusion detection: A review. *Comput. Secur.* **2011**, *30*, 353–375. [CrossRef]
23. Liang, D.; Tsai, C.-F.; Wu, H.-T. The effect of feature selection on financial distress prediction. *Knowl.-Based Syst.* **2015**, *73*, 289–297. [CrossRef]
24. Balogun, A.O.; Basri, S.; Abdulkadir, S.J.; Hashim, A.S. Performance analysis of feature selection methods in software defect prediction: A search method approach. *Appl. Sci.* **2019**, *9*, 2764. [CrossRef]
25. Tsai, C.-F.; Eberle, W.; Chu, C.-Y. Genetic algorithms in feature and instance selection. *Knowl.-Based Syst.* **2013**, *39*, 240–247. [CrossRef]
26. Huang, M.-W.; Chen, C.-W.; Lin, W.-C.; Ke, S.-W.; Tsai, C.-F. SVM and SVM ensembles in breast cancer prediciton. *PLoS ONE* **2017**, *12*, e0161501.
27. Kamel, S.R.; Yaghoubzadeh, R.; Kheirabadi, M. Improving the performance of support-vector machine by selecting the best features by Gray Wolf algorithm to increase the accuracy of diagnosis of breast cancer. *J. Big Data* **2019**, *6*, 1–15. [CrossRef]
28. Vidić, I.; Egnell, L.; Jerome, N.P.; Teruel, J.R.; Sjøbakk, T.E.; Østlie, A.; Fjøsne, H.E.; Bathen, T.F.; Goa, P.E. Support vector machine for breast cancer classification using diffusion-weighted MRI histogram features: Preliminary study. *J. Magn. Reson. Imaging* **2017**, *47*, 1205–1216. [CrossRef]
29. Wang, H.; Zheng, B.; Yoon, S.W.; Ko, H.S. A support vector machine-based ensemble algorithm for breast cancer diagnosis. *Eur. J. Oper. Res.* **2018**, *267*, 687–699. [CrossRef]

Review

A Systematic Review of Federated Learning in the Healthcare Area: From the Perspective of Data Properties and Applications

Prayitno [1,2], Chi-Ren Shyu [3,4], Karisma Trinanda Putra [1,5], Hsing-Chung Chen [1,6], Yuan-Yu Tsai [7], K. S. M. Tozammel Hossain [3,4], Wei Jiang [3,4] and Zon-Yin Shae [1,*]

1. Department of Computer Science and Information Engineering, Asia University, Taichung City 413, Taiwan; prayitno@polines.ac.id (P.); karisma@ft.umy.ac.id (K.T.P.); cdma2000@asia.edu.tw (H.-C.C.)
2. Department of Electrical Engineering, Politeknik Negeri Semarang, Semarang 50275, Indonesia
3. Institute for Data Science and Informatics, University of Missouri, Columbia, MO 65211, USA; shyuc@missouri.edu (C.-R.S.); hossaink@missouri.edu (K.S.M.T.H.); wjiang@missouri.edu (W.J.)
4. Department of Electrical Engineering and Computer Science, University of Missouri, Columbia, MO 65211, USA
5. Department of Electrical Engineering, Universitas Muhammadiyah Yogyakarta, Bantul 55183, Indonesia
6. Department of Medical Research, China Medical University Hospital, China Medical University, Taichung City 404, Taiwan
7. Department of M-Commerce and Multimedia Applications, Asia University, Taichung City 413, Taiwan; yytsai@asia.edu.tw
* Correspondence: zshae1@asia.edu.tw

Abstract: Recent advances in deep learning have shown many successful stories in smart healthcare applications with data-driven insight into improving clinical institutions' quality of care. Excellent deep learning models are heavily data-driven. The more data trained, the more robust and more generalizable the performance of the deep learning model. However, pooling the medical data into centralized storage to train a robust deep learning model faces privacy, ownership, and strict regulation challenges. Federated learning resolves the previous challenges with a shared global deep learning model using a central aggregator server. At the same time, patient data remain with the local party, maintaining data anonymity and security. In this study, first, we provide a comprehensive, up-to-date review of research employing federated learning in healthcare applications. Second, we evaluate a set of recent challenges from a data-centric perspective in federated learning, such as data partitioning characteristics, data distributions, data protection mechanisms, and benchmark datasets. Finally, we point out several potential challenges and future research directions in healthcare applications.

Keywords: federated learning; deep learning; artificial intelligence; healthcare; data privacy-preserving

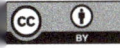

1. Introduction

Deep learning technology has shown promising results in smart healthcare applications to assist medical diagnosis and treatment based on clinical data. For instance, deep learning assists cancer diagnosis and prediction [1–3], brain tumor segmentation and classification from magnetic resonance image (MRI) [4–6], and text detection of medical laboratory reports [7,8]. Good performance of the deep learning model on smart healthcare applications highly depends on a diverse and vast amount of training data [9]. These training data were obtained from various clinical observations such as biomedical sensors, individual patients, clinical institutions, hospitals, pharmaceutical industries, and health insurance companies. However, acquiring the healthcare data required to develop a deep learning model may be challenging due to fewer patients and pathologies with a low incidence rate available in a single healthcare institution. Furthermore, Zech et al. [10] showed that deep learning models trained with single institutional data are vulnerable to institutional data bias, as shown in Figure 1a. This institutional data bias has been shown to have high accuracy when evaluated on the same clinical institution's data. However, it does not work well when applied to data from a different institution or even across departments within the same institution. Simultaneously, training deep learning models in a centralized data lake [11], as depicted in Figure 1b, is infeasible because of patient privacy and government regulations related to clinical data. Thus, to increase both the diversity and quantity of training data is through the collaboration of several healthcare institution to create a single deep learning model while maintaining patient privacy and confidentially.

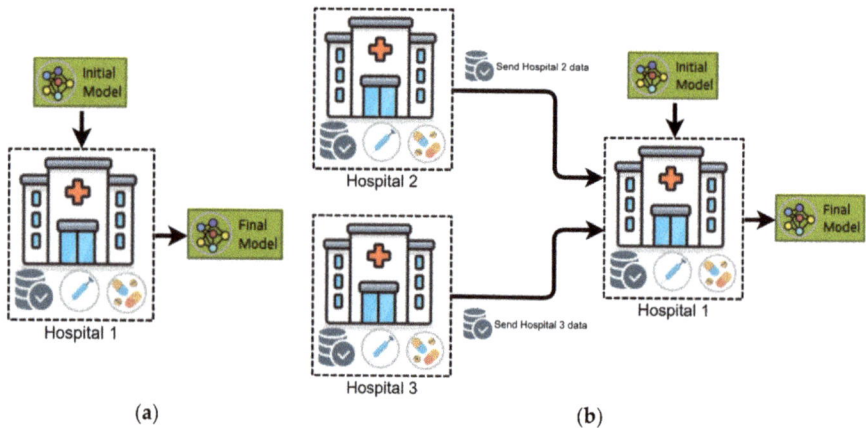

Figure 1. Single-institution and collaborative learning: (**a**) single-institution learning: machine learning model trained and validated with single institution dataset; (**b**) collaborative learning: machine learning model trained and validated with medical data collected from external institutions pooled in a central data lake.

Medical data are usually fragmented due to the complex nature of the medical system and processes. For instance, each medical institution may be able to access the medical data of their patients only. As protected health information (PHI), these medical data are only disclosed strictly regulated by law to third parties. The process of accessing and analyzing medical data is strictly regulated by laws and regulations, such as the Health Insurance Portability and Accountability Act (HIPAA) [12]. In addition, with an increasing number of data breaches at healthcare organizations, the prominence of data security and privacy protection has become a global consensus. For instance, in the American Medical Collection Agency (AMCA) recent healthcare data breach, the perpetrators have access to medical data, financial information, and payment details, affecting 11.9 million patients [13]. As a result, many countries around the globe are enacting stricter legislations to protect data security. For example, the General Data Protection Regulation (GDPR) went into effect in 2018 by the European Union to ensure users' privacy while protecting their data [14]. Under this GDPR, business entities must clearly explain why they need user data access and offer them the right to withdraw or delete their data. Business entities violating the regulation would face severe penalties. Many similar actions have taken place in the United States and Taiwan to protect individuals' privacy and security. For instance, Taiwan's Personal Data Protection Act (PDPA) and Cyber Security Management Act, enacted in 2018, prohibit online business entities from leaking or tampering with personal data details that they obtain [15]. This regulation enforces the business activities following the obligations of legal data protection. On the one hand, establishing these regulations will contribute to a more civil society's growth. On the other hand, these regulations introduce new challenges to data transaction and collaboration procedures for multi-institutional collaboration to train a deep learning model.

One recent approach to solving the problem of training a robust deep learning model from federated medical data while preserving patient privacy is federated learning

(FL) [16,17]. This method provides decentralized machine learning model training without transmitting medical data through a coordinated central aggregate server. Medical institutions, working as client nodes, train their deep learning models locally and then periodically forward them to the aggregate server. The central server coordinates and aggregates the local models from each node to create a global model, then distributes the global model to all the other nodes. It is worth noting that the training data are kept private to each node and never transmitted during the training process. Only the model's weight and parameters are transmitted, ensuring that medical data remain confidential. For these reasons, FL mitigates many security concerns because it retains sensitive and private data while enabling multiple medical institutions to work together. FL holds an excellent promise in healthcare applications to improve medical services for both institutions and patients—for instance, predict autism spectrum disorder [18], mortality and intensive care unit (ICU) stay-time prediction [19], wearable healthcare devices [20,21], and brain tumor segmentation [22]. However, FL algorithms face several challenges, mainly due to the properties of medical data, such as:

- **Data partitions:** FL technique aims to solve the limited sample size problem for training a secure collaborative machine learning model by aggregating a group of clients' data. However, choosing a data partition (horizontal or vertical) for FL is essential to solve the limited sample size, limited sample features, or both.
- **Data distribution (statistical challenge):** In developing a machine learning model in a centralized manner, the training data are centrally stored and balanced during training. However, with federated learning, each client generated the training data locally, remained decentralized, and cannot access the other clients' data. Thus, data distribution at one client can differ significantly from others, i.e., nonindependent and identically distributed (non-IID), impacting the performance of the federated learning model [23,24].
- **Privacy and security:** Data privacy and security are critical issues in medical applications. It is impossible to assume all of the clients in FL are reliable because the number of clients expected to participate is potentially thousands or millions. Thus, privacy-preserving mechanisms are needed to protect medical data from untrusted clients or third-party attackers.
- **Benchmark medical dataset:** Medical dataset quantity and quality have often limited the development of a robust solution to the FL algorithm. For various research purposes, the dataset used in FL experiments could vary significantly. For instance, some datasets focus on medical image classification and segmentation performance while others focus on network communication performance. However, the benchmark datasets have not already been compiled, specifically for medical datasets. Thus, a trusted benchmark is necessary to evaluate the performance of the FL that uses multiple medical data sources. Finally, we provide a comprehensive list of relevant medical datasets for future research on this topic.

Due to the ever-changing development in FL, several valuable studies on FL have been published in reputable publications from 2018 to 2021. Therefore, this paper aims to provide a recent review of federated learning in the medical domain. Specifically, this study describes the existing FL techniques related to solving the challenges inherent in medical data together with future research direction on FL for healthcare applications.

This study differs from existing reviews. General descriptions of FL are given in [16,17], while detailed discussions of recent challenges are presented in [25,26], security analysis [27], and personalization techniques [28]. Resumes of FL applications in edge computing [29], wireless networks [30], and healthcare [31,32] also have been published. However, none of the existing studies have explored the impact of medical data properties on the performance of FL in great detail. Moreover, it is necessary to provide a comprehensive overview related to benchmarking the FL in medical data. To fill the gap, this review presents a survey of FL from the perspective of data properties including data partitions, data distribution, data privacy, benchmarking, and its promising applications.

After a brief introduction of FL in this study, the rest of this paper is structured as follows. Section 2 describes the research method to conduct this study. Furthermore, in Section 3, we provide the search results from existing publications. Section 4 discusses our findings in data partition, data distribution properties, data privacy threats and protections, benchmark medical dataset, and open challenges applied in federated learning for medical applications. Finally, we have our paper's conclusion in Section 5.

2. Research Method

The Preferred Reporting Items for Systematic Reviews and Meta-Analyses (PRISMA) statement [33] was the research method to guide this study. PRISMA technique is a widely accepted standard for reporting evidence in systematic reviews that health-related organizations and journals have adopted [34]. PRISMA approaches provide several advantages, such as showcasing the review's quality, allowing readers to assess the review's strengths and flaws, replicating review processes, and structuring and formatting the review using PRISMA headings [33]. However, doing a systematic review and thoroughly publishing it may take time. Additionally, it can soon become out of date, thus it must be updated regularly to incorporate all newly published primary material since the project began.

2.1. Formulate Research Questions

We divide the research question into the following research questions.

- **RQ1**: What are the state-of-the-art FL methods in the healthcare area?
- **RQ2**: What are the FL methods proposed by scholars to solve challenging medical applications from a data properties perspective?
- **RQ3**: What are the research gaps and potential future research directions of FL related to medical applications?

The first research question (RQ1) aims to provide a comprehensive and systematic overview of all articles related to FL. Furthermore, RQ1 aims to provide evidence that the healthcare area can benefit by incorporating FL. Additionally, the second research question's (RQ2) motivation is to answer FL medical data settings challenges in FL such as data partition, statistic heterogeneity, and security. Finally, the third research question (RQ3) provides future directions for a researcher in the FL field primarily related to medical data challenges.

2.2. Data Eligibility and Analysis of the Literature

The article selection procedure uses the PRISMA flow diagram [33], as shown in Figure 2, which outlines papers' search, inclusion, and exclusion. There are three steps in the PRISMA flow diagram: identification, screening, and included. Firstly, in the identification step, we performed a comprehensive literature review between 1 January 2018 and 31 June 2021, using PubMed, Web of Science (WoS), Association of Computing Machinery Digital Library (ACM DL), Science Direct, and IEEEXplore digital libraries. We start from 2018 because we are interested in further implementation in the medical area one year after federated learning was proposed in 2017 [16]. The following search phrases were used in general are "Federate learning," and "Healthcare," and "data privacy protection." Because each publication database has its own set of filters for search queries, the specific query terms are specified in Appendix A Table A1. The initial result from digital libraries showed 197 articles satisfying the search criteria. Then, 28 articles were removed due to duplications, ending with 169 articles in the identification step.

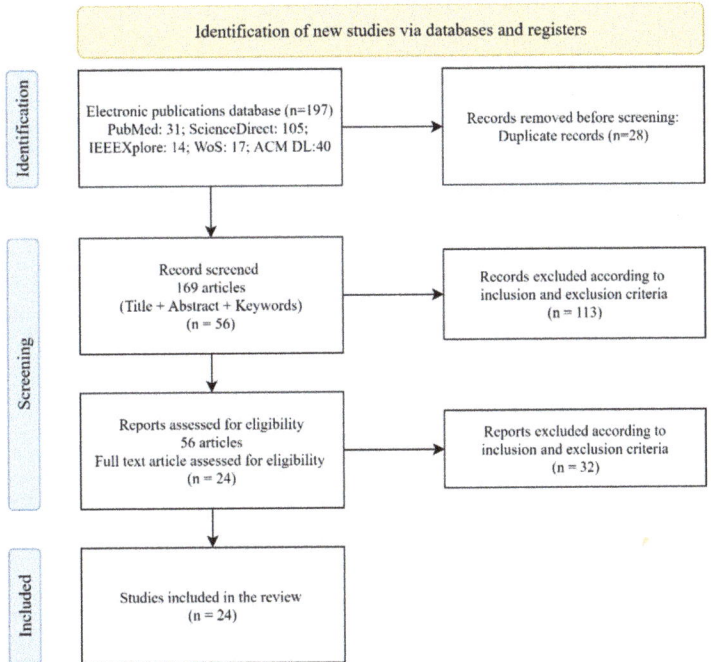

Figure 2. Study selection using PRISMA flow diagram method consisting of identification step, screening step, and included step.

While systematic reviews offer various advantages, they are prone to biases that obscure the study's objective results and should be evaluated cautiously [35]. Several approaches were used to eliminate bias and ambiguity in the research selection process, such as (i) conducting a dual review, (ii) defining clear and transparent inclusion and exclusion criteria, and (iii) tracing the resulting flow diagram using the PRISMA flow diagram. Firstly, two researchers independently analyzed the data and resolved inconsistencies through group discussion (P. and K.T.P). Then, the abstracts and complete texts of all relevant articles were carefully studied, and only those that fit the inclusion and exclusion criteria were chosen. Researchers then confirmed the selected papers and resolved any conflicts; if any disagreements persisted, third researchers were invited to discuss the matter, and the findings were appraised (Z.-Y.S., C.-R.S., and W.J.). There was no dispute over the papers included in this review.

This study should propose a good overview of FL for the healthcare sector and more in-depth about establishing FL's secure medical data mechanism. Thus, in the screening step, we define the inclusion and exclusion criteria. We included publications that (i) use FL to develop a model on a medical dataset, (ii) are published in well-known journals, and (iii) are published in English. Exclusion criteria were used to exclude the published studies that were not related, based on the following criteria: (i) articles that are not related to FL, (ii) FL for nonmedical application or not using medical dataset in the experiment, (iii) non-English language, (iv) review article, (v) proceeding or conference papers, (vi) arXiv preprints, and (vii) book, book chapter, book section.

Numerous considerations exist against the inclusion of conference papers in this study [36]. Firstly, conference proceedings usually contain various topics and much larger set of publications such that identifying suitable conferences, accessing their abstracts, and sifting through the frequent thousands of abstracts can be time-consuming and resource-consuming. Secondly, conference proceedings may lack sufficient information for systematic reviewers to evaluate the methods, risk of bias, and outcomes of the studies submitted at the conference due to their brevity. Finally, the reliability of the results is also in question especially in the healthcare area, partly because they are frequently preliminary or based on limited investigations undertaken in a position to meet conference deadlines. Thus, we do not include the conference papers in the inclusion criteria.

After applying inclusion and exclusion criteria from each study's title, abstract, and keywords, 56 articles were identified in the screening step. Next, 32 articles were excluded in the reports assessed for eligibility step due to exclusion criteria from full text in the article, ending with 24 articles. Finally, in the included step, 24 articles using FL in the healthcare application were selected for further analysis, and their results are discussed in this study. All of the 24 selected FL studies in the healthcare domain are listed in Table A2.

To provide a numerical description of the literature review, we gathered information from each article as follows: (i) paper information, such as author, title, year, and keywords; (ii) proposed methods, such as FL training algorithms and deep learning/machine learning models; (iii) data properties, such as medical datasets, data distribution techniques and challenges, data partition techniques, privacy attacks, and privacy mechanisms; and (iv) experiment results and discussion.

3. Results

We compiled the data properties in FL for healthcare applications from 24 published articles, as shown in Figure 3. The data scheme settings consisted of four layers: (i) data partitions such as horizontal federated learning (HFL), vertical federated learning (VFL), and federated transfer learning (FTL) (as discussed in Section 4.2); (ii) data distribution characteristics (non-IID) such as quantity skew, label distribution skew, feature distribution skew, and concept shift skew (as discussed in Section 4.3); (iii) possible data privacy attacks such as model inversion and membership inference attacks (as discussed in Section 4.4.1); (iv) additional data privacy protections such as differential privacy and homomorphic encryption (as discussed in Section 4.4.2). Above the medical data properties is the application task, where the task can be a classification or segmentation (as discussed in Section 4.6).

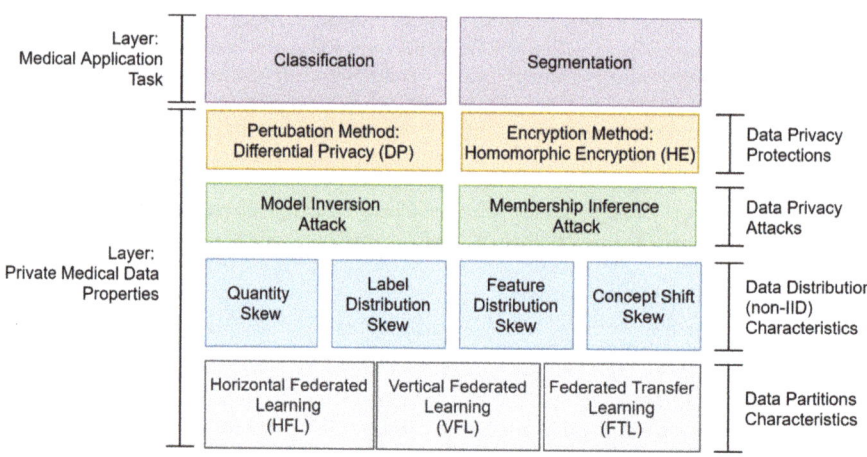

Figure 3. Medical data properties in federated learning for medical applications, consisting of data partitions, data distribution (i.e., non-IID) characteristics, possible data privacy attacks, and data privacy protections.

Numerical description. The following observations were made based on numerical analysis of the 24 included studies between 2018 and June 2021. Firstly, Figure 4a depicts the number of FL studies published in the medical application by year of publication. Since 2020, the number of articles published on FL has been continuously increasing. The number of papers published in 2021 should continue to increase linearly throughout the year. Secondly, Figure 4b shows the number of studies with data partition characteristics employed in FL.

According to the figure, most published FL studies use horizontal federated learning (HFL) as a medical data partition. Thirdly, Figure 4c shows the number of studies with various defense methods to protect from data privacy attacks. We can see that differential privacy is the most often employed type of data privacy protection. All of the possible data privacy protection methods will be discussed in Section 4.4. Based on Figure 4d, quantity skew is typical when dealing with multi-institutional medical data from FL experiments.

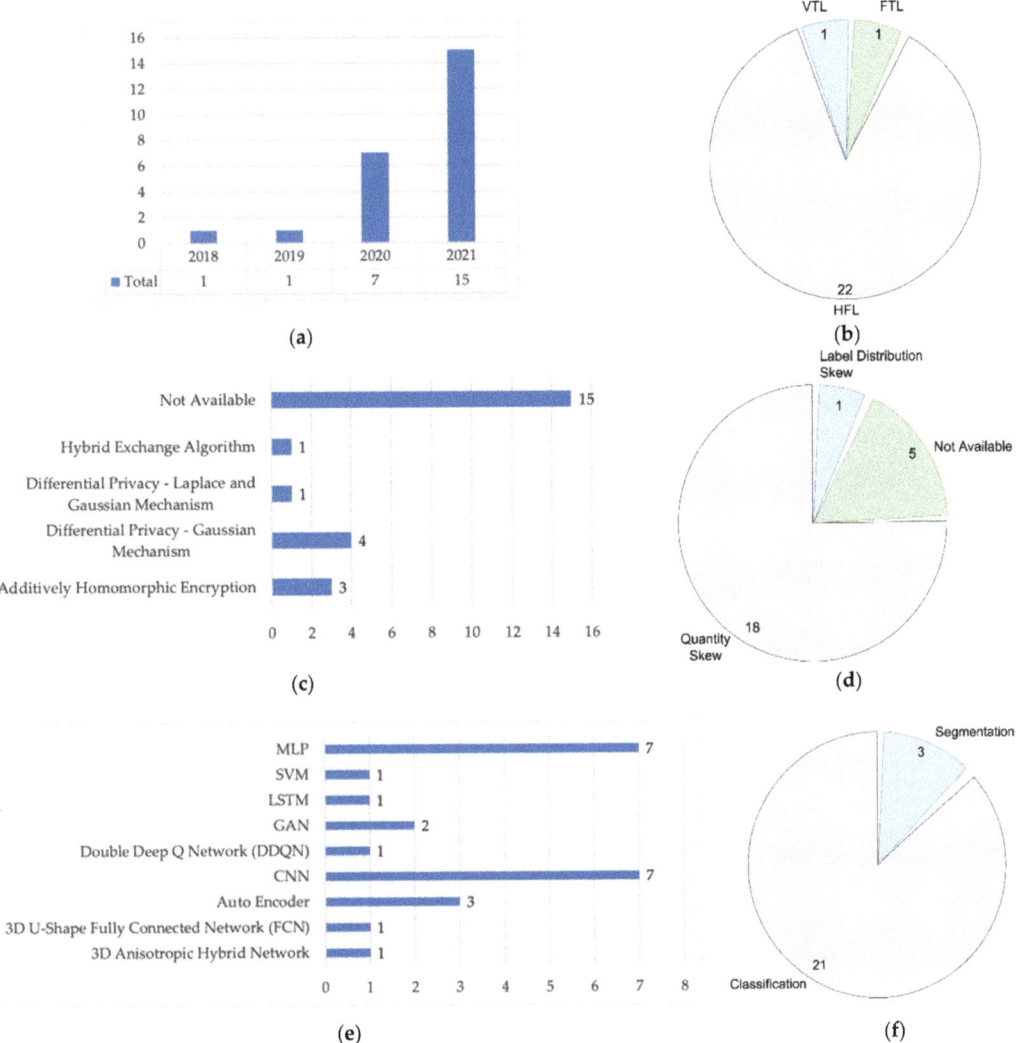

Figure 4. Numerical description of published articles in federated learning for medical applications. (a) The number of FL studies published in medical application included in the review, 2018–2021; (b) number of data partition characteristics employed in FL; (c) various data privacy algorithms employed in federated learning for the healthcare area; (d) number of non-IID characteristics discussed in FL studies published in the medical domain; (e) various machine learning models employed in federated learning for the healthcare area; (f) number of FL studies published in medical application included in the systematic review.

Machine learning algorithms. Additionally, we want to outline the machine learning models employed in the studies and evaluate their proposed FL algorithms. The outlined result of the machine learning model is shown in Figure 4e, where multilayer perceptron (MLP) is the most commonly used model when predicting with tabular medical datasets such as mortality prediction. Meanwhile, convolutional neural network (CNN) is the frequent model architecture used for medical image datasets. Other models include support vector machine (SVM) and autoencoder (AE) models. Additionally, we compile the machine learning task based on the 24 published articles, as shown in Figure 4f. There were 21 studies on classification tasks and three studies on segmentation tasks. Finally, we summarized in Table 1 the strengths and weaknesses of machine learning algorithms performing on federated learning.

Table 1. Summary of machine learning algorithms performing on federated learning, along with strengths and weaknesses.

ML Algorithms	Strength	Weakness	FL Study
AE	AE is mainly designed for dimensional feature reduction and denoising medical datasets via an unsupervised learning method. AE aims to recreate effective compact and effective feature representation.	An autoencoder may exclude essential information from a medical dataset's characteristics.	[19,21,37]
CNN	Performs well on medical image classification tasks such as prediction of COVID-19 using X-ray images	The training process of CNN that contains multiple layers will be time-consuming if the client in the FL environment does not have powerful computation resources.	[18,20,38–42]
GAN	Generate a synthetic sample of medical data for limited quantity in experiments datasets.	Training GAN is challenging due to the unstable training process, no standard metric evaluation, and numerous trial-and-error experiments required for effective outcomes.	[43,44]
LSTM	Performs well on time series or sequential medical datasets, for instance, detection of human activity recognition.	Due to the vanishing and exploding gradient challenges, training LSTM is difficult.	[45]
MLP	Good generalization performance on tabular medical datasets such as mortality prediction based on drug data	MLP is limited to learning elementary problems. Additionally, it is feature-scaling sensitive and involves setting numerous hyperparameters such as the number of hidden neurons and layers.	[46–51]
SVM	SVM is capable of modeling nonlinear decision boundaries and a variety of kernels are available. Additionally, it is highly resistant to overfitting, particularly in high-dimensional space.	SVM is memory-consuming, more difficult to modify because of critically selecting the appropriate kernel, and does not scale well to more extensive datasets.	[52]
U-Net	Achieve accurate results when performing segmentation tasks on medical image datasets, for example, when segmenting brain tumors disease using brain magnetic resonance medical images.	U-Net model development is time-consuming because the network must be operated independently for each patch, and redundancy due to overlapping patches. Additionally, a tradeoff exists between the precision of localization and the utilization of context.	[38,53]

AE: autoencoder; CNN: convolutional neural network; GA.: generative adversarial network; LSTM: long short-term memory; MLP: multilayer perceptron; SVM: support vector machine.

4. Discussion

RQ1: What are the state-of-the-art FL methods in the healthcare area?

4.1. Federated Learning Overview

FL is a technique to develop a robust quality shared global model with a central aggregate server from isolated data among many different clients. In a healthcare application scenario, assume there are K nodes where each node k holds its respective data $\mathcal{D}_k$ with n_k total number of samples. These nodes could be a healthcare wearable device, an internet of health things (IoHT) sensor, or a medical institution data warehouse. The FL objective is to minimize loss function given total data $n = \sum_{k=1}^{K} n_k$ and trainable machine learning weight vectors with d parameters $w \in R^d$ using Equation (1):

$$\min_{w \in R^d} F(w) = \sum_{k=1}^{K} \frac{n_k}{n} F_k(w) \text{ where } F_k(w) = \frac{1}{n_k} \sum_{x_i \in \mathcal{D}_k} f_i(w) \quad (1)$$

where $f_i(w) = \mathcal{L}(x_i, y_i; w)$ denotes the loss of the machine learning model made with parameter w. For instance, Huang et al. [19] used the categorical cross-entropy loss function to update the model parameters on the binary classification of patient mortality. In addition, Yang et al. [53] used the soft dice loss function for the COVID-19 region segmentation application.

In 2016, the basic concept of data parallelism in FL namely federated averaging (FedAvg) algorithm, was introduced by McMahan et al. [16]. As stated in the FedAvg algorithm, every communication round t consists of four phases. Firstly, the aggregate server initializes a global model with initial weights w_t^g, then shared with a group of clients S_t (medical nodes in our case), which was picked randomly with a fraction of $C \in \{0,1\}$. Secondly, each client $k \in S_t$, after received a global model w_t^g from the server, the client conducts local training steps with epoch E on minibatch $b \in B$ of n_k private data points. The local model parameters are updated with local learning rate η and optimized by minimizing loss function $\mathcal{L}(.)$. Thirdly, once client training is completed, the client k sends back its local model w_{t+1}^k to the server. Finally, after receiving the local model w_{t+1}^k from all selected groups of clients S_t, the aggregate server updates the global model w_{t+1}^g by averaging of local model parameters using Equation (2):

$$w_{t+1}^g \leftarrow \sum_{k=1}^{K} \alpha_k \times w_{t+1}^k \quad (2)$$

where α_k is a weighting coefficient to indicate the relative influence of each node k on the updating function in the global model, and K is the total nodes that participated in the training process. Choosing the proper weighting coefficient α_k in the averaging function can help improve the global model's performance (as discussed in Section 4.3.2 non-IID mitigation methods). The entire FL procedure is described in Algorithm 1.

Algorithm 1 FL with Federated Averaging (FedAvg) algorithm [16]

Input: T global round, C number of fractions for each training round, K number of clients, η learning rate at a local client, E number of epochs at a local client, B local minibatch at a local client.
01:     Initialize global model $w_{t=0}^g$
02:     **for** each round $t = 1, 2, \ldots, T$ **do**
03:         $m \leftarrow \max(C \times K, 1)$
04:         $S_t \leftarrow (m \text{ clients in a random order})$
05:         **for** each client $k \in S_t$ **do**
06:             $w_{t+1}^k \leftarrow ClientUpdate(k, w_t^g)$
07:         $w_{t+1}^g \leftarrow \sum_{k=1}^K \alpha_k \times w_{t+1}^k$
08:
09:     **ClientUpdate**(k, w_t^g):
10:         $w_k \leftarrow w_t^g$
11:         **for** each local epoch $e = 1, 2, \ldots E$ **do**
12:             **for** each local batch $b \in B$ **do**
13:                 $w_k \leftarrow w_k - \eta \nabla \mathcal{L}(b; w_k)$
14:         **return** local model w_k
Output: w_{t+1}^g a global model at round $t+1$

FL has differentiated from the standard collaborative learning in the following properties: (1) training is carried out across a vast number of many client nodes, and communication speed between the client nodes and the aggregate server is slow; (2) the central aggregate server does not have a control to individual nodes or devices, and full participation of all nodes is unrealistic because there are inactivate devices that do not respond to the server; (3) in real-world case scenario, data distribution is nonindependent and identically distributed (non-IID). Non-IID data distribution means that each node has a different distribution pattern from the other node. These properties are shown when the first proposed of FL algorithm is applied for mobile keyboard prediction [16,17]. However, these properties are different when FL is implemented in the healthcare area. First, the FL training is carried out across a limited number of healthcare nodes from 2 to 100 as listed in Table 2, and communication speed between healthcare participants and the aggregate server is usually reliable. Second, the aggregate server coordinates the participant nodes in the FL training scheme without exposing the participant's local data to the network; thus, data privacy and security can be guaranteed.

FL is divided into two categories based on the aggregation schema: (a) centralized FL and (b) decentralized FL. As shown in Figure 5a, for centralized FL, the central server selects a subset of nodes at the beginning of training and aggregates the model updates received from client nodes. As nodes, the medical institutions periodically communicate the local updates w_{t-1}^k with a central server to learn a global model w_t^g. The central server aggregates the updates and sends back the parameters of the updated global model. However, if the centralized server fails, the whole FL environment will collapse. This failure is one of the reasons that the decentralized FL was proposed. Specifically, all nodes coordinate themselves and work together from node to node to develop a global model in decentralized FL, as shown in Figure 5b.

RQ2: What are the FL methods proposed by scholars to solve challenging medical applications from a data properties perspective?

4.2. Data Partition Characteristics

This section discusses FL based on the healthcare data partition characteristics. Since FL uses data kept in various medical institutions, it is frequently presented in a feature matrix. Let matrix $\mathcal{D}_k$ denote medical data held by the medical institution k. Notably, a row in the matrix represents a patient index denoted by $\mathcal{I}$, a column represents a patient features diagnosis denoted by $\mathcal{X}$, and some data may contain a label data $\mathcal{Y}$. The complete training medical dataset $\mathcal{D}_k$ in a medical institution k is denoted by $(\mathcal{I}_k, \mathcal{X}_k, \mathcal{Y}_k)$. Thus, data partition in FL can be divided into horizontal federated learning (HFL), vertical federated learning (VFL), and federated transfer learning (FTL) [26].

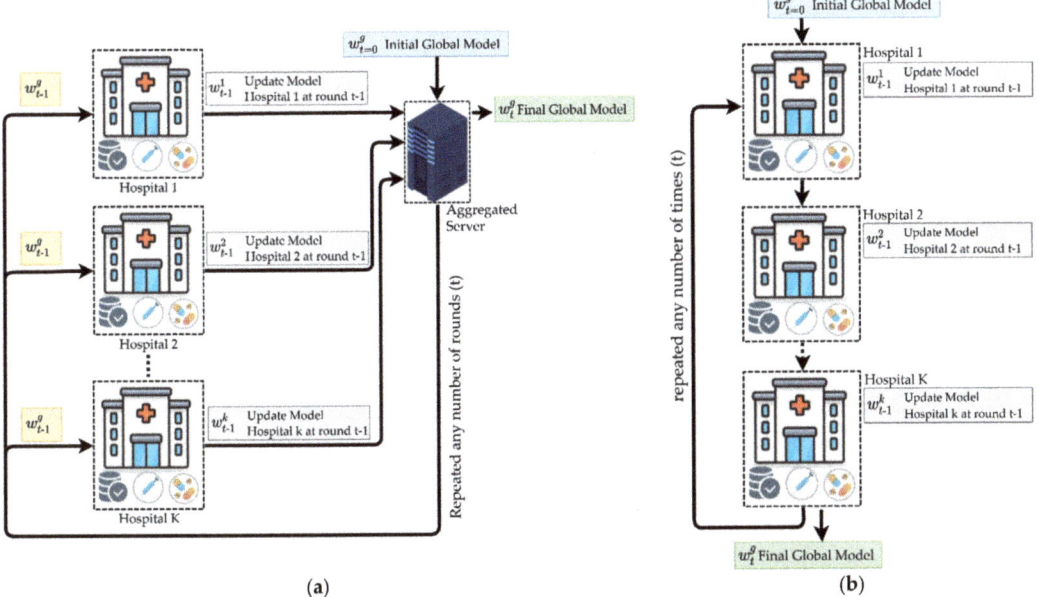

Figure 5. Federated learning framework for healthcare application based on aggregation schema. (**a**) Centralized FL: the central server selects the nodes, aggregates the updates, and sends back the updated global model parameters; (**b**) decentralized FL: to develop a global model, there is no central server to orchestrate all nodes.

4.2.1. Horizontal Federated Learning (HFL)

The horizontal federated learning (HFL) data partition, shown in Figure 6, is recommended in the case of limited sample size variability when developing a model. In this data partition setting, the nodes could be different health institutions or health data application providers. The HFL aims to develop a global model by integrating patients' sample data from different institutions without affecting patient privacy. Each node shares different patients' index $\mathcal{I}$ but has the same features $\mathcal{X}$ and labels $\mathcal{Y}$ information [26]. HFL is denoted as:

$$\mathcal{X}_j = \mathcal{X}_k, \quad \mathcal{Y}_j = \mathcal{Y}_k, \quad \mathcal{I}_j \neq \mathcal{I}_k, \quad \forall \mathcal{D}_j, \mathcal{D}_k, \quad j \neq k \qquad (3)$$

where D_i represents the dataset held by client i. For instance, two healthcare providers of the same business located in different countries would like to develop an AI model. User features of these two healthcare providers will mostly be the same because both operate the same business. However, the patient samples held by the two healthcare providers are different due to geographic locations. In this regard, we can use HFL to increase the total training sample by aggregating both of the healthcare providers' user samples in a privacy-preserving manner to enhance the model's performance. Therefore, the HFL data partition resolves the lack of sample size in data training because it combines all healthcare institutions' sample data.

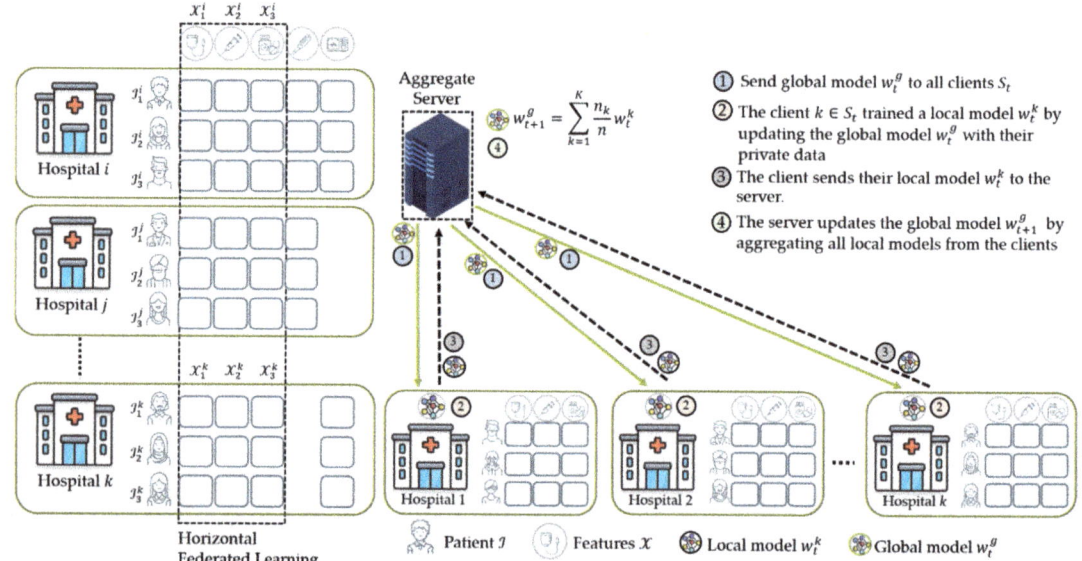

Figure 6. The typical medical data partitions scenario for horizontal federated learning (HFL). Each node is a medical institution data silo or wearable medical device. They share the same feature of medical diagnosis $\mathcal{X}_j = \mathcal{X}_k$ but have different patients index $\mathcal{I}_j \neq \mathcal{I}_k$.

HFL data partition is quite common in FL applied for medical applications. More than half of FL studies on medical applications implemented horizontal medical data partition in their experiment [18,19,21,37,39–49,51,52,54,55]. Unlike FL applied for nonmedical applications where training is carried out across many nodes, FL studies in medical applications only handle limited nodes from 2 to 100, as listed in Table 2. For instance, Li et al. [18] experimented with four medical institutions in different places for the autism spectrum disorder (ASD) prediction scenario. Each medical party shares the same user features generated by medical equipment and combines all patient samples from four medical nodes.

4.2.2. Vertical Federated Learning (VFL)

Data partition in vertical federated learning (VFL) is depicted in Figure 7. In this data partition setting, two nodes shared the same users' profile but different features information. The nodes could be different health institutions or health data application providers. VFL aims to develop a global model by integrating patient features from different institutions without directly sharing patient data. Each node shares different patients' features $\mathcal{X}$ and labels $\mathcal{Y}$ information but has the same sample data $\mathcal{I}$ [26]. VFL can be denoted as:

$$\mathcal{X}_j \neq \mathcal{X}_k, \; \mathcal{Y}_j \neq \mathcal{Y}_k, \; \mathcal{I}_j = \mathcal{I}_k, \; \forall \mathcal{D}_j, \mathcal{D}_k, \; j \neq k \qquad (4)$$

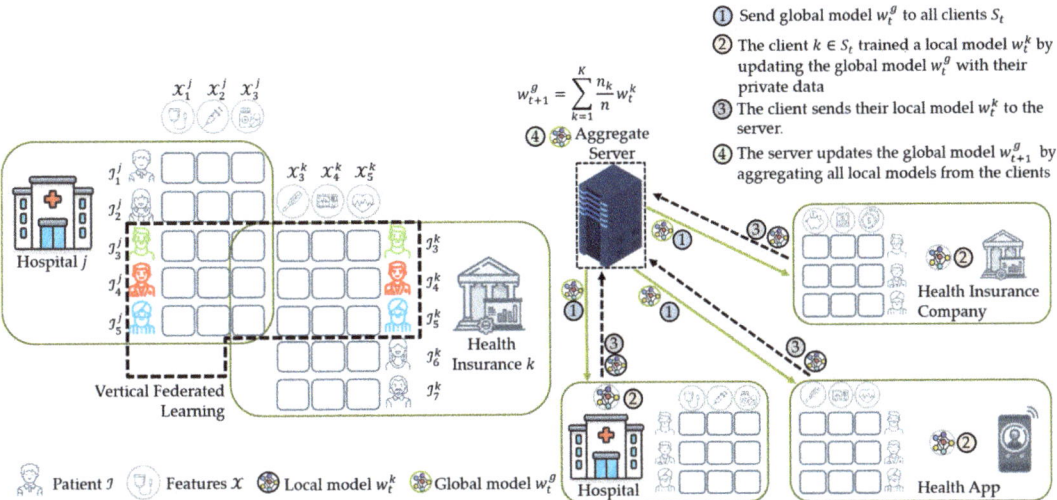

Figure 7. The typical medical data partitions scenario for vertical federated learning (VFL). Each node can be a different medical institution and application. They share the same patients' index $\mathcal{I}_j = \mathcal{I}_k$ but have different features of medical diagnosis $\mathcal{X}_j \neq \mathcal{X}_k$.

For example, two distinct healthcare organizations exist in the same region: one hospital and one health insurance company. Users of these two healthcare organizations may mostly be the same because they are the region's residents. However, the user features may not have anything in common because healthcare insurance records users' income and medical reimbursement, while hospitals keep users' medical treatment histories. VFL data partition securely combines different features sets to enhance the performance of the model. Thus, the VFL data partition increases feature dimension in data training.

In contrast to HFL, there are a few published VFL-based studies applied in medical applications. One such an example was proposed by Cha et al. [56]. The authors developed an autoencoder federated learning model for the vertically partitioned medical data. An autoencoder model is used for transforming user features in each client into a latent dimension. The proposed method does not share any raw medical data but latent dimensions as secure perturbed data. After receiving the clients' latent dimensions, the aggregate server concatenates all latent dimensions for training the global model. However, this approach is prone to reverse-engineering, which could discover the original medical data from the latent dimensions. In addition, the proposed method needs all the clients to perform data alignment, which means the user data has the same row indices in all data silos (first row data on clients k must be the same as client j).

4.2.3. Federated Transfer Learning (FTL)

Unlike the data configurations in HFL and VFL, data partition in federated transfer learning (FTL) considers the situation of multiple nodes shared neither the same users' profile nor features information, as shown in Figure 8. The main issue in this data partition configuration is that one node lacks labeled data. The nodes could be different health institutions or health data application providers located in different regions. Furthermore, each node shared different patients' features $\mathcal{X}$, labels $\mathcal{Y}$, and sample data index $\mathcal{I}$ [26]. FTL can be denoted as:

$$\mathcal{X}_j \neq \mathcal{X}_k,\ \mathcal{Y}_j \neq \mathcal{Y}_k,\ \mathcal{I}_j \neq \mathcal{I}_k,\ \forall \mathcal{D}_j, \mathcal{D}_k,\ j \neq k \quad (5)$$

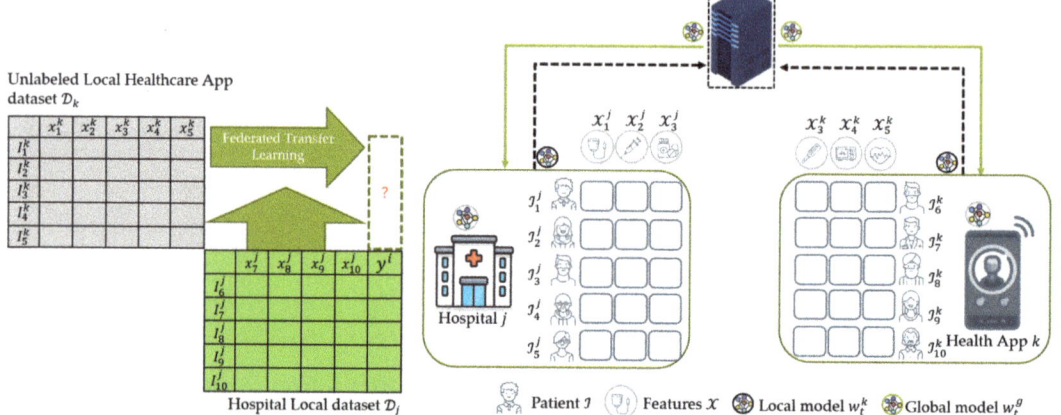

Figure 8. The typical medical data partitions scenario for federated transfer learning (FTL). One party is a medical institution, while the other is a healthcare application located in a different region. They share neither the patients' index $\mathcal{I}_j \neq \mathcal{I}_k$ nor features of medical diagnosis $\mathcal{X}_j \neq \mathcal{X}_k$.

For example, there are two distinct healthcare entities: one is a hospital in Taiwan, while the other is in the United States. Due to the geographical limitations, the two healthcare entities' user groups have little overlap, and the data features of the two entities datasets may slightly overlap. FTL addresses limited data sets and label samples in this scenario, thus increasing the model's performance while protecting user privacy.

The research in FTL is still in the early stages, and there is plenty of room for improvement. Chen et al. [20] proposed FedHealth assuming FTL data partition. FedHealth method collects data from several users/organizations using FL then offers a personalized model for each user/organization using transfer learning. First, the model learns to classify human activity and then extends the task to Parkinson's disease classification with transfer learning. In this case, FTL developed a global model for disease prediction in one task and then could be transferred to another task.

4.3. Data Distribution (Statistical Data Heterogeneity) Challenge

FL can solve the limited data quantity issue by combining data from each client without directly sharing each client's private data. However, FL also faces statistical data heterogeneity challenges due to data distribution at each client. The data distributions at each client are likely to be different, leading to poor global model performance [23,24]. Zhao et al. [23] demonstrated that the data distributions might considerably decrease FL model performance due to weight divergence induced by different population distributions. Within an FL environment, data distribution is frequently classified into IID and non-IID. Non-IID can result from an imbalance in the amount of data quantity, features, or labels. Non-IID is a common occurrence in the medical domain. Various medical tools manufacturers, different calibrated techniques, and different medical data acquisition techniques are the main reasons why each medical institution generates nonidentical data distribution. For instance, Li et al. [18] described how each medical institution uses various brain scanner manufacturers and instructions for each patient when taking autism brain imaging data. Specifically, during data acquisition, one medical site instructs patients to keep their eyes open while others instruct them to close their eyes during scanning. In the following subsection, we describe the non-IID characteristics and mitigation methods.

4.3.1. Non-IID Characteristics

The non-IID characteristics among healthcare nodes in the FL environment can take on four different forms such as (1) quantity distribution skew, (2) label distribution skew, (3) feature distribution skew, and (4) concept shift skew [24,25]. The non-IID characteristic summarized from 24 published FL studies applied for medical application is listed in Table 2.

Quantity skew (imbalance data) characteristic. Quantity skew characteristic in non-IID occurs when the class distribution of data instances $\mathcal{I}$ is not equal or far from equal across nodes in the FL scheme. An illustration of quantity skew is shown in Figure 9. In the IID scenario, the amount ratio of positive and negative instances is almost equal. For instance, in node two, the negative and positive amount ratios are 45% and 55%, respectively. In the non-IID case, the ratio of positive and negative instances is far from equal. For example, in node one, positive instances are around 5%, while negative ones are 95%. Krawczyk et al. [57] divided imbalance data categories into slight imbalance and severe imbalance. A slight imbalance is when the majority class is uneven by a small amount in the training dataset, and the ratio ranges from 1:4 up to 1:100. Severe imbalance data distribution is when the data distribution of the majority class is uneven by a vast amount in the training dataset, the ratio is more than 1:100. For example, the ratio of imbalance data in fraud detection tasks is up to 1:1000.

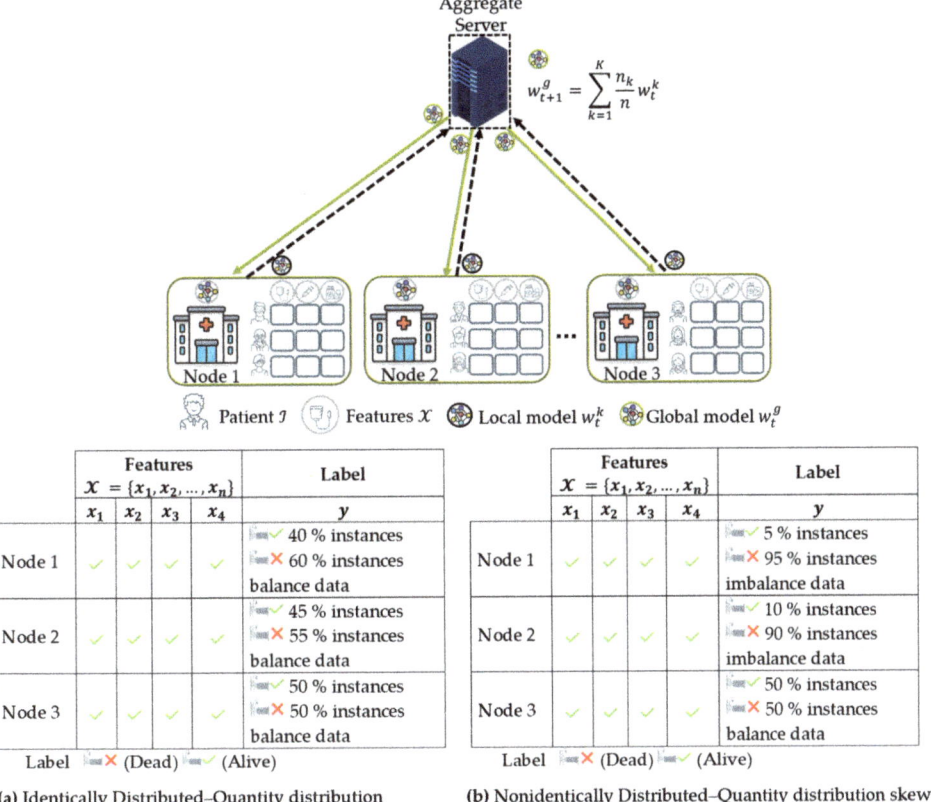

Figure 9. Non-IID from quantity skew (i.e., imbalanced dataset) characteristic. (**a**) IID: the amount ratio of positive and negative instances is equal or slightly equal; (**b**) non-IID: the ratio of positive and negative instances is far from equal. For example, the positive and negative instances ratio is 5% and 95% in node one, respectively.

Quantity skew characteristic exists in FL for medical application experiment datasets such as [18,19,46,52,53]. Quantity skew (i.e., imbalanced dataset) is common in the medical dataset since it is acquired from multiple healthcare institutions, and the number of instances in a class is not equally distributed for each institution. For instance, larger hospitals have more patient records than small clinics in rural areas. Huang et al. [19] tried to resolve this challenge by developing an imbalanced eICU dataset to predict patient mortality where the ratio is 5% and 95% for death and alive categories, respectively.

Label distribution skew characteristic. For label distribution skew, the distribution of labels $P(y_i)$ varies between different nodes. In the medical case, larger hospitals generally have more disease-related records than small clinics in rural areas. An illustration for label distribution skew characteristic is shown in Figure 10. In the IID setting, the distribution of labels $\mathcal{Y}$ is the same across all nodes. However, in the non-IID setting, the distribution of labels $\mathcal{Y}$ varies between each node. Specifically, there is a label y_i that only exists in one or several nodes in the FL environment. This label distribution skew characteristic was initially demonstrated in FedAvg's experiment [16]. Data samples with the same label are divided into subsets, and each client is assigned to no more than two subsets with distinct labels. Following FedAvg, this configuration is employed in published FL studies for medical applications [38].

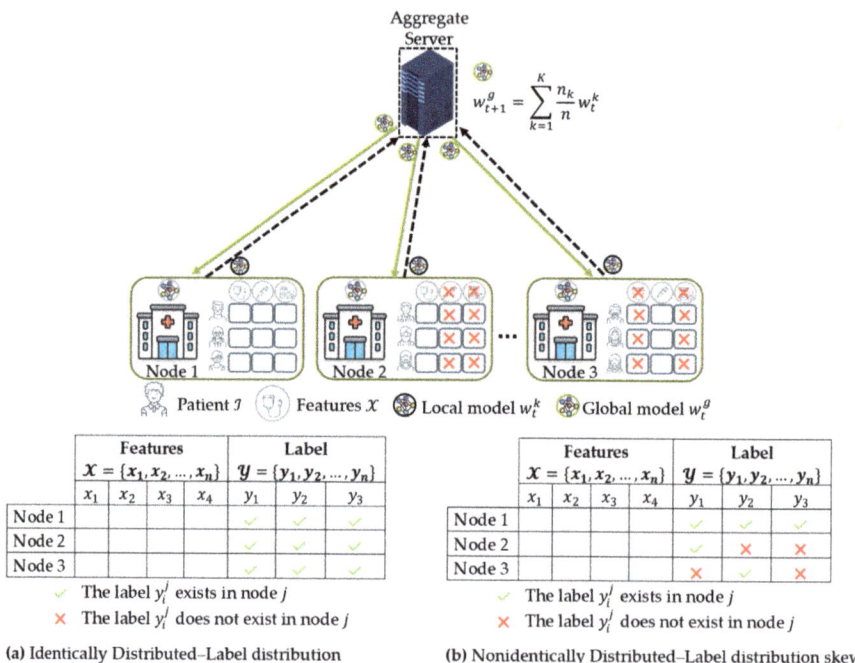

Figure 10. Non-IID from label distribution skew (prior probability shift) characteristic. (a) IID: The distribution of labels $\mathcal{Y}$ exists in all nodes; (b) non-IID: the distribution of labels $\mathcal{Y}$ varies between different nodes. For instance, node two does not have the labels y_2 and y_3 while node one has all labels.

Feature distribution skew characteristic. In the feature distribution skew characteristic, the distribution of features $P(x_i)$ varies between different nodes. An illustration of features distribution skew is shown in Figure 11. In the case of IID, the distribution of features $\mathcal{X}$ is the same across all nodes, while in the non-IID case, the distribution of features $\mathcal{X}$ varies between each node. Specifically, there is a feature x_i that only exists in one or several nodes in the FL environment. For instance, node two does not have the x_1

and x_2 features while other nodes have those features. Missing features or missing data is a common occurrence in medical datasets. For instance, missing features can be caused by failures of measurement on medical images. Measurement in medical image acquisition requires the images to be in focus. Medical images that are not in focus or blur can cause missing pixel values. The absence of some features in one or several nodes in the features distribution skew can be a problem in the FL training process. Data imputation techniques such as probability principal component analysis (PPCA) and multiple imputations using chained equations (MICE) can be employed to mitigate the problem [58].

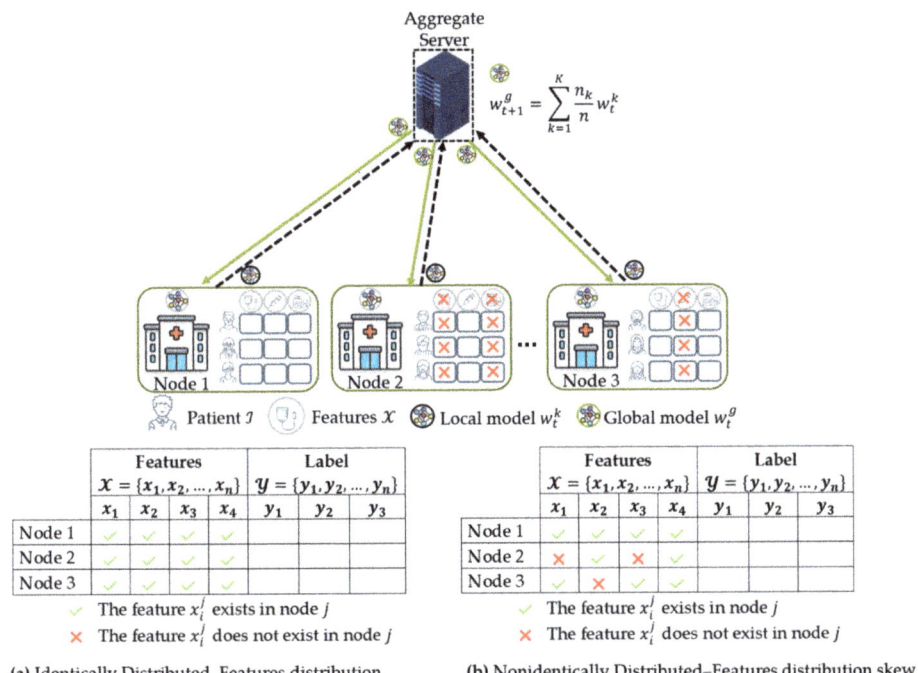

Figure 11. Non-IID from feature distribution skew characteristic. (a) IID case: the distribution of features $\mathcal{X}$ exists in all nodes; (b) non-IID case: the distribution of features $\mathcal{X}$ varies between each node. For instance, node two does not have the features x_1 and x_3 while the other nodes have those features.

Concept Shift Skew. There are two forms in the concept shift skew: the same label but different features $P(x|y)$ and the same features but different label $P(y|x)$. An illustration of concept shift skew is depicted in Figure 12. The same label but different features in non-IID characteristic is related to vertical federated learning data partition where each node shares the sample index $\mathcal{I}$ but have different features $\mathcal{X}$, while in the case of the same features but the different label in non-IID characteristics is not applicable in most FL studies.

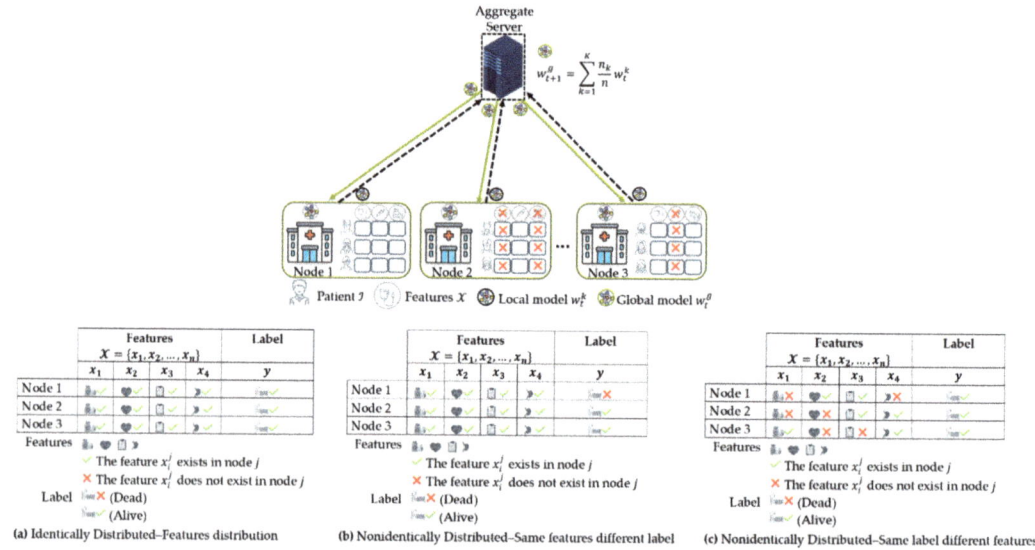

Figure 12. Non-IID from concept shift skew characteristic. (**a**) IID case; (**b**) non-IID same features but different label case; (**c**) non-IID same label but different features case.

4.3.2. Non-IID Mitigation Methods

Different non-IID characteristics may need different mitigating measures. There are three methods in the published FL for medical applications to improve the model performance with the non-IID dataset: (1) balancing the training dataset, (2) tuning the model hyperparameter in the FL algorithm, and (3) domain adaptation.

Balance the training dataset method. When dealing with quantity skew in non-IID characteristics, researchers balance the quantity of minority and majority classes in the training dataset with the synthetic data augmentation technique. It is important to note that the balancing method in the FL environment should keep the data secure and private. There are two methods to generate synthetic data augmentation in the FL environment: (1) local data augmentation and (2) server data sharing.

(1) The healthcare node generates a synthetic sample to balance the training dataset in the local data augmentation method. The synthetic minority oversampling technique (SMOTE) [21,49], generative adversarial method (GAN) [44], or geometric transformation [40,48,53] is employed to generate a synthetic sample in an FL environment. The SMOTE algorithm is an oversampling technique where the synthetic data are generated for the minority class. For instance, Wu et al. [21] and Rajendran et al. [49] employ SMOTE to balance the heavy imbalance in a fall detection and lung cancer training dataset, respectively. Zhang et al. [44] proposed secure synthetic COVID-19 data by combining the GAN and differential privacy method. Feki et al. [40], Duo et al. [48], and Yang et al. [53] applied geometric transformations such as random flipping, random rotation, and random translation to balance the quantity of minority class in their training dataset for the data augmentation method.

(2) The aggregate server securely shares a small portion of data to the healthcare node in the server data sharing method. For instance, Zhao et al. [23] proposed a global shared dataset partition to train non-IID data. The author demonstrated that by simply sharing 5% of data, they could get a 30% boost accuracy score. However, it raises model communication costs and is prone to data privacy attacks during the data sharing process.

Adaptive Hyperparameters Method. The adaptive hyperparameters method tries to find the proper FL hyperparameters values for each node during the training process. Each node can have different values of the FL hyperparameters, such as learning rate, loss score, and weighting coefficient. There are two published adaptive hyperparameters methods in the published FL studies for medical application: (1) weighting coefficient [16,19,20,45], and (2) adaptive loss function [46].

(1) The weighting coefficient α_k is a variable that indicates the relative influence of each node k on the aggregation equation in Equation (2) to update the global model. Initially, McMahan et al. [16] proposed FedAvg that the weighting coefficient is $\alpha_k = \frac{n_k}{n}$ as shown in Equation (6), where n_k and n are the private data points hold by node k and the total data from all nodes that participated during training, respectively. In this case, a node with significant data points has a considerable effect on the global model. This method worked well when dealing with label distribution skew characteristics experimented in their studies [16,20].

$$w^g_{t+1} \leftarrow \sum_{k=1}^{K} \frac{n_k}{n} \times w^k_{t+1} \tag{6}$$

In comparison, Chen et al. [20] proposed that the weighting coefficient is $\alpha_k = \frac{1}{K}$, where K is the total nodes participating in FL as shown in Equation (7). In this scenario, the author considered that each node would contribute equally to the aggregation function.

$$w^g_{t+1} \leftarrow \sum_{k=1}^{K} \frac{1}{K} \times w^k_{t+1} \tag{7}$$

Huang et al. [19] proposed that the weighting coefficient is $\alpha_k = \frac{m^c_k}{\sum_{c=1}^{C} m^c_k}$, as shown in Equation (8), where m^c_k and $\sum_{c=1}^{C} m^c_k$ are denoted as the clusters size in medical node k and the total number of clusters in community-based federated learning, respectively. In their method, the algorithm considers the weighted average from the cluster patient community.

$$w^g_{t+1} \leftarrow \sum_{k=1}^{K} \frac{m^c_k}{\sum_{c=1}^{C} m^c_k} \times w^k_{t+1} \tag{8}$$

Finally, Chen et al. [45] proposed that the weighting coefficient is $\alpha_k = \frac{n_k}{n} \times \left(\frac{e}{2}\right)^{-(t-timestamp^k)}$, as shown in Equation (9), where e is the natural logarithm number to denote the time effect and $timestamp^k$ is the round in the newest updated local model. Their proposed weighting coefficient considers not only the data samples held by node k shown by the portion of data $\frac{n_k}{n}$ but also the time required to update the global model in the local node.

$$w^g_{t+1} \leftarrow \sum_{k=1}^{K} \frac{n_k}{n} \times \left(\frac{e}{2}\right)^{-(t-timestamp^k)} \times w^k_{t+1} \tag{9}$$

(2) In addition, the adaptive loss function has the ability to change conditions based on the loss score function. The loss function was used to measure the model performance. The lower the loss score, the better a model was trained. Specifically, Huang et al. [46] proposed the LoAdaBoost method based on loss function in the FL environment for patient mortality prediction. In their proposed method, the adaptive loss function boosts the training process adaptively from the weak learners node. On each training step, the local node will send both the local model and training loss. If the training loss score is more than the loss threshold, it will be retraining again. Otherwise, it will send to the aggregate server.

Domain Adaptation Method. Domain adaptation (DA) is a subset of transfer learning in which a model developed in one or more "source domains" is applied to a new (but related) "target domain." DA is used when the source and target domains share the same feature space but different data representations and distribution [59]. In comparison, transfer learning is used when the target domain's feature is different from the source domain's feature. The goal of DA is to minimize discrepancies in data distributions. Li et al. [18] incorporated domain adaptation in their FL algorithm. The fundamental assumption is that DA approaches can increase the overall performance of multiple nodes in the FL environment with non-IID. Specifically, the author implemented a mixture of expert (MoE) and adversarial domain adaptation methods. The MoE implements adaptation near the model output layer, whereas the adversarial domain alignment implements adaptation on the data knowledge representation level.

Table 2. Summary of different data partition methods, number of nodes, non-IID characteristics, and non-IID mitigation employed in the published federated learning for healthcare applications.

Data Partition	Purpose	Number of Nodes	Non-IID Characteristics	Non-IID Mitigation	Studies/Year
HFL	Combining all samples from a group of selected nodes S_t to increase the sample size	10	Quantity Skew	Balancing the training dataset	Brismi et al., 2018 [52]
		50	Quantity Skew	Not Available	Huang et al., 2019 [19]
		20	Quantity Skew	Balancing the training dataset	Chen et al., 2020 [45]
		90	Quantity Skew	Adaptive Hyperparameters: Adaptive Loss Function	Huang et al., 2020 [46]
		4	Quantity Skew	Domain Adaptation: Mixture of Expert and Domain Adversarial	Li et al., 2020 [18]
		5	Quantity Skew	Not Available	Shao et al., 2020 [47]
		10	Quantity Skew	Not Available	Sheller et al. [38]
		5	Quantity Skew	Balancing the training dataset: SMOTE Algorithm	Wu et al., 2020 [21]
		10	Not Available	Not Available	Abdul Salam et al., 2021 [54]
		4	Quantity Skew	Balancing the training dataset: Geometric Transformation	Chhikara et al., 2021 [37]
		8	Quantity Skew	Not Available	Cui et al., 2021 [39]
		3	Quantity Skew	Balancing the training dataset: Geometric Transformation	Dou et al., 2021 [48]
		4	Quantity Skew	Balancing the training dataset: Geometric Transformation	Feki et al., 2021 [40]
		6	Quantity Skew	Not Available	Lee et al., 2021 [41]
		10	Quantity Skew	Balancing the training dataset	Liu et al., 2021 [42]
		2	Quantity Skew	Balancing the training dataset: SMOTE Algorithm	Rajendran et al., 2021 [49]
		3	Not Available	Not Available	Sarma et al. [50]
		5	Quantity Skew	Not Available	Vaid et al., 2021 [55]
		8	Not Available	Not Available	Xue et al., 2021 [51]
		8	Not Available	Not Available	Yan et al., 2021 [43]
		3	Quantity Skew	Balancing the training dataset: Geometric Transformation	Yang et al., 2021 [53]
		100	Label Distribution Skew	Balancing the training dataset: Generative Adversarial Network (GAN)	Zhang et al., 2021 [44]

Table 2. Cont.

Data Partition	Purpose	Number of Nodes	Non-IID Characteristics	Non-IID Mitigation	Studies/Year
VFL	Combining all features from a group of selected nodes S_t to increase features dimension	7	Not Available	Not Available	Cha et al., 2021 [56]
FTL	Improve the model performance with small data size and unlabeled samples	7	Quantity Skew	Balancing the training dataset	Chen et al., 2020 [20]

HFL: horizontal federated learning; VFL: vertical federated learning; FTL: federated transfer learning.

4.4. Data Privacy Attacks and Protections

Data security and privacy are critical issues in medical applications. In FL, it is usual for all nodes to calculate and upload their local model weights and parameters to an aggregate server. The steps of uploading and processing the weights and parameters may leak sensitive patient information contained in the medical data. The possible attacks include model inversion and membership inference attacks, which may leak patient data to an attacker. The common solutions for data privacy protection include differential privacy and homomorphic encryption [21] based techniques, which can guarantee the security of transferring the local weights and parameters in federated learning. In the following subsection, we describe the possible data privacy attacks and protections in FL.

4.4.1. Data Privacy Attacks on Federated Learning

There are two types of possible data privacy attacks on federated learning. The first attack is trying to recreate the input data, such as model inversion attack, and the second attack is to discover the training data such as membership inference attack.

Model Inversion (MI) Attack. The model inversion attack is an attack method for recreating data on which a machine learning model was trained [60]. In the case of federated learning for healthcare applications, this can leak the sensitive patient data used in the model's training process. Fredrikson et al. [60] demonstrated the MI attack that, given the machine learning model and several demographic data about a patient, an attacker could generate the patient's genetic markers. Specifically, the attack exploits the predicted output probability confidence score from the machine learning model when predicting the class given the features data. Given a machine model learning model as a function $\hat{y} = f(w; x_1, \ldots, x_n)$ where $\hat{y}$, w, and $\mathcal{X} = \{x_1, x_2, \ldots, x_n\}$ are predicted probability class, machine learning parameters, and features vector as an input, respectively. The model inversion attack aims to exploit a sensitive feature, for instance feature x_1, given some information about the other features $x_2, \ldots, x_n$ and the predicted output probability $\hat{y}$. One solution to overcome this threat is to use differential privacy mechanism which can be incorporated into the learning process to protect the data from inversion attacks, such as inferring model weights (discussed in Section 4.4.2).

Membership inference attack. Given a machine learning model $f(w; x_1, \ldots, x_n)$ and some sample instances, the membership inference attack task tries to discover whether the instance exists or not in the training dataset [61]. Membership inference attack poses a significant privacy issue as the membership can expose a person's private information. For instance, determining a person's presence in a hospital's clinical trial training dataset indicates that this patient was once a patient at the hospital. The patient and the hospital are the two key parties interested in defending against such membership inference attacks. The patients consider their memberships confidential and do not wish for their sensitive information to be made public. At the same time, the hospital does not want to be prosecuted for leaking patient data. Almadhoun et al. [62] demonstrated the first membership inference attack in the medical area that infers the personal information of the participants in a genomic dataset. Truex et al. [63] showed the threats of membership inference attack when the attacker is a member in the FL environment. The member could be the aggregation service or one of the client nodes. Their FL configuration is different from the one discussed above. Instead of pooling the weights to construct a new global model, each node trains their local model and contributes just the prediction probability when inferring a new instance. The process of membership inference attack consists of three steps [61]. Firstly, the attackers aim to develop a shadow dataset $\mathcal{D}'$ that mimics the target model training dataset $\mathcal{D}$. Secondly, the attacker create a shadow model using the shadow dataset $\mathcal{D}'$ which mimics the target model behavior. In this step, the attacker observed the shadow model behavior in response to instances known to have been provided during training against those that were not. This behavior is utilized to create an attack dataset that captures the different instances in the training data and data that have not been seen previously. Finally, this attack dataset is used to construct a binary classifier that predicts whether an instance was previously used in the target model output.

4.4.2. Data Privacy Protections for Federated Learning

There are two methods to protect data privacy from data leakage and attacker in the FL environment: perturbation and encryption. The perturbation method preserves private data and model privacy by adding a controlled random noise to the training data or the machine learning model parameters during the training process. For instance, differential privacy [18,43,44,55] and hybrid exchange parameters [39] algorithms are the perturbations techniques implemented in the FL studies published in medical applications. In comparison, the encryption method preserves private data and model privacy by encrypting the parameters exchanged and the gradients in the aggregation process in the FL environment, such as the homomorphic encryption algorithm [20,21,51].

Data Privacy Protections with Differential Privacy (DP) Method. Combining a deep learning model with privacy protection is an emerging research focus. For instance, many researchers use differential privacy (DP) methods to secure the deep learning model. Inspired by the successfully implemented DP in centralized learning, several researchers implemented DP in distributed training, especially in FL studies for medical application [18,43,44,55]. Dwork et al. [64] introduced differential privacy as a notion of privacy, ensuring that data analytics do not compromise privacy. It ensures that the effect of an individual's data on the model output is restricted. In other words, differential privacy aims for an algorithm's result to be nearly identical whether or not the dataset contains data about a specific individual. This technique can prevent the membership inference attack where the attacker tries to find if a specific individual is in the training dataset. Differential privacy is achieved by adding controlled statistical noise to the machine learning model's input or output. Whereas the addition of noise ensures that specific individual data contributions are hidden, it also provides insights into the entire population without compromising privacy. The quantity of added noise is called the privacy budget denoted by epsilon (ϵ). Gaussian and Laplace are two controlled random noise mechanisms implemented in differential privacy for the FL studies in medical applications. Differential privacy with Gaussian noise mechanism is a common technique used in FL studies [18,43,44,55]. For instance, in their training dataset, Li et al. [18] and Vaid et al. [55] incorporated the Gaussian noise in the model learning process to protect from model inversion attacks. In addition, Zhang et al. [44] and Yan et al. [43] proposed a differential privacy technique with a generative adversarial network (DPGAN) to generate private data samples at a medical node in a federated environment. Specifically, Zhang et al. [44] implemented controlled noise to the gradient value in the discriminator part of their generated adversarial network (GAN) for image sampling in federated learning, interfering with original data distribution. Their experiments showed that this method could address the lack of data availability and the non-IID issue in FL while keeping patient data private. In addition, Zhang et al. [44] evaluated that the smaller the Gaussian noise as part of DP will improve the model performance. Besides the Gaussian noise mechanism, differential privacy with the Laplace noise mechanism is implemented by Li et al. [18] in their studies. Li et al. [18] showed when the Laplace noise level was too high the deep learning model performance failed to classification task.

Data Privacy Protection with Homomorphic Encryption Method. Homomorphic encryption (HE) was used to ensure data privacy by encrypting the parameter exchanged in the gradient aggregation process. There are many recent FL studies for healthcare application that implemented HE during FL training [20,21,51]. Homomorphic encryption was categorized into fully homomorphic encryption (FHE) and additively homomorphic encryption (AHE) [65]. An FHE scheme is an encryption method that allows analytical functions to be run directly on the encrypted data while producing the same encrypted output as if the functions were executed in plaintext. In other words, if we perform an add or multiply operation on the ciphertext, the decryption result is the same as the actual result obtained by performing the same operation on the plaintext. In comparison, the AHE is an encryption method that allows only one type of operation to be run directly on the encrypted data and produces the same encrypted output as if the functions were executed in plaintext. In other words, the AHE scheme is intended for use with specific applications that require simple addition or multiplication operations. Formally, an encryption method is called homomorphic over an operation "+" if it supports Equation (10):

$$E\langle w_1 \rangle + E\langle w_1 \rangle = E\langle w_1 + w_2 \rangle \ \forall w_1, w_2 \in W \qquad (10)$$

where $E\langle . \rangle$ is the encryption method and W is the machine learning model parameters. For instance, in the AHE scheme, for parameters w_1 and w_2, one can obtain $E\langle w_1 + w_2 \rangle$ by using $E\langle w_1 \rangle$ and $E\langle w_2 \rangle$ without knowing w_1 and w_2 explicitly. Most of the FL studies for healthcare applications leverage the AHE rather than the FHE since FHE is computationally more expensive than AHE. For example, Chen et al. [20] and Wu et al. [21] incorporated the AHE in their local model parameters sharing and gradient aggregation between healthcare nodes and the aggregate server. Xue et al. [51] adopted two AHE schemes for a lightweight privacy module to prevent the patient EMRs' privacy leakage in the medical edge devices.

4.5. Benchmark Medical Dataset for Federated Learning

The dataset utilized in FL studies can vary depending on the task. For instance, some datasets concentrate on the performance of classification tasks, while others concentrate on segmentation tasks. There are datasets such as LEAF [66] and FedVision [67] for FL algorithm benchmarking. However, there is no specific open public medical dataset for FL algorithm benchmarking due to limited quantity, patient security, and privacy. Therefore, a comprehensive list of relevant medical datasets is compiled from published FL papers for future research on this topic. From 24 published FL papers in the healthcare area, 16 publications used the public dataset listed in Table 3. We exclude eight publications from the list because these papers use their institution/private dataset.

Besides benchmark medical datasets for federated learning, numerous scientific research communities and industries have developed various tools to accelerate the growth of federated learning. We summarized in Table 4 the federated learning tools based on data configuration challenges.

Table 3. Summary of public medical datasets in recent FL studies applied for a medical area for algorithm benchmarking.

	Dataset Type	Dataset Name	Description	FL Study
Healthcare dataset	Medical Image Classification	Autism Brain Imaging Data Exchange (ABIDE) I [68]	The ABIDE I is a consortium dataset openly sharing 1112 functional magnetic resonance imaging (fMRI) dataset from 539 patients with autism spectrum disorders.	[18]
		Public COVID-19 Image Data Collection [69]	The dataset consists of 108 healthy chest X-ray images and 108 confirmed with COVID-19 chest X-ray images taken from 76 patients.	[40,44,54]
		Facial Emotion Recognition (FER) 2013 [70]	The FER2013 dataset consists of 35,887 human facial emotion images. The dataset is labeled into seven emotions: neutral, anger, disgust, sadness, happiness, surprise, and fear.	[37]
	Medical Image Segmentation	Brain Tumor Image Segmentation Benchmark (BraTS) 2017 and 2018 [71]	The BraTs 2017 were collected from 13 institutions and consisted of 359 patients' brain tumor scans.	[38]
		SPIE-AAPM PROSTATEx dataset [72]	The PROSTATEx dataset consists of 343 MRI prostate image cancer from Siemens 3T MR scanners, the MAGNETOM Trio, and Skyra.	[43,50]
	Electronic Health Record	MobiAct [73]	The MobiAct dataset is human activity dataset taken from 57 volunteers (42 men and 15 women).	[21]
		Human Activity Recognition (HAR) [74]	The HAR dataset was collected from 30 volunteers. Each subject performed different activities such as walking, sitting, standing, and laying. There are 10,299 with 561 time-series features.	[20,45]
		WESAD (Wearable Stress and Affect Detection) [75]	The WESAD is a dataset for wearable effect and stress detection. Taken from 15 participants, the WESAD consists of 12 features with 63,000,000 time-series samples.	[42]
		Medical Information Mart for Intensive Care (MIMIC) III [76]	The MIMIC III dataset was collected from 40,000 patients during stayed in the ICU at Beth Israel Deaconess Medical Center between 2001 and 2012.	[46]
		The eICU collaborative research database. [77]	Critical care datasets consist of 200,859 patients data from 208 hospitals in the United States.	[19,39,56]
Nonhealthcare dataset	Image classification, sentiment analysis	LEAF Dataset [66]	The LEAF Dataset Benchmarking framework consists of images and text datasets such as EMNIST, Celeba, Shakespeare, and Synthetic datasets.	[66]
	Image Classification	FedVision—Real World image dataset for FL [67]	The FedVision dataset contains more than 900 real-world images generated from 26 street cameras. Precisely, it consists of 7 classes with a detailed bounding box. This dataset has non-IID properties reflecting a real-world data distribution.	[67]

ABIDE: autism brain imaging data exchange; BraTS: brain tumor image segmentation benchmark; eICU: electronic intensive care unit; FER: facial emotion recognition; FL: federated learning; fMRI: functional magnetic resonance imaging; HAR: human activity recognition; MIMIC: medical information mart for intensive care; MR: magnetic resonance; IID: independent and identical data distribution; WESAD: wearable stress and affect detection.

Table 4. Federated learning tools.

Framework Name	Creator	Supported Techniques				URL
		Data Partition	Data Distribution	Data Privacy Attack Simulation	Data Privacy Protection Methods	
PySyft	Open Mined	✓ HFL, VTL	✓ IID, non-IID	✗	✓ DP, HE	https://github.com/OpenMined/PySyft (accessed on 7 July 2021)
TFF	Google	✓ HFL	✗	✗	✗	https://www.tensorflow.org/federated (accessed on 7 July 2021)
FATE	Tencent	✓ HFL, VFL, FTL	✗	✗	✓ HE	https://github.com/FederatedAI/FATE (accessed on 21 July 2021)
Sherpa.ai	Sherpa.ai	✓ HFL	✓ IID, non-IID	✓ Data Poison	✓ DP	https://developers.sherpa.ai/privacy-technology/ (accessed on 27 August 2021)
LEAF	Sebastian Caldas	✓ HFL	✗	✗	✗	https://leaf.cmu.edu/ (accessed on 21 July 2021)

HFL: horizontal federated learning; VTL: vertical transfer learning; FTL: federated transfer learning; IID: independent and identically data distribution; DP: differential privacy; HE: homomorphic encryption.

4.6. FL Studies for Healthcare Applications

Published FL studies in medical applications mostly come with two tasks: classification and segmentation, as summarized in Table 5. In our selected papers, there are 24 studies. Out of these studies, 21 studies are on classification tasks, and three are on segmentation tasks. The following subsections describe the existing studies on FL for healthcare applications, organized by the application task type.

4.6.1. Classification Task in FL for Healthcare Applications

Classification is a common task tackled in the published FL applications in the medical domain. In machine learning, classification algorithms learn how to classify or annotate a given set of instances with classes or labels. There are several classification tasks that are studied in federated learning setting in healthcare, e.g., autism spectrum disorder (ASD) [18], cancer diagnosis [41,43,49], COVID-19 detection [40,44,48,54], human activity and emotion recognition [20,21,37,42,45], patient hospitalization prediction [52], patient mortality prediction [19,39,46,47,55,56], and sepsis disease diagnosis [51]. The summary of classification tasks in FL studies for medical application is listed in Table 5.

Cancer diagnosis. Recent studies show that researchers are employing FL technology to develop machine learning models for cancer diagnostic applications [41,43,49]. For instance, Lee et al. [27] proposed a CNN-based model to classify whether thyroid nodules were benign or malign. The training data were 8457 ultrasound images collected from six institutions. The results show that the performance of the FL-based method was comparable with centralized learning with accuracy, sensitivity, and specificity of 97%, 98%, and 95%, respectively. Similarly, Rajendran et al. [49] implemented FL with an MLP model for lung cancer classification using two independent cloud providers. The model initialized, trained, and transferred from one node to another node using a cloud repository. The model achieved 92.8% accuracy to classify cancer. Another study by Yan et al. [43] transformed all nodes' raw medical image data onto a common space via image-to-image translation without violating FL's privacy settings. The image-to-image translation was done using a cycle generative adversarial network (CycleGAN) model. The performance of the proposed method trained with eight medical nodes achieved 98% accuracy and 99% area under the curve (AUC) to classify prostate cancer.

Table 5. Summary of FL publications applied in medical applications.

ML Task	Clinical Tasks	Medical Input Data	Model Architecture	FL Study
Classification	Autism spectrum disorders (ASD) or Healthy control (HC)	fMRI	CNN	[18]
	Cancer diagnosis: - Prostate cancer - Thyroid cancer - Lung cancer	- MRI - Ultrasound images - Tobacco and radon data	- GAN - CNN - MLP	[43] [41] [49]
	COVID-19 detection	X-ray images	CNN	[40,44,48,54]
	Human activity	Wearable device	LSTM	[20,21,45]
	Human emotion	Wearable device	CNN	[37,42]
	Patient hospitalization	Patient EHR	SVM	[52]
	Patient mortality	Critical care data	MLP	[19,39,46,47,55,56]
	Sepsis disease	Patient EHR	Double Deep Q Network	[51]
Segmentation	Brain tumor	MRI	U-Net	[38]
	COVID-19 region	3D Chest CT	3D U-Net	[53]
	Prostate cancer	MRI	3D Anisotropic Hybrid Network	[50]

CNN: convolutional neural network; CT: computed tomography; EHR: electronic health record; fMRI: functional magnetic resonance imaging; GAN: generative adversarial network; MLP: multilayer perceptron; MRI: magnetic resonance imaging; SVM: support vector machine.

COVID-19 detection. For COVID-19 detection applications [40,44,48,54], FL is a potential approach for connecting medical images data from medical institutions, enabling them to develop a model while maintaining patient privacy. In this case, the model's performance is considerably enhanced from diverse medical datasets from several institutions. For instance, Abdul Salam et al. [54] experimented with different federated learning architectures for binary COVID-19 classification. Their results showed that the federated learning model with GAN architecture and stochastic gradient descent (SGD) optimizer had a higher accuracy while keeping the loss score lower than the centralized machine learning model. The model performance achieved accuracy and AUC of 98.30% and 9.63%, respectively. Similarly, Dou et al. [48] showed the efficacy of a federated learning system for detecting COVID-19-related CT anomalies using patients' medical data from one country hospital as training data, then validating the model with medical data from other countries. Specifically, the authors trained an MLP-model using 132 patients from three hospitals in Hong Kong and validated the model generalizability performance using the medical dataset from China and Germany. The system achieved 83.12% in terms of AUC. Feki et al. [40] showed that increasing the number of medical nodes will decrease the training round for the model to converge and increase the model performance in CT–X-ray COVID-19 prediction. The authors proposed the CNN-based model architecture and achieved a performance of 95.27% AUC score. Similar results were obtained by Zhang et al. [44], who proposed an FL framework that enables medical nodes to generate high-quality training data samples with a privacy-protection approach. Specifically, the proposed method solves the challenge of lacking COVID-19 medical training data in a federated environment. The GAN-based architecture was employed in the proposed system and achieved a comparable performance of 94.11% accuracy.

Human activity and emotion recognition. With increasing research on wearable technology and the internet of health things (IoHT), FL technology is one of the solutions to keep users' privacy while collaborating to develop a model for human activity and emotion recognition [20,21,37,42,45]. For example, Chen et al. [20] developed a deep learning model for human activity classification such as walking, sitting, standing, and laying. Then the author elaborates the trained CNN-based model with federated transfer learning to achieve a personalization model for each edge device. The system achieved 99.4% accuracy in classifying human activities. Similarly, Wu et al. [21] developed a cloud-edge federated learning infrastructure to create a patient privacy-aware deep learning model for in-home monitoring applications. The authors developed an autoencoder (AE) model architecture then deployed the model into five different healthcare nodes. The FL system achieved an accuracy of 95.41%. Chhikara et al. [37] combined the speech signal and facial expression to create an emotion index for monitoring the patient's mental health. Using the facial emotion recognition (FER) dataset collected from several data silos, the author employed a federated learning technique and AE-based architecture to create a secure machine learning model to classify a human emotion. The FL algorithm showed an AUC of 88%.

Patient mortality prediction. Similarly, FL enables early predictive modeling based on several sources, which can help to assist clinicians with extra information into the risks and benefits of treating patients earlier [19,46,47,51,52,55,56]. Huang et al. [19] used drug features to forecast critical care patients' mortality, and ICU stays time. Their algorithm based on AE architecture also addresses non-IID ICU patient data by grouping patients into clinically significant communities with shared diagnoses and geographical regions, then training one model per community. The proposed FL algorithm showed an AUC of 69.13%. In a similar study, Brismi et al. [52] proposed a method to forecast future patient hospitalizations with heart-related disorders by solving the L1-regularized sparse support vector machine (SVM) classifier in a federated learning environment. The proposed FL model performed an AUC of 77.47%. Shao et al. [47] proposed an MLP-based model framework to predict in-hospital mortality among patients admitted to the intensive care unit. Their findings indicate that training the model in a federated learning framework produces outcomes comparable to those obtained in a centralized learning environment with an AUC of 97.76%. Vaid et al. [55] demonstrated federated learning with an MLP-based model architecture to predict patient mortality with COVID-19 disease within seven days. Their experiment showed that the federated learning algorithm successfully produces a robust predictive model while preserving the patient's confidential information with an 82.9% AUC score.

Other healthcare areas. Besides the healthcare areas mentioned above, FL also applied for sepsis disease [51] and autism spectrum disorder classification [18]. Xue et al. [51] developed a fully decentralized federated framework (FDFF) that integrates a neural network model across edge devices to extract knowledge from internet-of-things for healthcare applications. The edge devices using FDFF can create a double deep Q-network (DDQN) that gives suggestions for sepsis treatment. In addition, Li et al. [18] proposed FL for multisite autism spectrum disorder (ASD) fMRI analysis.

4.6.2. Segmentation Task in FL for Healthcare Applications

Segmentation tasks with medical images have become an essential clinical task in healthcare applications. The medical image segmentation task is the process of identifying and selecting a region of interest within a medical image. Medical images can be in several forms, such as MRI or CT image scan. There are several published FL studies in medical image segmentation, namely brain tumor disease [38], COVID-19 region [53], and prostate cancer region [50]. The summary of published FL studies on segmentation tasks is listed in Table 5. Specifically, in brain tumor segmentation using brain MRI medical images, Sheller et al. [38]

applied the FL algorithm with CNN-based architecture for multi-institutional collaboration in brain tumor segmentation tasks while preserving the patient data. Compared to existing collaborative learning approaches, FL achieved the highest dice score of 85% and scaled more effectively as the number of collaborating institutions increases. Using multinational three-dimensional chest CT images from three countries, Yang et al. [53] applied federated semi-supervised learning with 3D u-shape fully connected layer model architecture to segment the COVID-19 disease region. Federated semi-supervised learning can assure good training performance even when some healthcare sites have a limited number of annotated data compared to unannotated data. Additionally, the semi-supervised environment may alleviate some of the strain associated with expert annotation, which is critical given the present pandemic crisis. Similarly, Sarma et al. [50] performed prostate segmentation with a 3D anisotropic hybrid network (3D AH-Net) model on MRI with collaboration from industry, public universities, and the federal institution. The proposed FL algorithm experimented with three medical nodes showed a dice score of 88.9%.

RQ3: What are the research gaps and potential future research directions of FL related to medical data?

4.7. Open Challenges

In this survey, we review the current progress on federated learning in the healthcare field. We highlight the comprehensive solutions to federated learning issues related to medical data configurations to provide a valuable resource for researchers. In what follows, we list some potential research directions or open questions when federated learning is applied in the healthcare area.

FL with Medical Data Stream. Medical data streams are collections of medical data that increase constantly and rapidly over time, generated during the treatment and monitoring of patients. For instance, in telemedicine or patient monitoring, the medical monitoring devices generate a large amount of time-sensitive data when monitoring patient vital signs such as temperature, heart rate, and blood pressure. This medical data is a stream of medical signals displayed for interpretation by physicians. Certain pieces of these data could be used in real-time to alert physicians about changes in patient circumstances. Medical data streams arrive periodically, and we would like to develop an analytic model that extracts meaningful patterns or risk factors in real-time. Federated learning incorporated with the medical data stream could improve training tasks and security performance, as inconsistencies in evolving medical datasets and the data transmission between the FL coordinator and participant nodes can be highly decreased [25]. However, the medical data streams are usually fast, large, and we must handle them in real-time. In addition, the medical data streams are dynamic, so our FL algorithm has to respond to these changes. Thus, it is essential to design an efficient federated learning algorithm to achieve good accuracy, low total memory, and minimum time in medical data streams.

FL with Hybrid Medical Data Partition. In the HFL data partition, the nodes share the same features $\mathcal{X}$ and label $\mathcal{Y}$ but have different data samples $\mathcal{I}$. Thus, the HFL aims to solve limited sample size variability by combining data samples from all nodes when developing a model, while for the VFL data partition the nodes share the same data samples $\mathcal{I}$ but have different features $\mathcal{X}$ and labels $\mathcal{Y}$. Therefore, the VFL aims to enrich the features by combining features from all nodes when developing a model. However, we need to simultaneously solve a limited sample size variability and enrich the features when developing a model in practice. For instance, a healthcare node may possess either partial features or data samples in healthcare insurance, which serves only a fraction of users and only has partial records. Incorporating both the HFL and the VFL data partition will result in a hybrid data partition. Compared to the HFL and the VFL, a hybrid FL data partition has its challenges. In HFL, each node shares neither its local data nor labels. In contrast, in VFL, the node shares the user's index to the server or is securely stored in one node as a key for aligning the features [56]. A hybrid FL data partition needs to deal with both types of nodes, so the FL training algorithm can run without requiring the aggregate server to access any data, including the users' index. New architecture and training algorithms in FL will be required to utilize the benefits of the hybrid data partition effectively.

FL with Incentive Mechanism for Good Data Contributor. The internet of health things (IoHT) uses internet of things (IoT) devices on e-health applications that enable the connection between healthcare resources and patients. The IoHT devices such as smartwatches and healthcare wearable trackers can record heart rate, body temperature, and blood pressure. These rich healthcare data are excellent for personal smartphone healthcare apps that can run on device federated learning. However, the IoHT nodes are burdened by significant computation and communication costs during the federated model training process. Without a proper incentive mechanism design, those IoHT nodes will be reluctant to participate in federated learning. In addition, a suitable incentive mechanism can have rewards and punishments. A good quality personal healthcare data contributor can obtain a good incentive, while harmful data contributors can receive a punishment. Thus, an effective and efficient incentive mechanism can attract good data contributors to join federated learning.

Limitation and future perspective. There are two limitations to the present study. The first limitation is that existing FL experiments focus exclusively on one of the non-IID properties, such as data imbalance or label skew. However, there are no comprehensive experiments in the medical dataset that examine multiple properties of non-IID. The future perspective will find additional algorithms for addressing the issues associated with hybrid non-IID features. The second limitation is the hyperparameter framework search for FL. Hyperparameter tuning is a critical yet time-consuming step in the machine learning workflow. Optimization of hyperparameters becomes considerably more difficult in federated learning, in which models are trained across a dispersed network of heterogeneous data silos. Thus, an automatic tool or framework to select the optimal hyperparameters in the FL model is critically needed in the future research.

5. Conclusions

We presented the advancement of federated learning growth in the context of healthcare applications over the last four years in terms of data properties such as data partition, data distribution, data privacy attack and protection, and benchmark datasets. We hope that this study stimulates additional research into FL in healthcare applications and eventually becomes a guideline for handling sensitive medical data. Several open challenges remain, including FL for the medical data stream, FL with medical data hybrid partitions, and incentive mechanisms for good medical data contributors. We envision the increased popularity of FL for medical purposes in the near future, resulting in more advanced protocols with security and privacy guarantees and the actual deployment of FL technology for solving real-world problems in the healthcare domain.

Author Contributions: Conceptualization, P. and Z.-Y.S.; methodology, P., Z.-Y.S. and C.-R.S.; software and validation, Y.-Y.T., K.T.P. and H.-C.C.; formal analysis, W.J. and K.S.M.T.H.; investigation, P. and K.T.P.; resources, P. and K.T.P.; data curation, P., Z.-Y.S. and C.-R.S.; writing—original draft preparation, P. and Z.-Y.S.; writing—review and editing, Z.-Y.S., W.J., Y.-Y.T., K.S.M.T.H. and C.-R.S.; visualization, P.; supervision, Z.-Y.S.; project administration, Z.-Y.S. and Y.-Y.T.; funding acquisition, Z.-Y.S. All authors have read and agreed to the published version of the manuscript.

Funding: This research was funded by the Ministry of Science and Technology of Taiwan under the grants MOST 110-2321-B-468-001 and MOST 110-2511-H-468-005.

Institutional Review Board Statement: Not applicable.

Informed Consent Statement: Not applicable.

Data Availability Statement: No new data were created or analyzed in this study. Data sharing is not applicable to this article.

Acknowledgments: This study was supported by the Ministry of Science and Technology of Taiwan under the project grants MOST 110-2321-B-468-001 and MOST 110-2511-H-468-005. Furthermore, the authors express their gratitude to the anonymous reviewers for their comments and recommendations, which significantly improved the original work.

Conflicts of Interest: The authors declare no conflict of interest.

Abbreviations

AI	Artificial intelligence
AMCA	American medical collection agency
AUROC	Area under the receiver operating characteristic curve
CNN	Convolutional neural network
CT	Computerized tomography image
DNN	Deep neural network
FCN	Fully connected network
FL	Federated learning
fMRI	Functional magnetic resonance image
GDPR	General data protection right
HIPAA	Health insurance portability and accountability act
IID	Independent and identical data distribution
LSTM	Long short-term memory
ML	Machine learning
MLP	Multilayer perceptron
MRI	Magnetic resonance image
PDPA	Personal data protection act
PHI	Protected health information

Appendix A

Table A1. Full query term in publication databases.

Scientific Database	Query	Studies Results #
PubMed	((federated learning AND ((fft[Filter]) AND (english[Filter]) AND (2018:2021[pdat]))) AND (healthcare OR hospital OR clinic AND ((fft[Filter]) AND (english[Filter]) AND (2018:2021[pdat])))) AND ("data quality" OR privacy protection OR non iid AND ((fft[Filter]) AND (english[Filter]) AND (2018:2021[pdat]))) AND ((fft[Filter]) AND (english[Filter])) AND ((fft[Filter]) AND (english[Filter]))	21
IEEE Xplore	("All Metadata":federated learning) AND ("All Metadata":healthcare OR "All Metadata":hospital OR "All Metadata":clinic) AND ("All Metadata":data quality OR "All Metadata":privacy protection OR "All Metadata":non iid)	14
Web of Science	"Healthcare OR Hospital OR Clinic" AND "federated learning" AND "Data Quality OR Privacy Protection OR non iid"	17
Science Direct	("federated learning") AND (healthcare OR hospital OR clinic) AND ("data quality" OR "privacy protection" OR "non iid")	105
ACM Digital Library	[All: "federated learning"] AND [[All: healthcare] OR [All: clinic] OR [All: hospital]] AND [[All: "data quality"] OR [All: "privacy protection"] OR [All: "non iid"]] AND [Publication Date: (1 January 2018 TO 30 June 2021)]	40

Table A2. Federated learning studies for medical applications.

Authors	Year	Title	Journal	FL Studies
Brismi et al.	2018	Federated learning of predictive models from federated electronic health records	International Journal of Medical Informatics	[52]
Huang et al.	2019	Patient clustering improves efficiency of federated machine learning to predict mortality and hospital stay time using distributed electronic medical records	Journal of Biomedical Informatics	[19]
Chen et al.	2020	FedHealth: A Federated Transfer Learning Framework for Wearable Healthcare	IEEE Intelligent Systems	[20]
Chen et al.	2020	Communication-Efficient Federated Deep Learning With Layerwise Asynchronous Model Update and Temporally Weighted Aggregation	IEEE Transactions on Neural Networks and Learning Systems	[45]
Huang et al.	2020	LoAdaBoost: Loss-based AdaBoost federated machine learning with reduced computational complexity on IID and non-IID intensive care data	PLOS ONE	[46]
Li et al.	2020	Multi-site fMRI analysis using privacy-preserving federated learning and domain adaptation: ABIDE results	Medical Image Analysis	[18]
Shao et al.	2020	Stochastic Channel-Based Federated Learning With Neural Network Pruning for Medical Data Privacy Preservation: Model Development and Experimental Validation	JMIR Formative Research	[47]
Sheller et al.	2020	Federated learning in medicine: facilitating multi-institutional collaborations without sharing patient data	Scientific Reports	[38]
Wu et al.	2020	FedHome: Cloud-Edge based Personalized Federated Learning for In-Home Health Monitoring	IEEE Transactions on Mobile Computing	[21]
Abdul Salam et al.	2021	COVID-19 detection using federated machine learning	PLOS ONE	[54]
Cha et al.	2021	Implementing Vertical Federated Learning Using Autoencoders: Practical Application, Generalizability, and Utility Study	JMIR Medical Informatics	[56]
Chhikara et al.	2021	Federated Learning Meets Human Emotions: A Decentralized Framework for Human–Computer Interaction for IoT Applications	IEEE Internet of Things Journal	[37]
Cui et al.	2021	FeARH: Federated machine learning with anonymous random hybridization on electronic medical records	Journal of Biomedical Informatics	[39]
Dou et al.	2021	Federated deep learning for detecting COVID-19 lung abnormalities in CT: a privacy-preserving multinational validation study	npj Digital Medicine	[48]
Feki et al.	2021	Federated learning for COVID-19 screening from chest X-ray images	Applied Soft Computing	[40]
Lee et al.	2021	Federated Learning for Thyroid Ultrasound Image Analysis to Protect Personal Information: Validation Study in a Real Health Care Environment	JMIR Medical Informatics	[41]
Liu et al.	2021	Learning From Others Without Sacrificing Privacy: Simulation Comparing Centralized and Federated Machine Learning on Mobile Health Data	JMIR mHealth and uHealth	[42]
Rajendran et al.	2021	Cloud-Based Federated Learning Implementation Across Medical Centers	JCO Clinical Cancer Informatics	[49]

Table A2. Cont.

Authors	Year	Title	Journal	FL Studies
Sarma et al.	2021	Federated learning improves site performance in multicenter deep learning without data sharing	Journal of the American Medical Informatics Association	[50]
Vaid et al.	2021	Federated Learning of Electronic Health Records to Improve Mortality Prediction in Hospitalized Patients With COVID-19: Machine Learning Approach	JMIR Medical Informatics	[55]
Xue et al.	2021	A Resource-Constrained and Privacy-Preserving Edge-Computing-Enabled Clinical Decision System: A Federated Reinforcement Learning Approach	IEEE Internet of Things Journal	[51]
Yan et al.	2021	Variation-Aware Federated Learning with Multi-Source Decentralized Medical Image Data	IEEE Journal of Biomedical and Health Informatics	[43]
Yang et al.	2021	Federated semi-supervised learning for COVID region segmentation in chest CT using multi-national data from China, Italy, Japan	Medical Image Analysis	[53]
Zhang et al.	2021	FedDPGAN: Federated Differentially Private Generative Adversarial Networks Framework for the Detection of COVID-19 Pneumonia	Information Systems Frontiers	[44]

References

1. Feng, Y.; Zhang, L.; Mo, J. Deep manifold preserving autoencoder for classifying breast cancer histopathological images. *IEEE/ACM Trans. Comput. Biol. Bioinform.* **2020**, *17*, 91–101. [CrossRef] [PubMed]
2. McWilliams, A.; Beigi, P.; Srinidhi, A.; Lam, S.; MacAulay, C.E. Sex and smoking status effects on the early detection of early lung cancer in high-risk smokers using an electronic nose. *IEEE Trans. Biomed. Eng.* **2015**, *62*, 2044–2054. [CrossRef]
3. Chen, S.; Yang, H.; Fu, J.; Mei, W.; Ren, S.; Liu, Y.; Zhu, Z.; Liu, L.; Li, H.; Chen, H. U-Net Plus: Deep semantic segmentation for esophagus and esophageal cancer in computed tomography images. *IEEE Access* **2019**, *7*, 82867–82877. [CrossRef]
4. Ge, C.; Gu, I.Y.; Jakola, A.S.; Yang, J. Enlarged training dataset by pairwise GANs for molecular-based brain tumor classification. *IEEE Access* **2020**, *8*, 22560–22570. [CrossRef]
5. Sultan, H.H.; Salem, N.M.; Al-Atabany, W. Multi-classification of brain tumor images using deep neural network. *IEEE Access* **2019**, *7*, 69215–69225. [CrossRef]
6. Noreen, N.; Palaniappan, S.; Qayyum, A.; Ahmad, I.; Imran, M.; Shoaib, M. A deep learning model based on concatenation approach for the diagnosis of brain tumor. *IEEE Access* **2020**, *8*, 55135–55144. [CrossRef]
7. Xue, W.; Li, Q.; Xue, Q. Text detection and recognition for images of medical laboratory reports with a deep learning approach. *IEEE Access* **2020**, *8*, 407–416. [CrossRef]
8. Harerimana, G.; Kim, J.W.; Yoo, H.; Jang, B. Deep learning for electronic health records analytics. *IEEE Access* **2019**, *7*, 101245–101259. [CrossRef]
9. Sun, C.; Shrivastava, A.; Singh, S.; Gupta, A. Revisiting unreasonable effectiveness of data in deep learning era. In Proceedings of the IEEE International Conference on Computer Vision (ICCV), Venice, Italy, 22–29 October 2017; pp. 843–852.
10. Zech, J.R.; Badgeley, M.A.; Liu, M.; Costa, A.B.; Titano, J.J.; Oermann, E.K. Variable generalization performance of a deep learning model to detect pneumonia in chest radiographs: A cross-sectional study. *PLoS Med.* **2018**, *15*, e1002683. [CrossRef]
11. O'Leary, D.E. Embedding AI and crowdsourcing in the big data lake. *IEEE Intell. Syst.* **2014**, *29*, 70–73. [CrossRef]
12. Moore, W.; Frye, S. Review of HIPAA, part 1: History, protected health information, and privacy and security rules. *J. Nucl. Med. Technol.* **2019**, *47*, 269–272. [CrossRef]
13. Mark Allen Group, Data breach at major healthcare firms. *Comput. Fraud. Secur.* **2019**, *2019*, 3–19. [CrossRef]
14. Voigt, P.; von dem Bussche, A. *The EU General Data Protection Regulation (GDPR)*; Springer: Cham, Switzerland, 2017.
15. Laws and Regulations Database of the Republic of China. Personal Data Protection Act. 2015. Available online: https://law.moj.gov.tw/ENG/LawClass/LawAll.aspx?pcode=I0050021 (accessed on 7 July 2021).
16. McMahan, H.B.; Moore, E.; Ramage, D.; Hampson, S.; y Arcas, B.A. Communication-efficient learning of deep networks from decentralized data. In Proceedings of the Artificial Intelligence and Statistics Conference, Fort Lauderdale, FL, USA, 20–22 April 2017; pp. 1273–1282.
17. Hard, A.; Rao, K.; Mathews, R.; Ramaswamy, S.; Beaufays, F.; Augenstein, S.; Eichner, H.; Kiddon, C.; Ramage, D. Federated learning for mobile keyboard prediction. *arXiv* **2019**, arXiv:1811.03604.

18. Li, X.; Gu, Y.; Dvornek, N.; Staib, L.H.; Ventola, P.; Duncan, J.S. Multi-site FMRI analysis using privacy-preserving federated learning and domain adaptation: ABIDE results. *Med. Image Anal.* **2020**, *65*, 101765. [CrossRef] [PubMed]
19. Huang, L.; Shea, A.L.; Qian, H.; Masurkar, A.; Deng, H.; Liu, D. Patient clustering improves efficiency of federated machine learning to predict mortality and hospital stay time using distributed electronic medical records. *J. Biomed. Inform.* **2019**, *99*, 103291. [CrossRef]
20. Chen, Y.; Qin, X.; Wang, J.; Yu, C.; Gao, W. FedHealth: A federated transfer learning framework for wearable healthcare. *IEEE Intell. Syst.* **2020**, *35*, 83–93. [CrossRef]
21. Wu, Q.; Chen, X.; Zhou, Z.; Zhang, J. FedHome: Cloud-edge based personalized federated learning for in-home health monitoring. *IEEE Trans. Mobile Comput.* **2020**. [CrossRef]
22. Li, W.; Milletarì, F.; Xu, D.; Rieke, N.; Hancox, J.; Zhu, W.; Baust, M.; Cheng, Y.; Ourselin, S.; Cardoso, M.J.; et al. Privacy-preserving federated brain tumour segmentation. In *Machine Learning in Medical Imaging*; Suk, H.-I., Liu, M., Yan, P., Lian, C., Eds.; Springer: Cham, Switzerland, 2019; Volume 11861, pp. 133–141.
23. Zhao, Y.; Li, M.; Lai, L.; Suda, N.; Civin, D.; Chandra, V. Federated learning with non-IID data. *arXiv* **2018**, arXiv:1806.00582. [CrossRef]
24. Hsieh, K.; Phanishayee, A.; Mutlu, O.; Gibbons, P.B. The non-IID data quagmire of decentralized machine learning. In Proceedings of the 37th International Conference on Machine Learning (ICML 2020), Virtual Event, 13–18 July 2020.
25. Kairouz, P.; McMahan, H.B.; Avent, B.; Bellet, A.; Bennis, M.; Bhagoji, A.N.; Bonawitz, K.; Charles, Z.; Cormode, G.; Cummings, R.; et al. Advances and open problems in federated learning. *arXiv* **2019**, arXiv:1912.04977.
26. Yang, Q.; Liu, Y.; Chen, T.; Tong, Y. Federated machine learning: Concept and applications. *ACM Trans. Intell. Syst. Technol.* **2019**, *10*, 1–19. [CrossRef]
27. Mothukuri, V.; Parizi, R.M.; Pouriyeh, S.; Huang, Y.; Dehghantanha, A.; Srivastava, G. A survey on security and privacy of federated learning. *Future Gener. Comput. Syst.* **2021**, *115*, 619–640. [CrossRef]
28. Wu, Q.; He, K.; Chen, X. Personalized federated learning for intelligent IoT applications: A cloud-edge based framework. *IEEE Open J. Comput. Soc.* **2020**, *1*, 35–44. [CrossRef] [PubMed]
29. Du, Z.; Wu, C.; Yoshinaga, T.; Yau, K.-L.A.; Ji, Y.; Li, J. Federated learning for vehicular internet of things: Recent advances and open issues. *IEEE Open J. Comput. Soc.* **2020**, *1*, 45–61. [CrossRef]
30. Putra, K.T.; Chen, H.-C.; Prayitno; Ogiela, M.R.; Chou, C.-L.; Weng, C.-E.; Shae, Z.-Y. Federated compressed learning edge computing framework with ensuring data privacy for PM2.5 prediction in smart city sensing applications. *Sensors* **2021**, *21*, 4586. [CrossRef]
31. Xu, J.; Glicksberg, B.S.; Su, C.; Walker, P.; Bian, J.; Wang, F. Federated learning for healthcare informatics. *J. Healthc. Inform. Res.* **2020**, *5*, 1–19. [CrossRef] [PubMed]
32. Pfitzner, B.; Steckhan, N.; Arnrich, B. Federated learning in a medical context: A systematic literature review. *ACM Trans. Internet Technol.* **2021**, *21*, 1–31. [CrossRef]
33. Page, M.J.; McKenzie, J.E.; Bossuyt, P.M.; Boutron, I.; Hoffmann, T.C.; Mulrow, C.D.; Shamseer, L.; Tetzlaff, J.M.; Akl, E.A.; Brennan, S.E.; et al. The PRISMA 2020 statement: An updated guideline for reporting systematic reviews. *BMJ* **2021**, *372*, n71. [CrossRef]
34. PRISMA. PRISMA Endorsers. Available online: http://www.prisma-statement.org/Endorsement/PRISMAEndorsers (accessed on 21 November 2021).
35. McDonagh, M.; Peterson, K.; Raina, P.; Chang, S.; Shekelle, P. Avoiding bias in selecting studies. In *Methods Guide for Effectiveness and Comparative Effectiveness Reviews*; Agency for Healthcare Research and Quality: Rockville, MD, USA, 2008.
36. Scherer, R.W.; Saldanha, I.J. How should systematic reviewers handle conference abstracts? A view from the trenches. *Syst. Rev.* **2019**, *8*, 264. [CrossRef]
37. Chhikara, P.; Singh, P.; Tekchandani, R.; Kumar, N.; Guizani, M. Federated learning meets human emotions: A decentralized framework for human–computer interaction for IoT applications. *IEEE Internet Things J.* **2021**, *8*, 6949–6962. [CrossRef]
38. Sheller, M.J.; Edwards, B.; Reina, G.A.; Martin, J.; Pati, S.; Kotrotsou, A.; Milchenko, M.; Xu, W.; Marcus, D.; Colen, R.R.; et al. Federated learning in medicine: Facilitating multi-institutional collaborations without sharing patient data. *Sci. Rep.* **2020**, *10*, 12598. [CrossRef]
39. Cui, J.; Zhu, H.; Deng, H.; Chen, Z.; Liu, D. FeARH: Federated machine learning with anonymous random hybridization on electronic medical records. *J. Biomed. Inform.* **2021**, *117*, 103735. [CrossRef] [PubMed]
40. Feki, I.; Ammar, S.; Kessentini, Y.; Muhammad, K. Federated learning for COVID-19 screening from chest X-ray images. *Appl. Soft Comput.* **2021**, *106*, 107330. [CrossRef] [PubMed]
41. Lee, H.; Chai, Y.J.; Joo, H.; Lee, K.; Hwang, J.Y.; Kim, S.-M.; Kim, K.; Nam, I.-C.; Choi, J.Y.; Yu, H.W.; et al. Federated learning for thyroid ultrasound image analysis to protect personal information: Validation study in a real health care environment. *JMIR Med. Inform.* **2021**, *9*, e25869. [CrossRef]
42. Liu, J.C.; Goetz, J.; Sen, S.; Tewari, A. Learning from others without sacrificing privacy: Simulation comparing centralized and federated machine learning on mobile health data. *JMIR mHealth uHealth* **2021**, *9*, e23728. [CrossRef]
43. Yan, Z.; Wicaksana, J.; Wang, Z.; Yang, X.; Cheng, K.-T. Variation-aware federated learning with multi-source decentralized medical image data. *IEEE J. Biomed. Health Inform.* **2021**, *25*, 2615–2628. [CrossRef]

44. Zhang, L.; Shen, B.; Barnawi, A.; Xi, S.; Kumar, N.; Wu, Y. FedDPGAN: Federated differentially private generative adversarial networks framework for the detection of COVID-19 pneumonia. *Inf. Syst. Front.* **2021**. [CrossRef]
45. Chen, Y.; Sun, X.; Jin, Y. Communication-efficient federated deep learning with layerwise asynchronous model update and temporally weighted aggregation. *IEEE Trans. Neural Netw. Learn. Syst.* **2020**, *31*, 4229–4238. [CrossRef]
46. Huang, L.; Yin, Y.; Fu, Z.; Zhang, S.; Deng, H.; Liu, D. LoAdaBoost: Loss-based AdaBoost federated machine learning with reduced computational complexity on IID and non-IID intensive care data. *PLoS ONE* **2020**, *15*, e0230706. [CrossRef]
47. Shao, R.; He, H.; Chen, Z.; Liu, H.; Liu, D. Stochastic channel-based federated learning with neural network pruning for medical data privacy preservation: Model development and experimental validation. *JMIR Form. Res.* **2020**, *4*, e17265. [CrossRef] [PubMed]
48. Dou, Q.; So, T.Y.; Jiang, M.; Liu, Q.; Vardhanabhuti, V.; Kaissis, G.; Li, Z.; Si, W.; Lee, H.H.C.; Yu, K.; et al. Federated deep learning for detecting COVID-19 lung abnormalities in CT: A privacy-preserving multinational validation study. *NPJ Digit. Med.* **2021**, *4*, 60. [CrossRef]
49. Rajendran, S.; Obeid, J.S.; Binol, H.; D'Agostino, R.; Foley, K.; Zhang, W.; Austin, P.; Brakefield, J.; Gurcan, M.N.; Topaloglu, U. Cloud-based federated learning implementation across medical centers. *JCO Clin. Cancer Inform.* **2021**, *5*, 1–11. [CrossRef]
50. Sarma, K.V.; Harmon, S.; Sanford, T.; Roth, H.R.; Xu, Z.; Tetreault, J.; Xu, D.; Flores, M.G.; Raman, A.G.; Kulkarni, R.; et al. Federated learning improves site performance in multicenter deep learning without data sharing. *J. Am. Med. Inform. Assoc.* **2021**, *28*, 1259–1264. [CrossRef]
51. Xue, Z.; Zhou, P.; Xu, Z.; Wang, X.; Xie, Y.; Ding, X.; Wen, S. A resource-constrained and privacy-preserving edge-computing-enabled clinical decision system: A federated reinforcement learning approach. *IEEE Internet Things J.* **2021**, *8*, 9122–9138. [CrossRef]
52. Brisimi, T.S.; Chen, R.; Mela, T.; Olshevsky, A.; Paschalidis, I.C.; Shi, W. Federated learning of predictive models from federated electronic health records. *Int. J. Med. Inform.* **2018**, *112*, 59–67. [CrossRef] [PubMed]
53. Yang, D.; Xu, Z.; Li, W.; Myronenko, A.; Roth, H.R.; Harmon, S.; Xu, S.; Turkbey, B.; Turkbey, E.; Wang, X.; et al. Federated semi-supervised learning for COVID region segmentation in chest CT using multi-national data from China, Italy, Japan. *Med. Image Anal.* **2021**, *70*, 101992. [CrossRef]
54. Abdul Salam, M.; Taha, S.; Ramadan, M. COVID-19 detection using federated machine learning. *PLoS ONE* **2021**, *16*, e0252573. [CrossRef]
55. Vaid, A.; Jaladanki, S.K.; Xu, J.; Teng, S.; Kumar, A.; Lee, S.; Somani, S.; Paranjpe, I.; De Freitas, J.K.; Wanyan, T.; et al. Federated learning of electronic health records to improve mortality prediction in hospitalized patients with COVID-19: Machine learning approach. *JMIR Med. Inform.* **2021**, *9*, e24207. [CrossRef]
56. Cha, D.; Sung, M.; Park, Y.-R. Implementing vertical federated learning using autoencoders: Practical application, generalizability, and utility study. *JMIR Med. Inform.* **2021**, *9*, e26598. [CrossRef]
57. Krawczyk, B. Learning from imbalanced data: Open challenges and future directions. *Prog. Artif. Intell.* **2016**, *5*, 221–232. [CrossRef]
58. Hegde, H.; Shimpi, N.; Panny, A.; Glurich, I.; Christie, P.; Acharya, A. MICE vs. PPCA: Missing data imputation in healthcare. *Inform. Med. Unlocked* **2019**, *17*, 100275. [CrossRef]
59. Tran, K.; Bøtker, J.P.; Aframian, A.; Memarzadeh, K. Artificial intelligence for medical imaging. In *Artificial Intelligence in Healthcare*; Elsevier: Amsterdam, The Netherlands, 2020; pp. 143–162.
60. Fredrikson, M.; Lantz, E.; Jha, S.; Lin, S.; Page, D.; Ristenpart, T. Privacy in pharmacogenetics: An end-to-end case study of personalized warfarin dosing. *Proc. USENIX Secur. Symp.* **2014**, *2014*, 17–32.
61. Shokri, R.; Stronati, M.; Song, C.; Shmatikov, V. Membership inference attacks against machine learning models. In Proceedings of the 2017 IEEE Symposium on Security and Privacy, San Jose, CA, USA, 22–24 May 2017; pp. 3–18.
62. Almadhoun, N.; Ayday, E.; Ulusoy, Ö. Inference attacks against differentially private query results from genomic datasets including dependent tuples. *Bioinformatics* **2020**, *36*, i136–i145. [CrossRef] [PubMed]
63. Truex, S.; Liu, L.; Gursoy, M.E.; Yu, L.; Wei, W. Demystifying membership inference attacks in machine learning as a service. *IEEE Trans. Serv. Comput.* **2019**. [CrossRef]
64. Dwork, C.; McSherry, F.; Nissim, K.; Smith, A. Calibrating noise to sensitivity in private data analysis. In *Theory of Cryptography*; Springer: Heidelberg, Germany, 2006; pp. 265–284.
65. Acar, A.; Aksu, H.; Uluagac, A.S.; Conti, M. A survey on homomorphic encryption schemes: Theory and implementation. *ACM Comput. Surv.* **2018**, *51*, 1–35. [CrossRef]
66. Caldas, S.; Meher Karthik Duddu, S.; Wu, P.; Li, T.; Konečný, J.; McMahan, H.B.; Smith, V.; Talwalkar, A. LEAF: A benchmark for federated settings. *arXiv* **2018**, arXiv:1812.01097.
67. Luo, J.; Wu, X.; Luo, Y.; Huang, A.; Huang, Y.; Liu, Y.; Yang, Q. Real-world image datasets for federated learning. *arXiv* **2021**, arXiv:1910.11089.
68. Di Martino, A.; Yan, C.-G.; Li, Q.; Denio, E.; Castellanos, F.X.; Alaerts, K.; Anderson, J.S.; Assaf, M.; Bookheimer, S.Y.; Dapretto, M.; et al. The autism brain imaging data exchange: Towards a large-scale evaluation of the intrinsic brain architecture in autism. *Mol. Psychiatry* **2014**, *19*, 659–667. [CrossRef]
69. Cohen, J.P.; Morrison, P.; Dao, L. COVID-19 image data collection. *arXiv* **2020**, arXiv:2003.11597.

70. Goodfellow, I.J.; Erhan, D.; Carrier, P.L.; Courville, A.; Mirza, M.; Hamner, B.; Cukierski, W.; Tang, Y.; Thaler, D.; Lee, D.-H.; et al. Challenges in representation learning: A report on three machine learning contests. In *Neural Information Processing*; Springer: Heidelberg, Germany, 2013; pp. 117–124.
71. Menze, B.H.; Jakab, A.; Bauer, S.; Kalpathy-Cramer, J.; Farahani, K.; Kirby, J.; Burren, Y.; Porz, N.; Slotboom, J.; Wiest, R.; et al. The multimodal brain tumor image segmentation benchmark (BRATS). *IEEE Trans. Med. Imaging* **2015**, *34*, 1993–2024. [CrossRef]
72. Litjens, G.; Debats, O.; Barentsz, J.; Karssemeijer, N.; Huisman, H. SPIE-AAPM PROSTATEx challenge data. *Cancer Imaging Arch.* **2017**. [CrossRef]
73. Vavoulas, G.; Chatzaki, C.; Malliotakis, T.; Pediaditis, M.; Tsiknakis, M. The MobiAct dataset: Recognition of activities of daily living using smartphones. In Proceedings of the International Conference on Information and Communication Technologies for Ageing Well and e-Health, Rome, Italy, 21–22 April 2016; pp. 143–151.
74. Anguita, D.; Ghio, A.; Oneto, L.; Parra, X.; Reyes-Ortiz, J.L. A public domain dataset for human activity recognition using smartphones. In Proceedings of the European Symposium on Artificial Neural Networks, Bruges, Belgium, 24–26 April 2013.
75. Schmidt, P.; Reiss, A.; Duerichen, R.; Marberger, C.; Van Laerhoven, K. Introducing WESAD, a multimodal dataset for wearable stress and affect detection. In Proceedings of the 20th ACM International Conference on Multimodal Interaction, Boulder, CO, USA, 16–20 October 2018; pp. 400–408.
76. Johnson, A.E.W.; Pollard, T.J.; Shen, L.; Lehman, L.H.; Feng, M.; Ghassemi, M.; Moody, B.; Szolovits, P.; Anthony Celi, L.; Mark, R.G. MIMIC-III, a freely accessible critical care database. *Sci. Data* **2016**, *3*, 160035. [CrossRef] [PubMed]
77. Pollard, T.J.; Johnson, A.E.W.; Raffa, J.D.; Celi, L.A.; Mark, R.G.; Badawi, O. The EICU collaborative research database, a freely available multi-center database for critical care research. *Sci. Data* **2018**, *5*, 180178. [CrossRef] [PubMed]

MDPI
St. Alban-Anlage 66
4052 Basel
Switzerland
Tel. +41 61 683 77 34
Fax +41 61 302 89 18
www.mdpi.com

Applied Sciences Editorial Office
E-mail: applsci@mdpi.com
www.mdpi.com/journal/applsci

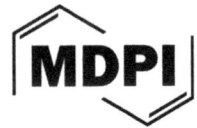

www.ingramcontent.com/pod-product-compliance
Lightning Source LLC
LaVergne TN
LVHW070740100526
838202LV00013B/1273